Outpatient Management
of HIV Infection

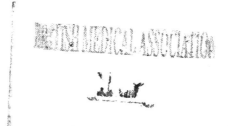

To my colleagues in the United States and abroad and to our patients.

Outpatient Management of HIV Infection

Fourth Edition

Joseph R. Masci, M.D.

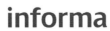

informa
healthcare

New York   London

Previous edition published in 2001 by CRC press.
This edition published in 2011 by Informa Healthcare, Telephone House, 69-77 Paul Street, London EC2A 4LQ, UK.

Simultaneously published in the USA by Informa Healthcare, 52 Vanderbilt Avenue, 7th Floor, New York, NY 10017, USA.

Informa Healthcare is a trading division of Informa UK Ltd. Registered Office: 37–41 Mortimer Street, London W1T 3JH, UK. Registered in England and Wales number 1072954.

©2011 Informa Healthcare, except as otherwise indicated

A CIP record for this book is available from the British Library.

Library of Congress Cataloging-in-Publication Data available on application

ISBN-13: 9781420087352

Orders may be sent to: Informa Healthcare, Sheepen Place, Colchester, Essex CO3 3LP, UK
Telephone: +44 (0)20 7017 5540
Email: CSDhealthcarebooks@informa.com
Website: http://informahealthcarebooks.com/

For corporate sales please contact: CorporateBooksIHC@informa.com
For foreign rights please contact: RightsIHC@informa.com
For reprint permissions please contact: PermissionsIHC@informa.com

Typeset by MPS Limited, a Macmillan Company.

Library of Congress Cataloging-in-Publication Data

Masci, Joseph R.
   Outpatient management of HIV infection / Joseph R. Masci. -- 4th ed.
      p. ; cm.
   Includes bibliographical references and index.
   ISBN 978-1-4200-8735-2 (hb : alk. paper) 1.   HIV infections -- Treatment. 2. Ambulatory medical care. I. Title.
   [DNLM: 1. HIV Infections -- therapy. 2. Ambulatory Care. WC 503.2]
   RC606.6.M37 2011
   616.97'92--dc22

                           2011006267

Preface

Remarkable advances have been made in the global battle against the acquired immune deficiency syndrome (AIDS). A proliferation of drugs in a variety of classes, some with novel mechanisms of action against the human immunodeficiency virus (HIV), the causative agent of AIDS, has brought a new era to the treatment of this massive global pandemic. A greater understanding of the pathogenesis of the disease, the genetics of resistance to antiretroviral agents, and the optimal timing of treatment has broadened the impact of therapy. For individuals living with HIV/AIDS who have ready access to modern therapy, the disease has been transformed into a chronic, typically manageable condition in which the immune dysfunction can be substantially reversed for decades.

Sadly, though, the advances in therapy and the reduction in death and suffering from HIV/AIDS have been largely confined to the developed world. As has been the case since the epidemic was first identified over 30 years ago, the regions most impacted, including many of the most impoverished countries of the world, have seen only modest progress in clinical outcomes. Despite inspired international efforts to broaden the impact of therapy, some of which are detailed in the final chapter of this book, consistent access to effective therapy remains the exception rather than the rule in most of the countries of sub-Saharan Africa in particular. Discouraging trends have also been seen in regions of the world previously only impacted to a limited degree by HIV/AIDS. The countries of Eastern Europe, including Russia, as well as South Asia and China have seen rising numbers of those infected and have struggled to create and maintain effective services. Parallel epidemics of tuberculosis and viral hepatitis have further complicated care in the same areas of the globe where HIV/AIDS has posed the greatest challenges to health care systems.

Even in environments where effective therapy for HIV itself is widely available, the news is not all favorable. Previously unrecognized and poorly understood complications of HIV infection involving a variety of organ systems have unmasked what may be a phenomenon of premature aging even among those who achieve immune reconstitution and sustained suppression of circulating levels of virus. In addition, new cases of HIV infection continue to occur in large numbers despite decades of education regarding risk behavior even in the wealthiest countries. The development of an effective vaccine, long seen as the ultimate answer to containment of the epidemic across all societies, remains frustratingly elusive.

As other calamities, both natural and man made, medical and political, have impacted the world's population since the dawn of the HIV/AIDS epidemic, the misery caused by this epic disease does not always receive the public attention that it once did. War, famine, climate change, financial instability, environmental disasters, terrorism, and other emerging or reemerging diseases such as pandemic influenza dominate the headlines as HIV/AIDS appears, at times, to have become an accepted addition to the long list of dilemmas faced by the human race.

Through the long and tragic history of this epidemic marked by both striking scientific advances and unimaginable suffering, dedicated workers in laboratories, hospitals, villages, rural clinics, harm reduction centers, governmental offices, academic institutions, and pharmaceutical company boardrooms have carried on the fight undeterred. The intention of this book is to provide a selective update of the global status of HIV/AIDS, highlighting old and new areas of discovery and challenge. Examples of strategies from around the world to contain, prevent, and treat HIV infection and its complications are offered. Some insights gained by the author in working in diverse systems of care are provided. It is hoped that this glimpse into the current state of the struggle against HIV/AIDS will offer a challenge to those wishing to begin or expand their involvement in this struggle—a struggle in which we can and must ultimately prevail.

Joseph R. Masci

Contents

SECTION III: ORGANIZATION OF CARE

1

The laboratory diagnosis of HIV infection

INTRODUCTION

Reliable testing techniques for antibody to HIV were established and made widely available in developed countries by the mid-1980s, not long after the discovery of the virus. Since that time, several important factors have affected strategies for HIV testing. First and perhaps most important, it was soon obvious that the majority of HIV-infected individuals were asymptomatic and that clinical criteria were inadequate to diagnose early infection. The public health implications of this fact have been far reaching, since HIV can be transmitted throughout the course of infection. Second, advances in antiretroviral therapy as well as counseling strategies to reduce transmission have made it imperative to detect HIV infection as early in the asymptomatic phase as possible. Third, antiretroviral therapy can dramatically reduce the risk of mother-to-child transmission during pregnancy, childbirth, and breast-feeding if HIV infection can be diagnosed in the mother by the second or third trimester. Fourth, only by an understanding of the distribution of HIV infection in the population through seroprevalence studies can allocation of resources for prevention and medical care be focused. Fifth, prevention of transmission of HIV infection to health care workers by means of needlestick injuries and other potential exposures is facilitated by the rapid testing of the source patient. For all of these reasons, HIV testing efforts are undergoing an expansion in an effort to increase testing of individuals regardless of presumed risk of infection and also targeted to pregnant women. In the United States, several states have established mandatory testing programs for pregnant women and neonates. Partner notification and contact tracing efforts have been enhanced in some areas. Public education campaigns intended to increase testing among high-risk populations have been expanded, and legal protections have been developed to reduce discrimination against the HIV infected.

Despite the widespread availability of HIV antibody testing and the high reliability of the test, a substantial proportion of HIV-infected individuals in the United States have not undergone testing and do not know that they carry the

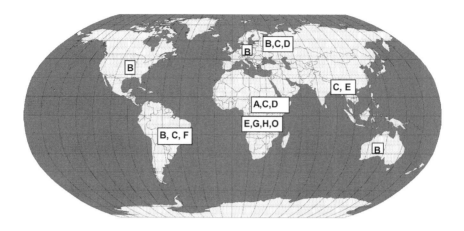

Figure 1.1 Global distribution of HIV-1 groups and subtypes. *Source*: Adapted from Ref. 2.

virus. Through 2004, approximately 950,000 persons had been diagnosed with AIDS in the United States, and 56% of these individuals died (1). Although roughly 40% of the U.S. population had been tested for HIV infection by 2002, an estimated 25% of the approximately one million HIV-infected individuals did not know that they were infected. The recognition that 200,000 to 300,000 of those infected were undiagnosed led to an extensive reevaluation of testing strategies and recommendations.

HIV-1 exists in several genetically distinct forms or clades as well as subtypes (Fig. 1.1). Three major phylogenetic groups, designated M, O, and N, have been identified. Most viral strains are in the M, or major, group. The subtypes are designated A through H and J. The vast majority of isolates from the United States and Western Europe have been subtype B. Types A, C, and D are common in Africa; E and C are the predominant strains in Southeast Asia and India, respectively. Increasingly, non-B subtypes are appearing in the United States as a result of the greater mobility of the world's population. In a study from New York City, nearly 5% of newly diagnosed were infected with non-B subtypes (3) by the mid-1990s. The types and subtypes of HIV-1 cannot be distinguished with standard antibody testing kits. HIV-1 genetic diversity has implications for measuring plasma viremia. Tests to measure plasma viral RNA may underestimate the viral load in patients infected with non-B strains of the virus (3).

PRINCIPLES OF TESTING PROCEDURES: UNITED STATES

Historically, HIV testing has been targeted, that is, largely directed, at those perceived to be at high risk of infection on the basis of established risk behaviors for transmission or clinical syndromes suggestive of HIV infection. The U.S. Centers for Disease Control and Prevention (CDC) has set and revised standards for strategies of HIV testing (1). Longstanding recommendations include the following:

HIV testing must be voluntary and free from coercion. Patients must not be tested without their knowledge.

HIV testing is recommended and should be routine for persons attending sexually transmitted disease (STD) clinics and those seeking treatment for STDs in other clinical settings.

Access to clinical care, prevention counseling, and support services is essential for persons with positive HIV test results.

Revised recommendations, published in 2006 (1), included the following:

Screening after notifying the patient that an HIV test will be performed unless the patient declines (opt-out screening) is recommended in all health care settings. Specific signed consent for HIV testing should not be required. General informed consent for medical care should be considered sufficient to encompass informed consent for HIV testing.

Persons at high risk for HIV should be screened for HIV at least annually.

HIV test results should be provided in the same manner as results of other diagnostic or screening tests.

Prevention counseling should not be required as a part of HIV screening programs in health care settings. Prevention counseling is strongly encouraged for persons at high risk for HIV in settings in which risk behaviors are assessed routinely (e.g., STD clinics) but should not have to be linked to HIV testing.

HIV diagnostic testing or screening to detect HIV infection earlier should be considered distinct from HIV counseling and testing conducted primarily as a prevention intervention for uninfected persons at high risk.

In a recent guidance statement (4), the American College of Physicians also recommended that HIV testing be routinely offered and patients be encouraged to undergo testing, leaving the frequency of repeat testing to be determined on a case-by-case basis.

Attempts to implement the CDC recommendations regarding opt-out testing have met with mixed results. In a large study in Denver, Haukoos and colleagues (5) found that when compared with targeted testing of individuals identified as at high risk for HIV infection, this form of testing yielded only a marginal increase in detected cases in an emergency department setting, and approximately 75% of patients declined testing. Furthermore, infection was not detected at earlier stages through the opt-out strategy. In contrast, studies of male and female prison inmates have yielded higher rates of acceptance of opt-out testing, particularly when it is offered within the first day of incarceration (6,7).

TESTING METHODOLOGY

Standard testing for HIV infection employs techniques to detect antibodies to the virus. This form of testing is used to detect chronic infection in adults and in children more than 18 months of age. Antibodies are typically detectable within 3 to 6 weeks after infection and almost always by 12 weeks. Occasionally, the appearance of detectable antibodies is delayed beyond this point for months or, very rarely, years. The initial testing procedures developed (conventional testing) were serum based and are typically carried out in specialized laboratories, and because of this, test results were often not available for several weeks. This delay necessitates second visits for individuals to receive the results even of preliminary screening tests. A large proportion of tested individuals, 31% in data gathered by the CDC in 2003, did not return for their test results (8). In recent years, highly sensitive and specific rapid testing techniques have been developed to facilitate point-of-care testing such that preliminary results can be available immediately. Subsequent testing by Western blot technique (see the following text) is still required for confirmation of positive results, but it is hoped that rapid testing programs will enable clinicians to inform individuals of their likely results within minutes. Although conventional testing is still carried out, rapid testing strategies have received increasing emphasis. It is hoped that such strategies will reduce the number of individuals who do not return for test results and will enable posttest counseling to be conducted promptly.

Antibody Testing

Infection with human immunodeficiency virus, type 1 (HIV-1) is typically diagnosed by detection of specific antibodies to the virus in the blood or oral fluid. The sensitivity and specificity of current blood tests for antibody exceed 99%. As noted above, however, an important limitation of the most widely used assays is that antibody is not detectable for weeks to months after infection has occurred. Although, as noted, most infected individuals test positive after three months, seroconversions occurring significantly later may be seen.

Despite the excellent reliability of HIV testing techniques, false-positive, false-negative, and inconclusive results are occasionally seen. False-positive results are encountered in less than 1% of tests conducted by enzyme immunoassay (EIA). This reflects the extremely high specificity of this technique and underscores both its value as a screening test as well as the requirement that positive results by this technique must be confirmed by Western blot (see the following text). Very rarely, false-positive tests by EIA reflect hypergammaglobulinemia or technical errors. False-negative tests by EIA are seen during the weeks after acute infection has occurred but before detectable antibody has appeared.

Profound hypogammaglobulinemia and, of course, technical errors may also result in false-negative results.

Conventional Testing Techniques

Screening Tests

Enzyme immunoassay. The standard screening blood test for HIV antibody is the enzyme-linked immunosorbent assay (EIA). The test employs HIV antigens on a solid phase, either beads or microtiter wells. Specimens of the patient's serum or plasma are incubated with the antigen preparation. If antibody to HIV is present in the specimen, it binds to the antigen. Antibody bound in this fashion is then detected by the addition of an antiglobulin-enzyme conjugate followed by a reagent, which reacts with the enzyme to produce a color change. When measured spectrophotometrically, the degree of color change is proportional to the amount of anti-HIV antibody present.

A less sensitive EIA, the so-called detuned EIA, has been used in epidemiologic studies to assist in determining the duration of infection in an HIV-positive individual. The test, conducted after routine HIV antibody testing is positive, detects only relatively high levels of antibody. Since antibody levels after acute infection rise to a maximum over a period of several months, individuals testing negative on "detuned" testing may be regarded as recently infected. The validity of this testing technique has not been established in clinical settings. Its primary role has been in epidemiologic research.

Confirmatory Tests

Western blot. Confirmatory testing is required on specimens testing positive by EIA. The confirmatory test in widest use is the Western blot, a more specific, though more labor-intensive, technique. The procedure is as follows:

1. The virus is disrupted, and viral proteins are separated by their molecular weight on a polyacrylamide gel and transferred onto a membrane.
2. The patient's serum is placed on the membrane, and antibodies, if present, bind to the viral proteins.
3. Specific patterns of antibody-protein binding are read visually.

Three major viral bands, p24, gp41, and gp120/160, detected in this fashion are used for diagnosis. If none of these bands is detected, the specimen is interpreted as nonreactive and is reported as negative for HIV-1, regardless of the result of the screening EIA. Specimens that demonstrate at least two of these three bands are reported as positive. If there is binding to any other combination of bands, the specimen is considered indeterminate. Under these circumstances, testing should be repeated after one month. Repeatedly indeterminate results should be evaluated further with further antibody or antigen testing.

Indirect immunofluorescence assay. A less commonly used confirmatory antibody test is the indirect immunofluorescence assay (IFA). Serum from the patient is exposed to HIV-infected cells and to control uninfected cells in wells for microscopic examination. A fluorochrome indicator is then used to detect antibody on the HIV-infected cells. The control wells are used to detect non-specific reactions.

Rapid Antibody Testing Techniques

As noted above, recent years have witnessed the advent of rapid testing techniques, which have permitted screening tests to be conducted and results provided at the point of care (POC). As of this writing, five rapid testing kits have been approved by the U.S. Food and Drug Administration. Two of these, the OraQuick ADVANCE Rapid HIV-1/2 Antibody Test (OraSure Technologies, Inc., Bethlehem, Pennsylvania, U.S.) and the Uni-Gold Recombigen HIV Test (Trinity Biotech, plc, Bray, Ireland), have received Clinical Laboratory Improvement Amendments (CLIA) waivers, permitting their use as POC tests. Either of these kits may be used to test whole blood or plasma; the OraQuick test may also be used to detect antibody in oral fluid.

Analyses of the OraQuick system have established that this technique has a high degree of sensitivity and specificity (9). This finding has been confirmed in postmarketing data (10), although rare clusters of false-positive results have occurred (11). It is hoped that removing the delay in obtaining the results of screening tests will result in more of those who are infected with HIV entering into care earlier, permitting antiretroviral therapy to be initiated if appropriate as well as educational interventions regarding transmission and partner notification.

Antigen Tests

Antigens of HIV-1 may be detected by several techniques.

Polymerase Chain Reaction for Viral RNA

At present, quantitative measures of viral RNA by polymerase chain reaction (PCR) have replaced older techniques such as p24 antigen detection, because of the clear relationship between RNA PCR, response to antiretroviral therapy, and prognosis. In this technique, levels of viral RNA in a specimen of plasma or other body fluids can be amplified by the annealing of complementary binders to various segments of denatured viral RNA followed by successive cycles of denaturation and annealing, which results in progressive amplification of the reaction, ultimately enabling the detection of minute amounts of viral RNA in the specimen. This assay is currently the only approved test for use in individuals testing positive for HIV-1 antibody for evaluation and monitoring of anti-retroviral therapy.

HIV RNA PCR tests are not as effective in detecting all subtypes of the virus as are antibody tests. Newer techniques capable of detecting non-B strains of the virus are under development and have met with mixed results (12). At present, patients from areas of the world where non-B subtypes are prevalent who have tested positive for HIV antibody but have an undetectable viral load by RNA PCR should be reevaluated using one of these techniques.

Branched-Chain DNA

Another quantitative method of testing for viral nucleic acid is the branched-chain DNA (bDNA) assay. This assay employs an ELISA-like system and does not involve PCR. An advantage of bDNA is that it is capable of detecting more viral subtypes than RNA PCR, although bDNA may be less sensitive in the detection of low levels of viremia (13).

p24 Antigen

An antigen-testing technique not based on nucleic acid is detection of the p24 core antigen of HIV. Although this test is relatively insensitive and has largely been replaced by the other antigen detection methods discussed, it is very specific and may be useful in detecting HIV infection during the window period after acute infection before the appearance of detectable antibody (14) and at advanced stages of infection.

VIRAL CULTURE

HIV-1 can be identified in culture by incubation of the patient's peripheral blood mononuclear cells (PBMC) with stimulated PBMC from an uninfected individual. The medium is then tested for the presence of reverse transcriptase or p24 antigen. The presence of either is indicative of a positive culture. Such culture techniques are utilized in research settings.

CLINICAL APPLICATIONS OF HIV TESTING

Although testing techniques for HIV infection have steadily improved and become more easily accessible in developed countries, the role of HIV testing in general medical care remains an area of debate. While testing can be used to diagnose both acute and chronic infection, the history of stigma associated with HIV infection and the resultant legitimate concerns regarding privacy and confidentiality cannot be easily ignored. HIV is a contagious, serious disease, which can be detected at a treatable stage with noninvasive techniques. Nonetheless, unlike screening tests for other chronic medical disorders, the discussion of HIV testing strategies has highlighted an often complex clash between public health concerns and patient autonomy and privacy issues. As a result, the most efficient and compassionate means of detecting and offering therapy to the large number of HIV-positive individuals who do not know that they are infected remains an open question. As noted above, current CDC recommendations seek to bring HIV testing into routine medical practice through an opt-out strategy. This approach has not yet been broadly implemented, and its ultimate effectiveness in identifying and bringing into care large numbers of previously undiagnosed HIV-infected individuals is being assessed. In light of this availability of rapid testing technology and the recommendations for significant expansion of HIV testing, the place of HIV testing in several types of settings is addressed in the following discussion.

Terminology (1)

Diagnostic Testing

Testing for HIV infection in persons with clinical signs or symptoms consistent with HIV infection.

Screening

Testing for HIV infection for all persons in a defined population rather than the general population, usually defined on the basis of behavioral, clinical, or demographic characteristics.

Opt-Out Screening

Performing HIV testing after notifying the patient that the test will be performed and that the patient may elect to decline or defer testing. Assent is inferred unless the patient declines testing.

Informed Consent

The process of communication between the patient and provider after which the patient can either choose to undergo testing or decline to do so. Informed consent typically involves providing oral or written information about HIV, the risks and benefits of testing, the implications of test results, how results will be communicated, and the opportunity to ask questions.

HIV Prevention Counseling

A process of identifying and assessing specific behaviors that increase the risk of contracting or transmitting HIV infection and developing a plan to reduce risk.

Laboratory Confirmation of Acute HIV Infection

An acute illness often occurs within the first few weeks after infection. The illness, which may occur in more than 90% of infected individuals, is seldom diagnosed because its nonspecific quality may cause clinicians to overlook the possibility of HIV infection, especially in absence of acknowledged risk behavior. Further, its often mild clinical features may not be sufficiently concerning to cause infected individuals to present for medical care at all. The syndrome, also referred to as the seroconversion illness is characterized by some or all of the following signs and symptoms:

Fever
Night sweats
Rash
Lympadenopathy
Pharyngitis
Headache
Myalgia
Arthralgia
Fatigue
Anorexia

Laboratory Diagnosis

The clinical manifestations of primary HIV infection almost always correspond temporally with the so-called "window period" during which antibodies to HIV are undetectable and only antigen tests can confirm the presence of infection. Routine laboratory tests such as complete blood count, basic metabolic panel, and liver function tests are typically normal or demonstrate only nonspecific abnormalities. Only antigen tests, particularly PCR, for viral RNA can confirm the diagnosis during this stage of infection. For this reason, the patient presenting with a clinical illness consistent with acute HIV infection should undergo both antibody testing and PCR. Antibody testing is indicated to exclude prior HIV infection and PCR to confirm acute infection.

Laboratory Confirmation of Chronic Infection

The clinical manifestations of HIV infection after the acute phase vary according to time since infection. As described in detail elsewhere in this book, acute infection is followed by a period of clinical latency during which specific signs and symptoms are absent. This period typically lasts for 10 years or more, although much shorter latency periods have been described. Most often, HIV infection is only suspected on clinical grounds after the onset of wasting or of conditions indicative of cellular immune dysfunction (e.g., oral candidiasis, localized varicella zoster infection). As noted above, a substantial proportion of HIV-infected individuals come to medical attention only after the onset of severe opportunistic infections characteristic of the acquired immune deficiency syndrome.

Who Should Be Tested?

Over the first two decades of the HIV/AIDS epidemic, testing for HIV infection in developed countries was largely conducted on the basis of perceived behavioral risk factors or clinical suspicion of infection. The recognition that targeting testing in this manner leaves large numbers of HIV-infected individuals undiagnosed (15) coupled with the success of programs to offer testing to pregnant women regardless of risk assessment (16) and the availability of rapid testing techniques has led to a reconsideration of the appropriate indications for testing. Since 2003, the U.S. CDC has recommended that voluntary HIV testing be conducted as a part of routine medical care for adults and adolescents (8). In 2006, this recommendation was expanded to include annual testing of individuals exposed to bloody needles, including intravenous drug use and those who are sexually active. In addition, in so-called opt-out testing, individuals aged 13 to 64 presenting for medical care would be informed that testing would be conducted unless they specifically declined. Further, the CDC recommended that no specific consent be required and that testing be routinely conducted for all pregnant women and repeat testing be performed for pregnant women aged 15 to 45 initially testing negative in areas of high or unknown prevalence (1).

Results of Rapid HIV Testing in Various Clinical Settings

As of this writing, the most recent strategies recommended by the CDC for implementation of rapid HIV testing and incorporating into routine medical care have not yet been widely adopted. New York City has conducted an expanded program of rapid HIV testing and referral into care over the past few years. However, data collected by the New York City Department of Health and Mental Hygiene (NYCDOHMH) indicated that only 11% were advised by physicians to undergo HIV testing in 2006 (New York City DOHMH) (28). Several other patterns were observed in this analysis.

> Individuals with low incomes were more likely to be tested than those with high incomes.
> Unmarried adults were more likely than married individuals to be tested.
> Less than half of New Yorkers at high risk of HIV infection were tested.
> Doctors had recommended testing in only 16% of men who have sex with men (MSM) and 14% of adults with multiple sexual partners.

Encouraging in this report was the fact that 78% of those who were advised to be tested indicated that they underwent testing because their doctor had recommended it.

Some additional insight into the potential effectiveness of these strategies can be gained from recent reports of testing in various clinical settings.

Emergency Departments

The results of three demonstration projects in which HIV testing (OraQuick Advance) was offered in emergency departments in New York City, Los Angeles, and Oakland, California suggested that testing was feasible and that routine testing appeared superior to testing on the basis of clinical risk assessment (17). In the New York City and Los Angeles sites, consent was obtained and pretest information, testing, and results were provided by trained HIV counselors. Using this model, testing was accepted by 98.3% and 84% of patients approached in the Los Angeles and New York sites, respectively. At the Oakland site, testing was offered by triage nurses to all patients who indicated that they were HIV negative or did not know their HIV status. ED staff then obtained consent for testing and provided pretest information and testing. A much larger proportion of patients were offered testing using this model (47.7% in Oakland vs. 3.6% and 2.1% in Los Angeles and New York, respectively), but the proportion agreeing to testing was significantly lower (38.5% in Oakland vs. 99.8% and 99.4% in Los Angeles and New York, respectively). Overall, HIV testing was offered to 18.6% (34,627 of 186,415) of patients at the three sites combined during the study period. The proportions testing positive were 0.8% in Los Angeles, 1.0% in Oakland, and 1.5% in New York. A total of 97 patients were newly diagnosed with HIV infection, and most (88%) were linked into care.

Despite the appeal of offering rapid HIV testing in emergency departments, periodic reports of low specificity and thus high rates of false-positive tests may indicate that current testing techniques are not fully suitable to such settings. Walensky and colleagues (18) reported on 39 patients testing positive by the OraQuick ADVANCE rapid oral test kit in the Brigham and Women's Hospital emergency department. Only 5 of these patients were confirmed to be positive by Western blot test, and 26 were found to be HIV negative (8 refused confirmatory testing). Although this extraordinarily high false-positive rate has not been reported from other centers, the use of oral testing has been associated with periodic and somewhat unexplained increased false-positive rates at the NYCDOHMH STD clinics (11). Since the results of rapid testing in emergency department settings may be used in diagnostic and treatment decisions prior to the availability of confirmatory test results, full acceptance of this testing strategy may require improved specificity of the oral test kits (19).

Sexually Transmitted Disease Clinics

Since HIV infection is sexually transmitted, clinics caring for patients with STDs have long been considered an appropriate site in which HIV testing should be made readily available and strongly encouraged (1). The NYCDOHMH has offered such testing in the 10 STD clinics, which it operates for many years. In 2003, prior to the widespread use of rapid testing techniques, approximately 33,000 tests were performed in these clinics, which see approximately 115,000 visits per years. In that year, 552 (1.6%) of tests were positive and 79% of all individuals tested received their results (11). In 2004, while rapid testing of finger-stick blood using the OraQuick tests, approximately 38,000 tests were performed, and the number of individuals receiving their test results rose to 88% of those testing positive and 86% of those testing negative. These results reinforce the assumption that rapid testing serves to reduce one barrier to HIV testing initiatives: the failure of patients to receive their results and, if appropriate, referred into further care because of the time delays inherent in conventional testing procedures. As noted in the previous discussion, however, occasional false-positive test results using oral testing techniques in STD clinics may reduce the effectiveness of this testing strategy, at least when compared with rapid testing of blood samples (11).

Prenatal Testing of Pregnant Women

One of the most important milestones in the struggle against the spread of HIV/ AIDS was the discovery that antiretroviral therapy during pregnancy and the perinatal period could dramatically reduce the risk of transmission of the virus from mother to child. This finding led to the recommendation for universal offering of voluntary testing for HIV infection early in pregnancy by U.S. Preventive Services Task Force (20) and the CDC. It is recommended that such testing be conducted using an opt-out approach (see above) and included in the routine panel of prenatal tests unless the woman specifically declines (1). No woman should be coerced into accepting HIV testing or tested without her knowledge. To facilitate streamlining of such testing, it is recommended that pregnant women receive information, in writing or verbally, explaining the need for testing and means of reducing transmission of HIV to their child but that no additional written documentation of informed consent be required beyond that which is required for routine prenatal care. If the woman declines testing, this fact should be documented in the medical record. It should be emphasized that these guidelines represent recommendations and that state and local regulations and strategies governing the testing of women during pregnancy should be consulted.

The prevention of maternal-to-child transmission (PMTCT) through screening, antiretroviral therapy to HIV-infected women and their newborns, Caesarian section in specific settings, and the avoidance of breast-feeding by infected mothers has been taken up in a variety of settings in the global fight against HIV/AIDS.

Rapid Testing During Labor and Delivery

Despite the effectiveness of prenatal testing in the PMTCT of HIV infection, women who did not receive prenatal care, who declined testing during pregnancy, or for whom testing was not accessible continue to present at term unaware of their HIV status. This scenario is less frequent in developed countries than in the developing world. Strategies to prevent vertical transmission under these circumstances have proceeded along several lines (21).

Inpatient Services

Although hospital inpatient services would appear to be a convenient location for implementation of rapid HIV testing, little data has yet been published on the yield of such testing. Lubelchek and colleagues (22) compared medical records of HIV-infected patients tested by rapid techniques prior to admission in the emergency department with those of individuals testing by conventional techniques during hospitalization at the same facility. Length of hospital stay was shorter among patients undergoing rapid testing, while a significantly larger group of patients tested by conventional means during their inpatient stay did not receive the results of testing prior to discharge and were delayed in attending the HIV clinic as outpatients. These findings would appear to indicate that the delay in obtaining results of conventional testing is followed by a delay in arrival into continuity care for HIV infection. Although not specifically addressed in this analysis, the indications for testing (i.e., risk based or routine) might be expected to be reflected in the length of hospital stay. If voluntary rapid testing is conducted in inpatient settings on a routine basis without regard to risk behavior or clinical findings, the great majority of individuals would be expected to test negative, even in high-prevalence areas of the United States, and the location of testing would not be expected to impact the length of hospital stay.

Community Settings

Rapid HIV testing techniques can be utilized outside of health care settings, since the results are available quickly so that tested individuals can be informed of their status and potentially undergo confirmatory testing, referred into care, counseled regarding transmission, and evaluated for the frequency of repeat testing if they test negative. Results of testing of individuals in community high-risk settings have been evaluated. An analysis of approximately 24,000 individuals tested in such community settings under the Advancing HIV Prevention demonstration project conducted in seven U.S. cities by the CDC found that 331 (1%) had a positive screening test. Two hundred and eighty-six of these individuals underwent confirmatory testing, and 267 of these (93%) were found to be true positives, and 200 (75%) received their confirmatory results. Despite the concerning rate of apparent false-positive rapid tests and the fact that a substantial proportion of those testing positive did not receive their confirmatory results, there were encouraging finding in this analysis in that 86% of those testing positive accepted referral into comprehensive care. Only 19 of the individuals with newly identified HIV infection in this community setting had visited a health care provider in the preceding year, and none of these had been offered HIV testing (23). This analysis lent support to the assumption that individuals at risk for HIV who have encounters with the health care system may be escaping detection and that community testing initiatives may play a key role in identifying the undiagnosed.

In further support of this premise, a smaller analysis of rapid testing efforts at gay pride events in a number of U.S. cities, also conducted under the auspices of the CDC, found that 6% of MSM who reported that they were HIV negative or did not know their status tested positive (24).

Cost-Effectiveness of HIV Testing

An analysis by Sanders and colleagues (25) indicated that widespread testing strategies, even among populations with a low seroprevalence of disease, perhaps as low as 0.05%, would be cost-effective. Paltiel and colleagues (26), using a computer simulation model of screening and treatment for HIV infection, provided additional evidence for the cost-effectiveness of screening. In what might be regarded as a relatively low-risk segment of the population, those between the ages of 55 to 75, Sanders and colleagues also found that HIV testing had a cost-effectiveness comparable to other screening tests for chronic disease if the screened individual had a partner at risk for HIV infection and if counseling procedures were streamlined (27).

The Potential Benefits of Early Detection of HIV Infection

Individual

As noted above, a substantial proportion of HIV-infected individuals in the United States, perhaps 25%, are unaware that they are infected. In addition, a large fraction of infected individuals continue to present for medical care after they have progressed to symptomatic HIV infection or AIDS. The proven survival advantages of antiretroviral therapy initiated before the advanced stages of HIV infection dictate that diagnosis of HIV infection prior to the onset of advanced-stage symptoms should be a high priority ranking with screening for cancer and cardiovascular disease.

Prevention of Transmission

In addition to the clinical advantages of early diagnosis of HIV infection, which are conferred to the individual, the potential impact on public health through reduction of transmission of HIV lends more support to early detection strategies. Partner notification and voluntary testing according to local laws can be carried out when individuals test positive. Furthermore, it has been demonstrated that a reduction in risk behavior often accompanies identification of HIV infection. The incorporation of routine testing into general medical care also creates an opportunity for discussion and counseling regarding risk behaviors even with individuals testing negative.

Changes in Testing Strategies: the Challenges

As is apparent from the discussion in this chapter, the approach to testing for HIV infection has undergone a radical transformation in recent years. The recognition that prior testing strategies left many HIV-infected individuals undiagnosed, even in areas where testing was easily available, coupled with the advent and expansion of rapid testing techniques, has raised hopes that the HIV epidemic can be more effectively addressed. Nonetheless, obstacles to fully realizing this goal remain. Historically, much time has been devoted to individual pretest counseling. This emphasis reflected the legitimate concerns regarding the stigma surrounding HIV infection, the earlier poor prognosis, confidentiality issues, and a variety of other issues. Individuals considering testing were informed of the implications of a positive or negative test.

Follow-up of individuals testing positive. To fulfill the purpose of expanded testing services, mechanisms for referral of individuals testing positive must be efficient and effective. The immediate availability of preliminary results through rapid testing should facilitate direct referral for evaluation and care by knowledgeable providers.

Follow-up of individuals testing negative. A single negative antibody test for HIV infection does not of course indicate that an individual will not subsequently become infected. In addition, as noted above, a negative screening test may be encountered in those recently infected with HIV. For this reason, a specific plan of repeat testing should be individualized based on the individual. As noted, the CDC currently recommends a minimum of annual repeat testing for those perceived to be at ongoing risk of infection. For this reason, an understanding of each tested individual's possible risk behavior is needed even if universal opt-out testing strategies are fully implemented. Theoretically, follow-up testing should virtually never be required for those not at ongoing risk of infection (except those who are acutely infected and have not yet developed an antibody response), but establishing risk patterns and future likelihood of HIV infection has been a difficult challenge for HIV care providers since the early days of the AIDS epidemic. Of course it is this very difficult challenge that has led to the recommendation for more widespread, routine testing, which is not based on perceived risk.

The role of pre- and posttest counseling. For the above reasons, counseling remains an important component of HIV testing. Although the current recommendations appropriately deemphasize the previously time-consuming pretest counseling procedures, the value of posttest counseling is more difficult to dismiss. For those testing positive, of course referral into care becomes a paramount goal of posttest counseling. For all individuals who remain at risk, whether they test positive or negative, however, HIV testing represents an opportunity for counseling regarding the reduction of risk behavior. The effectiveness of such counseling in reduction of risk behavior and transmission of HIV infection has not been consistently demonstrated, however.

HUMAN IMMUNODEFICIENCY VIRUS, TYPE 2

Infection with the human immunodeficiency virus, type 2 (HIV-2) is rarely encountered in the United States, and most screening tests for HIV-1 detect only approximately 70% of HIV-2 infections. For this reason, both conventional and rapid antibody tests are often a combination of EIA for both HIV-1 and HIV-2, and four of the six available rapid tests can detect both viruses. In contrast to HIV-1 infection, no confirmatory test for HIV-2 has yet been licensed in the United States, and such testing is currently available only in research laboratories. Since HIV-2 infection has remained largely confined to the countries of West Africa, individuals who had sexual or needle-sharing contact with persons in or from Angola, Mozambique, Togo, Senegal, Cape Verde, Ivory Coast, Gambia, Guinea-Bissau, Sao Tome, Niger, Liberia, Benin, Burkina Faso, Ghana, or Guinea should be evaluated for testing for HIV-2. In addition, persons with symptoms of HIV infection who test negative for HIV-1 should also be considered potentially infected with HIV-2, and appropriate testing should be offered.

FREQUENTLY ASKED QUESTIONS

Who Should Be Tested for HIV Infection?

There is no debate that individuals known to be at risk for HIV infection should undergo voluntary HIV testing. These include individuals with signs or symptoms of HIV infection, current or former injection drug users, men who have a history of sex with other men, female partners of men known to be at risk, health care workers who have received a percutaneous injury from an instrument used on an infected individual victims of sexual assault, and children born to women known to be HIV infected or whose status is unknown. Pregnant women should undergo voluntary testing early in pregnancy. As noted in the discussions in this chapter, expansion of voluntary testing has been advocated by the CDC and many experts. See above for details. The ultimate goal of making HIV testing a component of infection has been set by the CDC.

How Reliable Is HIV Testing?

Conventional testing by EIA with confirmation by Western blot (see above) has a sensitivity above 99%. Rapid testing techniques used for screening purposes generally have had comparable reliability, although several reports of false-positive tests, particularly with oral specimens, have raised concerns (see above). Confirmatory testing should always be performed on all initially positive specimens.

What Is the Advantage of Rapid Testing?

Rapid testing either of oral specimens or of blood can be performed at the POC and in diverse settings. This form of testing permits the results to be known within approximately 20 minutes so that infected individuals can be referred directly for confirmatory testing and care. By conventional testing procedures in which both screening and confirmatory tests are performed in specialized laboratories, results are frequently available only after several days to a week or two, and this delay may cause the infected patient to be lost from care.

Why Has Routine Testing Been Advocated?

In the United States, it has been noted that a substantial proportion of HIV-infected individuals are being diagnosed only after the onset of AIDS-related illness and are thus not conferred the advantages of antiretroviral therapy in a timely fashion. This fact also strongly suggests that HIV transmission is occurring at an unacceptably high rate because many infected persons are not aware of their status. Traditional testing based on perceived risk behavior and/or clinical signs suggestive of HIV infection has not changed this high proportion of individuals coming into care late.

What Form of Counseling Is Needed Before and After Testing?

Counseling requirements before and after HIV testing currently vary from state to state. In general, the recent trend has been toward less detailed and time-consuming pretest counseling with continued focus on posttest counseling and referral into care. Opt-out testing will require no pretest counseling at all other than to inform patients that testing will be conducted unless they specifically decline. Posttest counseling is important both for those testing negative and for those testing positive. For those testing negative, a review of risk behaviors and in high-risk situations, a plan for repeated testing are warranted. In primary HIV infection where antibody testing would typically yield a negative result, quantitative measurement of HIV RNA is indicated. For individuals testing positive, a number of points require emphasis and follow-up. Notification of sexual and/or needle-sharing partners, past and present, is required in many states, and arrangements for this notification to take place and be documented should be made. Rapid and efficient plans for referral into care by a provider trained in HIV medicine must also be made. Perhaps most importantly, individuals testing positive should be given ample opportunity to express their emotional reaction to their test results. The providers who discuss the results with the patients, whether they are trained counselors or not, must take into account the possibility of a devastating emotional crisis and be prepared to address this or have access to referral to mental health professionals. In most instances, the posttest discussion with an individual testing positive should take place over more than one session. The initial session to provide information regarding care and an opportunity to address immediate concerns regarding partner notification, privacy safeguards, and emotional issues should be followed after the patient has entered care with a more detailed discussion of treatment options and prognosis. Although remarkable advances in antiretroviral therapy have taken place in recent years, individuals learning that they are infected with HIV for the first time are unlikely to be aware of the improved prognosis and may regard the news essentially as a death sentence.

In What Settings Is HIV Testing Best Conducted?

As noted previously, HIV testing has been successfully conducted in a variety of health care and community settings. Ideally, testing should be made available in the emergency department, the inpatient wards, and the clinics of hospitals. While the scale-up of rapid testing proposed by the CDC is under way, the most productive settings for detecting unsuspected HIV infection are the emergency department and the inpatient service. Other venues in which high-risk individuals may present for care include STD, urology, dermatology, and women's health clinics as well as, perhaps, adolescent clinics.

REFERENCES

1. Centers for Disease Control and Prevention (CDC). Revised recommendations for HIV testing of adults, adolescents and pregnant women in health care settings. MMWR Morb Mortal Wkly Rep 2006; 55(RR14):1–17.
2. Hu DJ, Dondero TJ, Rayfield MA, et al. The emerging genetic diversity of HIV: the importance of global surveillance for diagnostics, research and prevention. JAMA 1996; 275:210.
3. Irwin KL, Pau CP, Lupo D, et al. Presence of HIV-1 subtype A infection in a New York commmunity with high HIV-1 prevalence: a sentinel site for monitoring HIV genetic diversity in North America. J Infect Dis 1997; 176:1629.
4. Qaseem A, Snow V, Shekelle P, et al. for the Clinical Efficacy Assessment Subcommittee of the American College of Physicians. Screening for HIV in health care settings: a guidance statement from the American College of Physicians and HIV Medicine Association. Ann Intern Med 2009; 150:125–131.
5. Haukoos JS, Hopkins E, Conroy AA, et al. Routine opt-out rapid HIV screening and detection of HIV infection in emergency department patients. JAMA 2010; 304: 284–292.
6. Kavasery R, Maru DS, Sylla LN, et al. A prospective controlled trial of routine opt-out HIV testing in a men's jail. PLoS One 2009; 25(11):e8056.

7. Kavasery R, Manu DS, Cornman-Homonoff J, et al. Routine opt-out HIV testing strategies in a female jail setting: a prospective controlled trial. PLoS One 2009; 4(11):e7648.

8. Centers for Disease Control and Prevention (CDC). Advancing HIV prevention: new strategies for a changing epidemic—United States, 2003. MMWR Morb Mortal Wkly Rep 2003; 52(15):329–332.

9. Delaney KP, Branson BM, Uniyal A, et al. Performance of an oral fluid rapid HIV-1/2 test: experience from four CDC studies. AIDS 2006; 20:1655–1660.

10. Wesolowski LG, MacKellar DA, Facente SN, et al. for the Post-marketing surveillance team. AIDS 2006; 20:1661–1666.

11. Centers for Disease Control and Prevention (CDC). False-positive oral fluid rapid HIV tests—New York City, 2005-2008. MMWR Morb Mortal Wkly Rep 2008; 57 (early release):1–5.

12. Holquin A, Lopez M, Molinero M, et al. Performance of three commercial viral load assays, Versant human immunodeficiency virus type 1 (HIV-1) RNA bDNA v3.0, Cobas AmpliPrep/Cobas TaqMan HIV1, and NucliSens HIV-1 EasyQv1.2, testing HIV1 non-B subtypes and recombinant variants. J Clin Microbiol 2008; 46(9): 2918–2923.

13. Lubelchek RJ, Max B, Sandusky CJ, et al. Reliability at the lower limits of HIV-1 RNA quantification in clinical samples: a comparison of RT-PCR versus bDNA assays. PloS One 2009; 4(6):e6008.

14. Brust S, Duttmann H, Feldner J, et al. Shortening of the diagnostic window with a new combined HIV p24 antigen and anti-HIV-1/2/0 screening test. J Virol Methods 2000; 90(2):153–165.

15. Begier EM, Bennani Y, Forgione L, et al. Undiagnosed HIV infection among New York City jail entrants, 2006: results of a blinded serosurvey. J Acquir Immune Defic Syndr 2010; 54(1):93–101.

16. Birkhead GS, Pulver WP, Warren BL, et al. Progress in prevention of mother-to-child transmission of HIV in New York State: 1988-2008. J Public Health Manag Pract 2010; 16(6):481–491.

17. Centers for Disease Control and Prevention (CDC). Rapid HIV testing in emergency departments—three U.S. sites, January 2005-March 2006. MMWR Morb Mortal Wkly Rep 2007; 56(24):597–601.

18. Walensky RP, Arbelaez C, Reichmann WM, et al. Revising expectations from rapid HIV tests in the emergency department. Ann Intern Med 2008; 149:153–160.

19. Pilcher CD, Hare CB. The deadliest catch: fishing for HIV in new waters. Ann Intern Med 2008; 149:204–205.

20. Chou R, Smits AK, Huffman LH, et al. U.S. Preventive Services Task Force. Prenatal screening for HIV: a review of the evidence for the U.S. Preventive Services Task Force. Ann Intern Med 2005; 143(1):38–54.

21. Lampe M, Branson B, Paul S, et al. Rapid HIV-1 antibody testing during labor and delivery for women of unknown HIV status. A practical guide and model protocol. Centers for Disease Control and Prevention (CDC), 2004:44.

22. Lubelchek R, Kroc K, Hota B, et al. The role of rapid vs conventional human immunodeficiency virus testing for inpatients: effects on quality of care. Arch Intern Med 2005; 165(17):1956–1960.

23. Centers for Disease Control and Prevention (CDC). Rapid HIV testing among racial/ethnic minority men at gay pride events—nine U.S. cities, 2004-2006. MMWR Morb Mortal Wkly Rep 2007; 56(24):602–604.

24. Centers for Disease Control and Prevention (CDC). Rapid HIV testing in outreach and other community settings—United States, 2004-2006. MMWR Morb Mortal Wkly Rep 2007; 56(47):1233–1237.

25. Sanders GD, Bayoumi AM, Sundaram V. Cost-effectiveness of screening for HIV in the era of highly active antiretroviral therapy. N Engl J Med 2005; 352:570–585.

26. Paltiel AD, Weinstein MC, Kimmel AD, et al. Expanded screening for HIV in the United States—an analysis of cost-effectiveness. N Engl J Med 2005; 352:586–595.

27. Sanders GD, Bayoumi AM, Holdniy M, et al. Cost-effectiveness of HIV screening in patients older than 55 years of age. Ann Intern Med 2008; 148:889–903.

28. New York City Department of Health and Mental Hygiene. HIV testing in New York City. NYC Vital Signs 2008; 7(4):1–4.

2

General approach to HIV infection

INTRODUCTION

Beginning in the late 1980s, testing for human immunodeficiency virus (HIV) infection became commonplace. As a result of greater public awareness of acquired immunodeficiency syndrome (AIDS) and increasingly easy access to counseling and testing services, many individuals perceiving themselves to be at risk of infection underwent voluntary testing. Widespread prenatal testing programs as well as mandatory testing of military recruits, applicants for immigration, and many persons applying for life or health insurance have identified individuals who were unaware of their risk. In recent years, as rapid testing for antibody to HIV has become more accessible and efforts have focused increasingly on the "routinization" of HIV testing as an important component of primary care of adults and adolescents, additional individuals have been identified with symptomatic or asymptomatic HIV infection at all stages of diseases. Simultaneously, as discussed in chapter 5, advances in therapy and preventive strategies for certain AIDS-related opportunistic infections have provided a strong medical indication for identifying HIV infection in its earliest stages.

These trends have resulted in large numbers of HIV-positive patients seeking medical care before the onset of AIDS. Many primary care physicians, including some practicing in areas where HIV infection is common, lack familiarity with HIV-related disorders and with relevant laboratory diagnostic tests. Sexual counseling and/or substance abuse treatment of patients at risk of HIV infection may vary greatly among practitioners. Nonetheless, as testing efforts intensify, increasing numbers of individuals will present for care.

General guidelines for the care of all HIV-infected patients are provided in this chapter. Although the information included is oriented toward the asymptomatic patient, however, much of the overall approach to initial assessment and follow-up care is equally applicable to patients in symptomatic phases of the disease. General health maintenance for the aging HIV-infected adult is discussed in detail in chapter 9. Issues of special importance in the care of women are presented in chapter 10. Evaluation of specific symptoms and signs is reviewed in chapter 4. Therapy of specific HIV-related disorders is discussed in chapter 6. It is recognized that many of the diagnostic and screening tests recommended for evaluation of the HIV-infected individual entering care may not be available in resource-deprived areas.

OVERALL MANAGEMENT STRATEGY

Issues in Medical Management

Medical management of HIV-infected individuals involves several elements.

Clinical and immunologic staging.

Appropriate antiretroviral therapy if indicated.

Prevention of opportunistic infections.

Screening for conditions highly associated with HIV infection, such as tuberculosis, viral hepatitis, and sexually transmitted diseases.

Provision of immunizations according to established guidelines.

General health maintenance including screening for hypertension and hypercholesterolemia, counseling regarding smoking cessation in all patients and age-appropriate colon cancer, as well as screening for prostate cancer in men and for breast and cervical cancer in women. In addition, referral for substance abuse treatment, nutritional and dental assessment, psychiatric evaluation, and subspecialty services are frequently necessary.

Throughout the longitudinal care of the patient, repeated assessments of adherence to therapy and counseling regarding risk behavior remains an essential element.

These services should be integrated as much as possible to maximize convenience and to reduce the risk of medication interactions, duplication of services, and accurate maintenance of records to maintain and periodically assess the quality of care delivered. The provider coordinating care should be trained, experienced, and knowledgeable in the care of HIV-infected individuals at all stages of disease.

Clinical Staging

Although the traditional stages of HIV infection continue to have a place in international treatment guidelines, the distinction between AIDS and HIV infection without AIDS has become somewhat less important because laboratory markers including CD4 lymphocyte count and viral load are more precise and specific indicators of disease stage, response to therapy, and prognosis. Nonetheless, the distinction between symptomatic and asymptomatic HIV infection continues to have relevance. For example, symptomatic infection, other than the acute retroviral syndrome, is universally considered an indication for antiretroviral therapy regardless of laboratory parameters. For this reason, each patient should be carefully screened for HIV-related symptomatic disorders as discussed below.

Immunologic Staging

Immunologic staging by means of lymphocyte subset analysis is essential for adequate evaluation and management of HIV infection. The CD4+ lymphocyte count provides invaluable guidance to the clinician and, to a large extent, dictates the approach to therapy and monitoring. CD8+ lymphocyte counts and CD4+/CD8+ ratios are of substantially less utility in forming the basis of management decisions.

Lymphocyte analysis should be performed as part of the initial assessment of all patients. The analysis should be repeated at regular intervals, typically every three to four months, and as dictated by immunologic stage and clinical events. For those with initial counts between 200 and 500 cells/mm^3 or those changing or initiating therapy, however, reevaluation at more frequent intervals may provide valuable information regarding the rate of rise or fall. The pattern of this "trajectory" may be of clinical value in identifying indications for either initiation of or change in antiretroviral therapy and in interpreting clinical syndromes, which might represent immune reconstitution (see chap. 6). When the count is below 200 cells/mm^3 or if such symptoms as nonspecific fever, oral candidiasis, weight loss, diarrhea, or neurologic manifestations of HIV infection develop at any immunologic stage, the lymphocyte subset analysis may be especially helpful in determining when to initiate or alter antiretroviral therapy.

Screening for HIV-Related Complications

The patient should be questioned thoroughly about current and prior medical conditions. Disorders that are particularly suggestive of HIV infection include tuberculosis, bacterial pneumonia, severe or disseminated Herpes zoster infection, oral candidiasis, severe seborrheic dermatitis, and unexplained, persistent, generalized lymphadenopathy. Persistent, unexplained fever, prolonged diarrhea, and significant (>10%), unintentional weight loss should be considered symptoms of HIV infection.

Mental Illness

Psychiatric disorders (1) and, perhaps, early cognitive decline (2) are common among HIV-infected individuals. The early recognition of depression, anxiety disorders, borderline personality, and other conditions may permit them to be addressed before or during the initiation of therapy for HIV if indicated. Any history of diagnosed mental illness should be ascertained and thoroughly explored. Symptoms of depression (insomnia, anorexia, psychomotor retardation, frequent crying, etc.) and anxiety should be sought. The routine use of an abbreviated standardized depression scale may be used as a means of identifying individuals in need of early referral to mental health professionals.

Assessing Likelihood of Treatment Adherence

Although antiretroviral therapy has become considerably less cumbersome in recent years, adherence to likely lifelong therapy for HIV infection is very difficult for many and requires not only a commitment on the part of the patient but also an understanding of potential obstacles in the patient's life, which, unless addressed, may make compliance with a regimen of medications, whether complex or simple.

Living Conditions

Stable living conditions greatly enhance the likelihood that an individual will be able to comply with therapy. Homelessness, with limited access to water and no ability to store medications properly, is particularly devastating and must be addressed before there can be any reasonable hope of maintaining an individual on antiretroviral therapy. Persons living in marginal housing may find it difficult to tolerate even minor side effects of the medications because of lack of heat, air conditioning, or ventilation or the need to walk up many stairs. Institutionalized patients, whether in temporary shelters or in more long-term facilities, may have medications confiscated or lost or may be forced to reveal their HIV status to obtain appropriate care.

Substance Abuse

Active substance abuse, including alcoholism, while not necessarily incompatible with effective HIV therapy (see chap. 7), reduces the likelihood of the high level of treatment adherence to antiretroviral therapy required for successful long-term management. Each patient must be screened for this, and if active or past substance abuse is identified, it must remain an issue of active discussion for the primary care provider at each encounter with the patient. Appropriate referrals should be made, and care should be monitored closely. Individuals who live within a network of other substance abusers cope less well with the impact of HIV infection (3), even if they have stopped drug use. Structured HIV treatment programs may seek to provide peer counselors as well as group and individual therapy sessions to provide a more supportive social structure for such individuals.

Comprehension

Outdated attitudes regarding HIV infection persist, and many patients become discouraged and frightened because of the assumption that treatment is fraught with intolerable side effects and is ultimately ineffective. Despite the dramatic advances seen in recent years in the convenience and efficacy of antiretroviral therapy, often patients are not prepared for the need to maintain a strict timetable for taking medications. Frequent encouragement and an optimistic attitude on the part of the provider may be essential for some. Reminding patients, whether newly diagnosed or heavily treatment experienced, that realistic and feasible therapeutic options are very likely to be available can foster their resilience. Careful instruction regarding side effects and their management and strategies to maintain compliance can be critically important and should be undertaken whenever therapy is initiated or changed. For those who have difficulty keeping to a complex therapeutic schedule, it is often helpful to provide labeled containers for medications separated by individual doses as a reminder. Social status is not a necessary and effective predictor of medications compliance, and it should be recognized that individuals who are employed and out of the house during the day may have as much or more difficulty in maintaining complex medication schedules as those who are homebound. In multidisciplinary programs, the presence of a clinical pharmacist and adherence team can be indispensible in maintaining patients on appropriate therapy. In resource-deprived areas, these functions can be taken on in part by any practitioner involved in the patient's care.

Dietary Patterns

Because some antiretroviral agents must be taken on an empty stomach and others must be taken with meals to maximize drug levels, many patients need assistance in creating a schedule for their medications. To be sure, this issue is magnified among people who are homeless or who lead disordered or chaotic lives for any reason. The importance of the proper timing of meals should be discussed clearly whenever antiretroviral therapy is initiated or changed.

Commitment

Each patient who is to initiate antiretroviral therapy must feel committed to maintaining a high level of adherence. Since the advent of multidrug therapy, concern about the potential side effects of medications, particularly the protease inhibitors, has been expressed in many quarters. It is not unusual that patients have been exposed to these concerns in an unbalanced manner through the vast amount of information available through the Internet and other sources and do not fully appreciate the potential benefits of effective therapy. Reservations about therapy may not be voiced by the patient for fear of insulting or angering the provider. For this reason and since nearly perfect compliance with treatment is necessary to achieve durable suppression of viral replication, it is essential that the patient be given the opportunity to express any concerns or misgivings they may feel about beginning treatment. An accepting atmosphere must be provided for this discussion so that the provider is better able to understand and respond to concerns about the safety or effectiveness of treatment. If an individual decides against beginning therapy, it is usually best to accept the decision with the plan of revisiting it at a later time. Antiretroviral therapy is seldom indicated on an urgent basis, and incomplete compliance due to patient reservations or confusion can rapidly lead to the emergence of drug resistance and a limitation of future treatment options as well as discouragement on the part of the patient and the provider in pursuing effective therapeutic strategies.

Assessing the Impact of the Diagnosis

Patients who have received appropriate counseling should be questioned about their understanding of the disease, routes of transmission, and recommended changes in their sexual practices and lifestyle.

When informed of a positive HIV test result, patients may react with a range of feelings, including denial, anger, guilt, depression, and apparent indifference. Although individual practitioners' styles differ, questions designed to explore such reactions should be asked in an understanding, accepting manner, and patients should be encouraged to discuss their feelings.

Many asymptomatic patients do not initially believe that they are infected and question the validity of positive test results. In such cases, the meaning of the test result should be reviewed and discussed (see chap. 1), and if doubt remains, repeat testing should be considered.

Most asymptomatic patients presenting themselves for medical care are young adults with little or no history of significant health problems, although as HIV testing becomes a more routine component of general medical care, an increasing number of older individuals may now enter (see chap. 9). It is important for the primary care practitioner to determine the impact of HIV infection on the patient's daily life. Disruption of family support mechanisms and, in some cases, worsening of existing alienation from family and friends are common. Employment, housing, and financial concerns may become paramount for some individuals. Appropriate questioning about these areas may lead the physician to arrange family counseling or social service intervention and demonstrate to the patient that there is an interest in providing assistance and support.

Patients presenting themselves for initial assessment may be confused about the distinction between HIV infection and AIDS. The relatively long natural history that HIV-related disease usually pursues should be explained and emphasized. Questions about prognosis are often asked by the patient at the first encounter. Although specific predictions are unwise and likely to be inaccurate, an atmosphere of both realism and hope should be established. After immunologic staging has been completed, the short-term risk of AIDS-related complications should be more easily assessed.

Assessing Family Structure

The provider should understand the patient's family structure to anticipate problems in appointment and medication compliance as well as to assist the individual in coping with the diagnosis of HIV infection. In a large-scale assessment of factors influencing access to health care among HIV-infected women in New York (4), it was found that home responsibilities, particularly child care, may have a significantly negative impact on a woman's ability to comply with medications and appointments. Some women were found to be essentially neglecting their own care in favor of their children, HIV infected or not. In addition, patients with children may be extremely concerned about the possibility that their children are also HIV infected or about planning for the children's care if they themselves should require hospitalization, be incapacitated, or die. It is also important to have an awareness of the adult support system available to the patient so that coping strategies involving close friends or relatives can be explored. Important issues such as the patient's wishes regarding their own confidentiality within their family and household must be clarified.

Permanency Planning

Patients differ in their understanding of and concern for long-range planning. Some are concerned almost immediately after learning that they are HIV infected about the impact on their loved ones if they were to die. Others may wish to defer a discussion of such issues until they themselves understand more about the disease and their own prognosis. The provider should guide this discussion in a manner that takes into account the clinical and immunological stages of the patient, comorbidities, and the likelihood of response to antiretroviral therapy. In general, the prognosis of most patients has improved substantially since the advent of combination antiretroviral therapy. For this reason, the provider discussing long-term issues should be very knowledgable in the natural history of HIV infection and the impact of therapeutic advances. Certain areas should be discussed with virtually all HIV patients as well as patients with other serious chronic medical conditions. These include advance directives, designation of a health proxy, and creation of a will, especially if the patient has dependents.

Family Planning

HIV-infected women or the female sexual partners of HIV-infected men may inquire about the safety and advisability of childbearing. Counseling should be provided regarding the potential risk of vertical transmission and measures that must be taken to reduce this risk (see chap. 10). The possible risk of premature delivery, intrauterine growth retardation, and death in utero should also be discussed in an objective manner. The potential risks, both known and unknown, to the fetus of antiretroviral therapy or other medications that the mother needs to take during pregnancy or breast-feeding should be explained. The possible implications of raising a child while under treatment for HIV infection should be pointed out, and the potential impact on the child of early loss of one or both parents must be faced objectively. Although the risk of vertical transmission has been reduced considerably by perinatal antiretroviral therapy, it is not possible to completely reassure an individual woman that she would not transmit HIV infection to her child even if her viral load is undetectable, her CD4 lymphocyte count is normal, and she receives appropriate therapy to reduce maternal-to-child transmission.

MEDICAL HISTORY

A carefully obtained medical history of a patient with HIV infection can provide the clinician with many important insights. Because HIV infection is largely a disease of young adults, patients in an early, asymptomatic stage may commonly feel well and have no significant chronic illnesses. Many patients doubt that they are infected at all, particularly those referred for medical assessment simply because of a positive screening test result. This attitude stems in part from the popular misconception that HIV infection and AIDS are synonymous terms and represent a rapidly progressive, debilitating disease. In later stages of the disease, some patients may be inclined either to deny or to exaggerate somatic complaints. Cognitive defects, perhaps reflection of the AIDS dementia complex, may interfere with some patients' ability to accurately relate their medical history or their current complaints.

HIV-infected individuals are regarded as asymptomatic only if there is no history of AIDS-related opportunistic infections or malignancies and symptoms compatible with the direct effects of HIV infection. What follows are several goals that should be borne in mind when obtaining the medical history.

Evaluation of the patient's reaction to the diagnosis of HIV infection
Evaluation for symptoms of HIV Infection
Evaluation for current or previous evidence of immunodeficiency
Assessment of the risk of specific HIV-related disorders
Assessment of immunization status
General medical history
Assessment of past and current behaviors and the likely impact of testing positive on future risk behavior
Country of birth, upbringing
Significant travel (including military)
Medications
Allergies

PHYSICAL EXAMINATION

The physical examination should be thorough and appropriate for the patient's age and medical history. In addition, it should be specifically directed toward identifying HIV-related abnormalities. The differential diagnosis and recommended diagnostic workup of abnormal physical findings are discussed in chapter 4.

VITAL SIGNS

Orthostatic changes in heart rate or blood pressure may indicate volume depletion, autonomic neuropathy, or adrenal insufficiency. An increase in respiratory rate or resting heart rate may suggest congestive heart failure resulting from HIV cardiomyopathy. Fever, even if low grade, should prompt a thorough evaluation for infection.

SKIN

HIV-infected individuals, especially those with significant immunodeficiency, frequently have abnormalities of the skin, hair, and nails. Common mucocutaneous disorders such as seborrheic dermatitis, xerosis, psoriasis, and folliculitis are generally easily recognized. Herpes simplex oral or genital infections are often present as ulcerating lesions on the lips, anterior oral cavity, perineum, penis, or perirectal region. Occasionally, herpes simplex may produce more disseminated infection with ulcerating lesions on the trunk, face, and extremities.

Varicella zoster virus may produce any of its typical manifestations, including primary varicella (chicken pox), dermatomal zoster (shingles), and disseminated zoster. Dermatomal zoster may manifest as a severe infection, sometimes leaving permanent scarring, years before the onset of AIDS.

Several opportunistic infections may become evident as papular or pustular skin lesions. These include cryptococcosis, tuberculosis, histoplasmosis, bacillary angiomatosis, and pneumocysosis. Molluscum contagiosum is seen frequently in HIV-infected patients at all stages of immunodeficiency and may appear on the face, neck, trunk, or extremities. The lesions are smooth, dome-shaped papules and often have an umbilicated center containing a waxy plug.

The lesions of Kaposi's sarcoma may be evident on any part of the body but most commonly occur on the face, particularly the tip of the nose and the ears, the trunk, and the extremities. Subcutaneous lesions may resemble cellulitis. Mucous membrane involvement is particularly common, and lesions are often seen on the gingival surfaces, palate, and peritonsillar areas.

LYMPHOID SYSTEM

A careful assessment for lymphadenopathy should be made by examining all lymph node beds systematically at each visit. Although generalized lymph node enlargement is a common finding, particularly in patients who have not yet become profoundly immunosuppressed, asymmetric lymphadenopathy or rapidly enlarging nodes in one or more areas may be a clue to the presence of a lymphadenopathic infection or malignancy. The cervical (anterior and posterior), jugular, supraclavicular, axillary, epitrochlear, inguinal, and femoral areas should be palpated, and the size and character of any palpable nodes should be carefully documented.

EYES

The eyes should be examined at each visit. Annual thorough examination by an ophthalmologist is advisable, particularly for patients with low CD4 lymphocyte counts below $50/mm^3$ (5) and always if symptoms are present. The conjunctival sacs should be carefully examined. Petechiae detected here may be a clue to the presence of systemic emboli, as may be seen in infective or thrombotic endocarditis. The fundoscopic examination should be emphasized and performed at each visit. Detecting fundal hemorrhages or exudates may provide evidence of retinitis, caused by cytomegalovirus, *Toxoplasma gondii*, or other pathogens and should prompt a thorough examination by an ophthalmologist. Visual field defects suggest focal neurologic disorders such as toxoplasmosis of lymphoma and justify neurologic referral and appropriate brain imaging studies. The periorbital area is a common location for cutaneous and subcutaneous Kaposi's sarcoma lesions.

OROPHARYNX

The examination of the oropharynx in HIV-infected patients must be especially thorough because abnormalities are often found. Common lesions include thrush (appearing as a cheesy exudate that typically occurs on the dorsum of the tongue, buccal mucosa, or palate), hairy leukoplakia (white streaks and patches on the sides of the tongue), herpes simplex (painful ulcers, vesicles, or generalized erythema), aphthous stomatis (painful ulcers), or Kaposi's sarcoma. Rarely, lymphoma, histoplasmosis, cryptococcosis, and tuberculosis may present with oral ulcers or mass lesions. Dental caries should be noted, and the patient should be referred annually at least for dental evaluation and care.

SINUSES

The examiner should palpate for tenderness over the paranasal sinuses and mastoids. Both symptomatic and asymptomatic sinusitis are encountered commonly at all stages of HIV infection.

CHEST

Breathlessness, tachypnea, and a dry cough exacerbated by deep inspiration often signal the presence of HIV-related pulmonary disorders or congestive heart failure. However, the chest examination may be normal in a patient with early respiratory infection or malignancy.

Bronchial breath sounds, dullness to percussion, or other signs of consolidation suggest bacterial pneumonia. Localized wheezing may indicate airway compression by tumor or an obstructing endobronchial lesion due to Kaposi's sarcoma.

Findings compatible with pleural effusion may suggest tuberculosis, pulmonary Kaposi's sarcoma, congestive heart failure, or bacterial or fungal pneumonia.

HEART

Because of the high incidence of HIV-related myocardial and pericardial disease, evidence of left ventricular dysfunction (e.g., third heart sound) or pericardial effusion should be carefully sought.

Valvular disease is particularly common among patients with a history of intravenous drug use and previous endocarditis, but noninfectious, thrombotic endocarditis may also occur in patients in other high-risk groups.

ABDOMEN

Enlargement of the liver or spleen may be encountered early in the course of HIV infection or may reflect late involvement with opportunistic infection or malignancy. Isolated splenomegaly may be an indication of portal hypertension and advanced cirrhosis. Localized upper abdominal tenderness may indicate biliary or pancreatic disease. Lower abdominal tenderness may suggest colitis (e.g., cytomegaloviral or antibiotic associated), appendicitis, or ileitis (related to tuberculosis, histoplasmosis, or other localized intestinal infection). Intra-abdominal lymphoma often causes nonspecific, diffuse abdominal pain with or without mass lesions. The diagnostic approach is dictated by the stage of HIV infection and associated findings.

GENITOURINARY SYSTEM

A careful examination of the genital area should be conducted to identify lesions associated with sexually transmitted diseases (ulcers, vesicles, urethral discharge, genital warts). Bimanual and speculum vaginal examination should be performed in women, and Pap smear should be obtained. Palpation of the testicles and prostate should be performed in men.

RECTAL EXAMINATION

Anorectal carcinoma is seen with increased frequency among HIV-infected homosexual men. For this reason, a careful rectal examination should be performed periodically (e.g., as part of the annual assessment). The role of anal Pap smears and anoscopy with biopsy as a means of screening for anal cancer is discussed in chapter 6. Fecal occult blood testing and/or sigmoidoscopy should be conducted as a routine screening test for all patients aged 50 or greater as well as for those at particularly high risk of colon cancer (see chap. 16).

EXTREMITIES

The extremities should be examined for edema and cyanosis as well as for muscle atrophy and joint inflammation or deformity. Venous thrombosis may be seen in association with HIV infection because of both immobility and, perhaps, hypercoagulable states such as the antiphospholipid syndrome.

NERVOUS SYSTEM

A thorough neurologic assessment directed toward detecting evidence of peripheral neuropathy (motor and sensory examination and deep tendon reflexes), focal neurologic deficits, and evidence of myelopathy, as well as a careful evaluation of mental, is important at any stage of HIV infection. Subtle cognitive deficits can be detected in a large proportion of patients. An effort should be made to identify and characterize problems as memory loss and difficulty concentrating.

INITIAL DIAGNOSTIC STUDIES

Diagnostic studies at intake are conducted to screen for undiagnosed medical disorders and to assess for potential side effects of therapy.

COMPLETE BLOOD COUNT

Because of the high incidence of anemia, thrombocytopenia, and white blood cell abnormalities, a complete blood cell count should be part of the initial evaluation and routine follow-up screening in all patients.

BIOCHEMICAL PROFILE

A number of abnormalities may be detected in asymptomatic patients at various stages of HIV infection on routine biochemical tests. Common among these disorders are hyponatremia, liver function abnormalities, elevation of bilirubin, and abnormalities of creatinine and urea nitrogen. Fasting lipid studies should be obtained in all patients and repeated as necessary according to national guidelines (see chap. 3). Special attention must be paid to the potential onset of dyslipidemia and/or insulin resistance manifested as new-onset hyperglycemia in patients beginning antiretroviral therapy, especially with protease inhibitors but in all patients at regular intervals.

LIVER FUNCTION TESTS

Liver enzymes and indicators of hepatic synthetic function, such as albumin, may provide the first indication of acute or chronic liver disease. Establishing the presence of disorders such as chronic viral hepatitis, cirrhosis, and biliary inflammation or obstruction is critical in the selection of medications and the targeting of screening efforts for hepatitis B and C.

TOXOPLASMA ANTIBODY

The presence of antibody to *T. gondii* identifies the patient at risk for reactivation of toxoplasmosis during the latter stages of immune deficiency.

HEPATITIS SEROLOGY

The natural history of both hepatitis B and C appears to be accelerated by coinfection with HIV. Identification of individuals infected with hepatitis B virus (HBV) allows further evaluation for disease activity and potential therapy. Individuals with negative HBV serologies should be immunized. In the case of either hepatitis B or hepatitis C, individuals with antibody should be further evaluated for disease activity with viral load studies and serial liver enzyme measurements (see chap. 8). Although there is currently no vaccine to prevent hepatitis C virus (HCV), patients who have evidence of chronic infection should receive hepatitis A and hepatitis B vaccines (if not immune) because of the potential for more rapid progression including fulminant hepatitis in HCV-infected patients coinfected with either of these viruses.

SYPHILIS SEROLOGY

Syphilis is more common among HIV-infected individuals than in the general population. Manifestations of disease may be more severe in coinfected individuals, and the natural history of syphilis in its progression through primary, secondary, latent, and tertiary stages may be accelerated dramatically in some individuals. Active screening and appropriate therapy are especially important for these reasons.

CHEST X RAY

In HIV-infected patients with respiratory symptoms, the value of the chest radiograph is clear. The yield of screening radiographs performed in cases of asymptomatic HIV infection, however, may be low. Nonetheless, evidence of healed or active tuberculosis, enlargement of thoracic lymph nodes, pleural disease, and interstitial infiltrates may be detected on radiographic examination in the absence of symptoms. A chest X ray should be obtained for the individual with a positive tuberculin skin test or other test indicative of latent tuberculosis (see below).

PAP TEST

The relatively high incidence of cervical neoplasia (see chap. 6) in women infected with HIV necessitates an organized approach to screening with pelvic examinations, Pap tests, and, in some high-risk individuals, colposcopy (see chaps. 6 and 10).

TUBERCULIN SKIN TEST

Because of the high rate of coinfection with *Mycobacterium tuberculosis* in HIV-infected individuals, tuberculin skin tests should be performed at intake, and in individuals with negative tests, it should be performed annually thereafter. Since active tuberculosis may be remarkably occult in some individuals and since preventive therapy appears to be quite effective in tuberculin-positive patients, whether coinfected or not, the approach to testing should be organized and diligent. Induration of 5 mm or greater is considered positive in HIV-infected individuals. Anergy testing is not recommended. Interferon-γ releasing assays (IGRAs), where available, offer a more specific means of identifying individuals with latent tuberculosis (see chap. 8).

MEASUREMENT OF VIRAL LOAD

Plasma viral load, measured by RNA-PCR, should be conducted as early in the initial assessment process as feasible. Such information aids in early identification of patients with meeting indications for antiretroviral therapy (see chap. 5) and appropriate triage for frequency of follow-up visits.

VIRAL RESISTANCE TESTING

It has been recommended that even patients who have never received antiretroviral therapy undergo viral resistance testing because of the increasing prevalence of circulating resistant strains (5).

TROPISM ASSAY

The CCR5 coreceptor blocking agent maraviroc is effective only when circulating virus is tropic for this coreceptor (see chap. 5). Whether or not therapy with maraviroc is contemplated, the tropism assay may be of benefit since later addition of the drug to augment an antiretroviral regimen may prove advantageous at a time when there is insufficient circulating virus to perform the assay.

IMMUNIZATIONS

Pneumococcal Vaccine

Pneumococcal infection, particularly pneumonia, is seen with increased frequency in HIV-infected individuals, even prior to the onset of severe immune deficiency (see chap. 4). Vaccination is recommended for all symptomatic and asymptomatic HIV-infected patients, although response to the vaccine may be suboptimal. Revaccination after five years should be considered.

Influenza Vaccine

Influenza may be severe in the setting of HIV infection. Secondary bacterial pneumonia may also be life threatening. For this reason, annual immunization during influenza season is recommended for all HIV-infected patients.

Hepatitis A Vaccine

Individuals with antibody to HCV who lack antibody to hepatitis A virus (HAV) should be immunized against hepatitis A because of the increased risk of fulminant hepatitis in HCV-positive patients who contract hepatitis A.

Hepatitis B Vaccine

Individuals lacking surface antibody to HBV should be vaccinated against HBV.

Haemophilus influenzae Type B Vaccine

This vaccine, now commonly administered to infants in developed countries, should be considered for individuals with a history of recurrent *Haemophilus* infection or those who are functionally asplenic.

Human Papillomavirus Vaccine

Consider for administration to females, aged 9 to 26, preferably before they have become sexually active.

Varicella Vaccine

Consider for administration to individuals with CD4 count below 200 cells/mm^3 who are nonimmune to varicella (5).

PREVENTION OF OPPORTUNISTIC AND OTHER INFECTIONS

Early in the history of the HIV/AIDS epidemic, it was recognized that prevention of certain opportunistic infections prolongs overall survival in HIV/AIDS (6). As a result, this strategy has been a cornerstone in the care of HIV-infected patients. Prophylaxis directed at *Pneumocystis carinii* pneumonia (PCP), toxoplasmosis, and *Mycobacterium avium* complex infection has been considered the standard of care for selected patients, based on CD4 cell counts, for years (7). These guidelines were developed on the basis of data from before the widespread use of current antiretroviral multidrug regimens. Patients responding to this therapy often have significant return of cellular immune function. Because of this, since the advent of highly active antiretroviral therapy (HAART), abundant evidence has accumulated that the incidence of most AIDS-related opportunistic infections has decreased, especially among patients with significant restoration of cellular immune function and control of viral replication (8).

PNEUMOCYSTIS CARINII PNEUMONIA

Patients with a history of AIDS-related opportunistic infection or malignancy and those with a CD4+ lymphocyte count below 200 cells/mm^3 are at extraordinarily high risk for the development of PCP. At particularly high risk are those with a prior episode of PCP. In one prospective study prior to the advent of modern antiretroviral therapy, 16 of 30 patients with Kaposi's sarcoma who received no prophylaxis developed PCP within approximately two years (9). One-third of early patients with an initial CD4+ lymphocyte count of 200 cells/mm^3 or less developed PCP by 36 months in the Multicenter AIDS Cohort Study. Approximately 80% of patients receiving zidovudine but no specific PCP prophylaxis had recurrences within 24 months (9). On the basis of these and other data, routine administration of therapy to revent PCP has been an accepted standard of care since the early days of the AIDS epidemic and is considered a mandatory component of care.

Four agents, trimethoprim-sulfamethoxazole (TMP-SMX), pentamidine, dapsone, and atovaquone, have been shown to provide protection against the development of PCP and are in wide use.

Trimethoprim-Sulfamethoxazole

A large number of studies have demonstrated that TMP-SMX confers excellent primary and secondary protection against PCP. It is currently regarded as the agent of choice. None of 142 patients with CD4+ lymphocyte counts below 200 cells/mm^3 developed PCP while receiving daily TMP-SMX (80 mg TMP/400 mg SMX or 160 mg TMP/800 mg SMX) as primary prophylaxis over a mean follow-up period of 264 days (10). In secondary prophylaxis, Hardy and colleagues (11) found an 11.4% rate of recurrence over a median period of follow-up of 17.4 months among patients receiving TMP-SMX (160 mg/800 mg daily). Lower-dose regimens with intermittent dosing (twice or thrice weekly) appear to be approximately as effective as daily therapy.

TMP-SMX also confers protection against cerebral toxoplasmosis and certain bacterial infections.

Dapsone

Dapsone is a sulfone antibiotic long used in the treatment of leprosy. In several dosing regimens, both alone and in combination with pyrimethamine, it has been shown to confer varying degrees of protection against the development of PCP in high-risk, HIV-infected patients. In a large, prospective study, dapsone (100 mg by mouth twice weekly) was found to be effective in prophylaxis, with an overall failure rate of 18% over a mean period of follow-up of 42 weeks (12).

Atovaquone

Atovaquone (1500 mg daily) represents another alternative for patients intolerant of TMX-SMP. Its effectiveness in preventing PCP is approximately equivalent to that of dapsone (13), although it is considerably more expensive and has variable absorption.

Discontinuing Prophylaxis for PCP

Primary (14) and secondary (15) prophylaxis directed against PCP can be safely discontinued among patients whose CD4+ cell counts have risen to levels above $200/mm^3$ for three months.

MYCOBACTERIUM AVIUM COMPLEX

Preventive therapy with either clarithromycin (500 mg twice daily) or azithromycin (1200 mg weekly) is recommended for individuals with CD4 cell counts of less than $50/mm^3$.

Discontinuing Prophylaxis for MAC

Prophylaxis may be safely discontinued in patients whose CD+ cell count has risen above $100/mm^3$ for at least three months and who have had sustained viral suppression (16).

TOXOPLASMOSIS

Primary prophylaxis of toxoplasmosis is recommended for individuals with CD4+ cell counts less than $100/mm^3$ or, if other opportunistic infections are present, less than $200/mm^3$ (17).

Effective regimens include the following:

TMP-SMX (one double-strength tablet daily)
Dapsone (50 mg once daily) + pyrimethamine (50 mg weekly) + leucovorin (25 mg weekly)
Dapsone (200 mg weekly) + pyrimethamine (75 mg weekly) + leucovorin
Atovaquone (1500 mg daily) +/− pyrimethamine (25 mg daily) + leucovorin (10 mg daily)

Discontinuing Prophylaxis for Toxoplasmosis

As is the case for PCP prophylaxis, it is considered safe to discontinue primary prophylaxis of toxoplasmosis if the CD4+ rises above 200 cells/mm^3 for at least three months (18).

SECONDARY PROPHYLAXIS: SPECIAL CONSIDERATIONS

Relatively little data are available addressing the need for continuing lifelong suppression (so-called secondary prophylaxis) of established opportunistic infections, with the exception of CMV retinitis, after viral suppression and immune reconstitution has been accomplished with antiretroviral therapy. Several studies have demonstrated that secondary prophylaxis of CMV retinitis may be suspended, at least for a while, among patients who have had a good virologic and immunologic response to antiretroviral therapy HAART therapy (19,20). Current guidelines reflect this observation and allow for the discontinuation of CMV antiviral therapy for patients who do not have sight-threatening disease and maintain increases of CD4 cell counts of 100 to 150 cells/mm^3 for three to six months (16).

Limited data suggest that secondary prophylaxis for PCP, MAC, toxoplasmosis, and cryptococcal infection might be safely discontinued under certain circumstances. This issue is addressed for individual opportunistic infections in chapter 6.

OTHER MEASURES TO AVOID INFECTIOUS COMPLICATIONS

Patients should be instructed in effective hand washing and encouraged to maintain personal hygiene. Specific risks of contagion should be considered (16).

Occupational Exposures

Patients should be counseled about potential risk of occupational exposure to opportunistic pathogens (16). The risk of uncontrolled exposure to *M. tuberculosis* should be eliminated for individuals working in health care facilities, homeless shelters, and diagnostic laboratories. Patients living in areas endemic for histoplasmosis should avoid heavy exposure to soil, bird or bat droppings, and construction sites. Contact with farm animals may increase the risk of cryptosporidiosis, salmonellosis, and toxoplasmosis. The risk of infection with cytomegalovirus, HAV, and cryptosporidium may be increased in child day care facilities.

Pet-Related Infections

Contact with cats increases the risk of toxoplasmosis, bartonellosis, and cryptosporidiosis. Cats in close contact with the patient should be in good health.

Litter boxes should be cleaned frequently and, if possible, by an HIV-negative, nonpregnant individual. Strict hand washing should be observed after any contact with cat droppings or litter and after any handling of the cat. Cat scratches should be avoided if possible and, if they occur, washed thoroughly to reduce the risk of bartonellosis. If illness, particularly diarrhea, develops in the cat, a veterinarian should be consulted promptly.

Reptiles should be avoided to reduce the risk of salmonellosis. Gloves should be worn when cleaning fish tanks to avoid infection with atypical mycobacteria. Exotic pets should be avoided.

Travel

Several issues should be considered by the HIV-infected traveler.

Travel to developing countries increases the risk of exposure to enteric pathogens, tuberculosis, and, depending on the itinerary and anticipated activities, other potentially dangerous infections such as histoplasmosis, leishmaniasis, and strongyloidiasis.

Access to medical care may be limited.

HIV infection is a contraindication to most live-virus vaccines, such as those to prevent yellow fever or measles. Some of these vaccines are recommended for travel to certain areas.

Foods

To reduce the risk of salmonellosis, poultry should be cooked until no longer pink in the middle, and foods containing raw eggs should be avoided. Water from rivers, lakes, streams, etc., may transmit cryptosporidiosis. As with all travelers, HIV-infected persons should avoid drinking tap water or eating fresh vegetables or fruits that may have been washed in tap water to avoid enteric pathogens associated with traveler's diarrhea, such as *Escherichia coli.*

ANTIRETROVIRAL THERAPY

Guidelines for the initiation and management of antiretroviral therapy are discussed in chapter 5.

FOLLOW-UP CARE

Routine Care

A plan of care should be formulated for each patient, taking into account clinical and immunologic stages and viral load. Because of the high frequency of both minor medical complaints and medication side effects, provision should be made for walk-in visits if feasible.

Urgent and Emergency Care

Patients should be provided with a means of rapidly contacting a provider with access to their medical records in the event of a sudden change in their condition. No universally accepted guidelines for triage and emergency management of HIV-infected patients have been created. However, certain common symptoms should prompt urgent evaluation and care. These include the following:

Acute shortness of breath
High fever
Severe headache
Focal neurological findings or change in mental status
Focal or generalized seizure
Severe diarrhea, vomiting, or abdominal pain
Severe skin rash

Patients should be routinely instructed that they should go to the emergency room or seek immediate care from their provider if any of these symptoms develops.

Other symptoms should be evaluated within a few days but do not necessarily require emergency care. Among these are the following:

Mild to moderate vomiting or diarrhea
Persistent cough without high fever or shortness of breath
Mild skin rash
Low-grade fever (less than 102°) without rigors

Patients should receive clear instructions on accessing care under any circumstances. A telephone triage system with a provider (e.g., a nurse) knowledgable in HIV care should be considered in any practice or clinic caring for a large number of patients. A medication list should be provided to each patient so that treatment decisions can be made when the full medical record is not available.

Treatment Adherence

Adherence to treatment is critically important for patients taking antiretroviral therapy and medications to prevent or suppress opportunistic infections. Methods to evaluate and improve adherence to treatment are discussed in this chapter and in chapter 5.

REFERENCES

1. Ances BM, Letendre SL, Alexander T, et al. Role of psychiatric medications as adjunct therapy in the treatment of HIV associated neurocognitive disorders. Int Rev Psychiatry 2008; 20(1):89–93.

2. McArthur JC, Steiner J, Sacktor N, et al. Human immunodeficiency virus-associated neurocognitive disorders: mind the gap. Ann Neurol 2010; 67(6):699–714.
3. Brook JS, Brook DW, Win PT, et al. Coping with AIDS. A longitudinal study. Am J Addict 1997; 6:11–20.
4. Lang L, Bernstein K, Nagi N, et al. HIV-infected women: treatment, 5th Internal Congress on Drug Therapy in HIV Infection, Glasgow, October 22–26, 2000.
5. Aberg JA, Kaplan JE, Libman H, et al. Primary care guidelines for the management of persons infected with human immunodeficiency virus: 2009 update by the HIV Medicine Association for the Infectious Diseases Society of America. Clin Infect Dis 2009; 49:651–681.
6. Osmond D, Charlebois E, Lang W, et al. Changes in AIDS survival time in two San Francisco cohorts of homosexual men. JAMA 1994; 271:1083.
7. USPHS/IDSA Prevention of Opportunistic Infections Working Group: 1997 USPHS/ IDSA guidelines for prevention of opportunistic infections in persons infected with human immunodeficiency virus: disease specific recommendations. Clin Infect Dis 1997; 25(suppl 3):S313.
8. Powderly WG. Prophylaxis for opportunistic infections in an era of effective anti-retroviral therapy. Clin Infect Dis 2000; 31:597.
9. Fischl MA, Dickinson GM, LaVlie L. Safety and efficacy of sulfamethoxazole and trimethoprim chemoprophylaxis for *Pneumocystis carinii* pneumonia in AIDS. JAMA 1988; 259:1185.
10. Schneider MM, Hoepelman AI, Eeftinck Schattenkerk JK, et al. A controlled trial of aerosolized pentamidine or TMP-SMX as primary prophylaxis against *Pneumocystis carinii* pneumonia in patients with human immunodeficiency virus infection: the Dutch AIDS Treatment Group. N Engl J Med 1992; 327:1836.
11. Hardy WD, Feinberg J, Finkelstein DM, et al. A controlled trial of trimethoprim-sulfamethoxazole or aerosolized pentamidine for secondary prophylaxis of Pneu-mocystis carinii pneumonia in patients with the acquired immunodeficiency syn-drome. AIDS Clinical Trials Group Protocol 021. N Engl J Med 1992; 327 (26):1842–1848.
12. Torres RA, Barr M, Thorn M, et al. Randomized trial of dapsone and aerosolized pentamidine for the prophylaxis of *Pneumocystis carinii* penumonia and toxoplasmic encephalitis. Am J Med 1993; 95:573.
13. El-Sadr WM, Murphy RL, Yurik TM, et al. Atovaquone compared with dapsone for the prevention of *Pneumocystis carinii* pneumonia in patients with HIV infection who cannot tolerate trimethoprim, sulfonamides or both. N Engl J Med 1998; 339:1889–1895.
14. Furrer H, Egger M, Opravil M, et al. Discontinuation of primary prophylaxis against *Pneumocystis carinii* pneumonia in HIV-1-infected adults treated with combination antiretroviral therapy. Swiss HIV Cohort. N Engl J Med 1999; 340(17):1356–1358.
15. Lopez Bernaldo de Quiros JC, Miro JM, Pena JM, et al. A randomized trial of the discontinuation of primary and secondary prophylaxis against *Pneumocystis carinii* pneumonia alter highly active antirretroviral therapy in patients with HIV infection. Grupo de Estudio del SIDA 04/98. N Engl J Med 2001; 344(3):159–167.
16. Centers for Disease Control and Prevention. USPHS/IDSA guideline for the pre-vention of opportunistic infections in persons infected with human immunodefi-ciency virus. Morbid Mortal Weekly Rep 1999; 48(RR-10):59.

17. Leport C, Chene G, Morlat P, et al. Pyrimethamine for primary prophylaxis of TE in patients with human immunodeficiency virus infection: a double-blind, randomized trial. J Infect Dis 1996; 173:91–97.
18. Mussini C, Pezzotti P, Govoni A, et al. Discontinuation of primary prophylaxis for *Pneumocystis carinii* pneumonia and TE in human immunodeficiency virus type 1-infected patients" The changes in opportunistic prophylaxis study. J Infect Dis 2000; 181:1635–1642.
19. Tural C, Romeu J, Sirera G, et al. Long-lasting remission of cytomegalovirus retinitis without maintenance therapy in human immunodeficiency virus-infected patients. J Infect Dis 1998; 177:1080.
20. MacDonald JC, Torriani FJ, Morse LS, et al. Lack of reactivation of cytomegalovirus (CMV) retinitis after stopping CMV maintenance therapy in AIDS patients with sustained elevation in CD4 T cells in response to highly active antiretroviral therapy. J Infect Dis 1998; 177:1182.

3

Overview of HIV-related disorders

INTRODUCTION

Infection with the human immunodeficiency virus (HIV)-1 leads to a complex multisystem disease. Opportunistic infections and malignancies resulting from the progressive immunologic impairment that is central to the disorder may involve any organ system. However, a more direct relationship between HIV infection and end organ dysfunction also exists. Such clinical syndromes as dementia, cardiomyopathy, and nephropathy, which are commonly seen in HIV-infected patients, appear to be caused by the virus itself in many cases.

Many of the clinical manifestations of HIV infection occur early in the course of the disease, before the onset of opportunistic infections and malignancies. Some infections, including pneumococcal pneumonia, oral candidiasis, human papillomavirus infection, and other sexually transmitted diseases, viral hepatitis, and tuberculosis, although seen with greater frequency in HIV-infected individuals, are not considered AIDS-defining conditions because they occur frequently in the general population as well. Similarly, many idiopathic disorders, such as autoimmune thrombocytopenia and Reiter's syndrome, are also seen more commonly but not exclusively in patients with HIV infection and are therefore not considered diagnostic of AIDS.

Highly active antiretroviral therapy (HAART) has dramatically reduced the incidence of many of the complications of HIV infection, both those due to immune deficiency as well as direct end organ syndromes caused by the virus itself. Such progress, while vitally important for patients in care, does not impact a large proportion of HIV-infected individuals who present for care late in the course of their disease after the onset of opportunistic infections or other HIV-related disorders in developed countries and vast numbers of individuals living in resource-limited settings. The spectrum of opportunistic infections seen in the setting of HIV infection represents a graphic illustration of the impact of effective antiretroviral therapy (ART). In the early years of the HIV/AIDS epidemic in the United States and currently in the developing world, a relatively small number of life-threatening opportunistic infections accounted for most of the morbidity and mortality of HIV/AIDS. The ongoing phenomenon of patients presenting with opportunistic infections at advanced stages of AIDS even in the United States where HIV testing has been widely available for decades led to the current guidance by the Centers for Disease Control and Prevention that HIV testing should become part of routine health care for persons between the ages of 13 and 64 (see chap. 1).

It is therefore important that providers caring for HIV-infected patients maintain their abilities in the diagnosis and management of these "traditional" AIDS-related disorders even in the era of HAART.

In recent years, a number of disorders, particularly involving the cardio-vascular system, have been newly recognized to result from HIV infection. The primary care provider must thus be prepared to recognize and evaluate a great diversity of clinical manifestations of HIV infection. Distinctions between AIDS-defining disorders and other clinical syndromes associated with HIV infection, although important for surveillance purposes, often become somewhat artificial in practical management.

In the developing world, HIV and its treatment may impact on the man-ifestations of other endemic infections, such as histoplasmosis (1) and malaria (2). Although insufficient data has been published regarding potential inter-actions between HIV and many tropical infections, the impact of HIV infection on the natural history of leprosy, for example, appears to be insignificant (3), while immune reconstitution resulting from effective treatment of HIV appears to be associated with reversal reactions among individuals with leprosy (4).

Research over the past decade has pointed to the important role of anti-retroviral therapy (ART) for the prevention of serious opportunistic infections (5). In some instances, most notably perhaps *Pneumocystis carinii* pneumonia (6) but including other serious infections such as pulmonary tuberculosis (7), the early institution of ART confers a distinct survival advantage. ART itself may effect dramatic improvement on certain HIV-related infections, including progressive multifocal leukoencephalopathy (PML) (8) and cryptosporidiosis (9), for which other therapies are inadequate or unavailable and may result in regression of Kaposi's sarcoma (KS) (10). It should be noted that early ART has not been shown to be beneficial in tuberculous or cryptococcal meningitis (11). The rec-ognition of the so-called immune reconstitution inflammatory syndromes (IRIS), which result in activation or reactivation of latent infections during a period of immune restoration resulting from ART, have also received increasing attention.

As in other sections of this text, the emphasis in this chapter will be on the manifestations of HIV/AIDS as they present in adults. Guidelines addressing the recognition and management of pediatric patients have been recently updated, and the reader is referred to these for additional information on the unique features of disease and management consideration in children (12).

This chapter provides an overview of major HIV-related disorders, whether AIDS-defining or not, arranged by organ system. Detailed discussions of the diagnosis and treatment of various disorders will be found in subsequent chapters.

SKIN DISORDERS

Dermatologic manifestations of HIV infection are present in most patients and are common at all stages of disease. Although not life threatening, disorders such as seborrheic dermatitis, psoriasis, xerosis, and alopecia are often extremely disturbing to the patient. Other processes involving the skin represent serious, potentially fatal complications. These include KS and cutaneous manifestations of opportunistic infections such as cryptococcosis, pneumocystosis, tuberculosis, histoplasmosis, and herpes simplex or varicella zoster infection. An increase in the severity of dermatologic symptoms may be associated with overall clinical progression (13).

Seborrheic Dermatitis

Severe and refractory seborrheic dermatitis is a common sequela of HIV infection, especially among dark-haired men.

Ichthyosis

Dry skin is frequently seen in association with HIV infection. Flaking and pruritis, which may be extreme, are often very troubling to patients.

Herpesvirus Infections

Localized or disseminated infection with herpes simplex is common in HIV-infected individuals and may take a variety of forms (14). Localized infection most typically occurs in the perianal or genital region and, unlike genital herpes in non-HIV-infected individuals, may cause chronic, destructive, ulcerating lesions, which may erode into the rectum, scrotum, or other adjacent structures. Herpes simplex infection may also be seen as nonhealing mouth or lip ulcers or as disseminated ulcerating lesions. Varicella zoster virus may cause severe primary infection (chicken pox) in nonimmune patients or may reactivate as localized (shingles) or generalized herpes zoster. Shingles in the setting of HIV infection is often quite severe and destructive lesions and severe postherpetic pain (15).

Bartonella Infections

Infection with bacteria of the genus *Rochalimaea* (*Rochalimaea henselae* and *Rochalimaea quintana*) has been described in association with a generalized rash highly associated with HIV infection (16). Typical lesions are red papules that may bleed when traumatized, although crusted, scaling plaques, subcutaneous nodules, and a variety of other lesions have been described (17). The infection may involve a wide variety of visceral sites, especially bone and liver (hepatic peliosis) (18). Differentiation from KS and other disseminated bacterial or fungal infections may be impossible without biopsy. In 1993, the genus *Rochalimaea* was reclassified and included in the genus *Bartonella*. These organisms are associated with cat scratch disease (CSD) in normal hosts. This condition, which typically presents with self-limited regional lymphadenopathy in the axillary, supraclavicular, or cervical region, may also be encountered as the cause of a similar syndrome in HIV individuals or may result in more widespread lymphadenopathy.

Rhodococcus equi Infections

R. equi, a bacterium previously associated only with pulmonary infection in horses, has been described as a respiratory and soft-tissue pathogen in a small number of HIV-infected individuals. Typically nodular, sometimes cavitating pulmonary densities are associated with these infections.

SKIN MANIFESTATIONS OF SYSTEMIC OPPORTUNISTIC INFECTIONS

Cryptococcosis

A variety of skin lesions have been associated with cryptococcal infection. Most often, papules resembling molluscum contagiosum have been described (19), although cellulitis and nodular lesions may also be seen.

Mycobacterial Infections

Cutaneous manifestations of mycobacterial infection may include nonhealing ulcers, nodules, pustules, and papules (20).

Histoplasmosis

Histoplasmosis may present as papular or ulcerative lesions, either localized or generalized, involving either the epidermis or the mucosal areas. Similar lesions may be seen in association with other so-called geographically restricted fungal infections, including coccidioidomycosis and blastomycosis.

SKIN MANIFESTATIONS OF MALIGNANCIES

Kaposi's Sarcoma

KS, a cutaneous, systemic neoplasm, was among the first disorders recognized to be associated with AIDS. Among patients with AIDS, KS occurs most frequently in individuals who acquired HIV infection through sexual contact, particularly male homosexuals (21). It has been observed that the incidence among male homosexuals has declined steadily since the beginning of the AIDS epidemic, although the reasons for this decline are unclear. Over the past two decades, strong evidence has implicated human herpesvirus 8 (HH8) as the causative agent of KS (22). This virus may lead to KS most rapidly among men who acquire HHV-8 infection after HIV infection (23).

AIDS-related KS differs from classic KS in its tendency to produce multiple lesions and visceral involvement. In addition to the skin, frequent sites of involvement include mucous membranes, gastrointestinal and respiratory tracts, lymph nodes, and spleen (24,25). Involvement of the liver, heart (26,27), and other unusual sites has also been described.

There has been a dramatic decline in the incidence of KS since the advent of potent ART in the mid-1990s, and regression of Kaposi's skin lesions may be seen in individuals receiving such therapy. Visceral involvement with KS may also be seen, most typically in the oropharynx, gastrointestinal tract, and lungs. ART alone is less effective in visceral disease, and chemotherapy is typically required.

Melanoma

Malignant melanoma may occur more frequently in the setting of HIV infection (28). The course may be particularly aggressive (29).

NEUROLOGICAL DISORDERS

HIV has a marked predilection for the central nervous system (CNS), and involvement in the form of aseptic meningitis may be evident during primary infection. Evidence of so-called HIV encephalopathy was seen in the majority of AIDS patients at autopsy in an early study (30). The CNS is also a frequent site of HIV-related opportunistic infections and malignancies. The term AIDS dementia complex is used to characterize the direct clinical and pathologic results of HIV infection of neural tissue typically occurring at advanced stages of immunodeficiency. Peripheral neuropathy is also frequently seen in these patients and, like dementia and myelopathy, may become extremely debilitating as well as demoralizing. As in the case of other complications of advanced HIV infection, CNS disease, both HIV-related and opportunistic, has decreased in incidence since the advent of ART (31).

CENTRAL NERVOUS SYSTEM

Since the earliest days of the AIDS epidemic, it has been recognized that infection of the nervous system by HIV may be associated with aseptic meningitis (32), myelopathy (33), peripheral neuropathy (34), and dementia (35).

CENTRAL NERVOUS SYSTEM FOCAL DISORDERS

Toxoplasmosis

Cerebral toxoplasmosis, caused by the protozoal parasite *Toxoplasma gondii*, was the initial manifestation of AIDS in approximately 2% of patients in early statistics (36), although the widespread use of trimethoprim-sulfamethoxazole for prevention of *Pneumocystis* infections has, in addition to the development of effective ART, reduced the incidence of symptomatic toxoplasmosis. Nonetheless, it remains a frequent cause of focal neurological disease, particularly among individuals with previously undiagnosed advanced HIV infection or those not receiving effective prophylaxis. Focal abnormalities, including hemiparesis, aphasia, ataxia, visual field deficit, cranial nerve palsies, and movement disorders, are evident in most cases. However, such nonfocal findings as lethargy, confusion, psychosis, and coma are also encountered and may lead to diagnostic uncertainty. The incidence of seizures in cerebral toxoplasmosis has been reported to be approximately 16% (35), comparable to that seen in AIDS dementia.

Although only tissue examination (biopsy or autopsy) can establish a diagnosis of cerebral toxoplasmosis with certainty, imaging studies of the brain, either computed tomography (CT) or magnetic resonance imaging (MRI), may be suggestive enough to allow for a presumptive diagnosis. Mass lesions are almost always demonstrated by these techniques. Lesions of toxoplasmosis are typically located in the basal ganglia and hemispheric conticomedullary junction (37) and are usually, but not always, bilateral. On contrast CT, lesions characteristically show a peripheral pattern of uptake, so-called ring enhancement. Single photon imaging computed tomography (SPECT) and positron emission tomography (PET) can aid in the distinction between cerebral toxoplasmosis and a common mimicker, lymphoma (38). Lymphoma typically produces isotope uptake in the mass lesion, while toxoplasmosis does not. No imaging study has completely replaced brain biopsy for diagnosis in ambiguous cases.

Serologic studies also may aid in the distinction between toxoplasmosis and AIDS dementia or other CNS disorders. Immunoglobulin G (IgG) antibody to *T. gondii* is present in the serum of 97% to 99% of AIDS patients with cerebral toxoplasmosis (36). A finding of a higher titer of antibody in the CSF than in the serum is particularly suggestive of cerebral toxoplasmosis. Serologic testing is of limited utility, however, because most adults in the general population have *T. gondii* antibody and cerebral toxoplasmosis can occur in the absence of antibody.

A therapeutic trial with sulfadiazine and pyrimethamine is appropriate in cases with suggestive radiographic and clinical features and is the approach taken by most clinicians. Clinical and radiographic responses may often be evident within several weeks. Such empirical therapy, if successful, provides indirect supporting evidence for the diagnosis of toxoplasmosis. The response rate of patients treated on the basis of clinical and radiographic findings is comparable to that of patients with biopsy confirmation (39). Nonetheless, histologic examination of brain tissue remains the only definitive means of diagnosis and is occasionally necessary, particularly when the response to therapy is inadequate.

Lymphoma

Primary CNS lymphoma is the initial manifestation of AIDS in fewer than 1% of cases overall but occurs with increasing frequency at advanced stages of HIV infection. Most patients have clinical and radiographic findings of one or more intracerebral mass lesions and may have biomarkers of Epstein-Barr virus (EBV) infection in the cerebrospinal fluid (40). Focal lesions with contrast enhancement, often indistinguishable from toxoplasmosis, are typically seen on CT. Multiple lesions are seen less commonly than in toxoplasmosis, but distinguishing between these two disorders on clinical and radiographic examination is often impossible. As noted above, PET and SPECT have been shown to aid in the distinction between CNS lymphoma and nonneoplastic disorders in AIDS.

Histologic examination of the brain provides conclusive evidence of lymphoma and should be strongly considered for patients with characteristic not responding to therapy for toxoplasmosis as the two conditions may completely mimic each other clinically (41).

Progressive Multifocal Leukoencephalopathy

PML caused by human JC polyomavirus is a progressive demyelinating disease, which may be present in association with a variety of immunodeficiency states or, in rare instances, in normal hosts. PML was reported in early series to occur in 2% to 5% of AIDS patients (42) and can present at higher CD4 cell counts than other common severe opportunistic infections (43). Typical symptoms include personality change, memory loss, and language disturbances. However, focal neurologic abnormalities may also occur, facilitating the distinction between PML and AIDS dementia.

Definitive diagnosis of PML requires histologic confirmation by brain biopsy or autopsy. However, the diagnosis may occasionally be made presumptively on the basis of brain imaging studies. Lesions of PML typically appear as areas of lucency within the white matter, rarely exerting mass effect. CT scans may be normal in PML, however, and double-dose contrast studies or MRI may improve the diagnostic yield.

Tuberculosis

Tuberculosis involving the CNS can present as a lymphocytic meningitis with or without cranial nerve involvement or as a mass lesion, which may be difficult to distinguish from other, more common entities such as toxoplasmosis and lymphoma. Enhancement of the basilar meningitis and hydrocephalus may also be seen. The diagnosis of focal infection of the brain with *Mycobacterium tuberculosis* normally requires tissue examination. Tuberculous meningitis should be suspected in cases, acute or subacute, of lymphocytic meningitis, especially among persons born in areas of the world where tuberculosis is highly endemic. Low CSF glucose and high protein in the absence of another cause are also suggestive. See chapter 8 for additional information regarding tuberculosis.

Nocardiosis

Nocardiosis is seen rarely in the setting of AIDS. Infection may involve the lungs, skin, brain, or a variety of other sites. Brain lesions are typically focal and demonstrate enhancement similar to that seen in toxoplasmosis and several other disorders (see the previous text). Diagnosis can be confirmed by demonstration of the organism in tissue specimens or abscess fluid.

NONFOCAL DISORDERS

Cryptococcal Meningitis

Early in the epidemic in the United States, CNS infection with the yeast *Cryptococcus neoformans* was the initial opportunistic infection in 7% of reported cases of AIDS (44). It is unclear at present if improvements in ART have had an effect on the relative incidence of this infection. Among patients with undiagnosed HIV infection, however, cryptococcosis remains a common presenting complication, although most cases occur among individuals with CD4 cell counts below $50/mm^3$ (45).

Fever and headache are the most common features of infection. Although the neurological examination is typically nonfocal, a great variety of focal abnormalities may be seen in occasional patients. These include hemiparesis, blindness, deafness, and seizure, among others. Brain imaging studies are usually normal or demonstrate only widening of the sulci and ventricular enlargement. The diagnosis is confirmed by examination of the CSF. India ink stain of the CSF is positive for yeast cells in more than 70% of cases (46), and culture and cryptococcal antigen assays are positive in more than 90%. The cellular response in the CSF is usually modest, with fewer than 20 mononuclear cells per cubic millimeter, although higher cell counts may be seen. The CSF protein level is elevated, and the glucose level is depressed in the minority of cases.

Cytomegaloviral Encephalitis

Histologic findings of cytomegalovirus (CMV) infection were present in the brains of 24% of patients in one early study (47). A number of specific neurologic syndromes have been associated with CMV infection in AIDS. These include diffuse encephalitis (48), a characteristic ventriculoencephalitis marked by cranial nerve palsies, gaze-directed nystagmus and decreased CSF glucose concentration (49), and a polyradiculomyelopathy (50). CNS involvement by CMV is seen more among patients with CMV retinitis, which, fortunately, has become less common since the advent of effective ART. The diagnosis of these syndromes, which tend to be rapidly progressive, is usually made on clinical grounds, although encephalitis may be associated with characteristic periventricular lesions seen on CT or MRI (48), and CMV may be detected in the CSF by in situ hybridization (51).

Herpes Simplex Encephalitis

Herpes simplex virus a common cause of encephalitis in normal hosts and can occur in association with HIV infection, although it appears to be uncommon. Onset of symptoms is usually abrupt with fever and headache. Rapid progression to focal neurological abnormalities is the rule, and grand mal seizures are common. Occasionally, these features are absent, however, and the presentation is one of a nonfocal, diffuse cerebritis. CT of the brain may demonstrate focal hemorrhagic areas, typically in the temporoparietal regions, either unilaterally or bilaterally. Initial imaging studies may be normal on occasion, however, and should be repeated if the diagnosis is in doubt. Cutaneous lesions and other extraneural manifestations of herpes simplex infection are usually absent.

HIV Encephalopathy

Dementia caused by HIV infection may become evident before or after the onset of AIDS-defining opportunistic infections or malignancies but typically becomes evident in advanced, symptomatic stages of disease and immune system depression, particularly among patients not receiving effective ART. Symptoms of dementia may remain stable for long periods or suddenly worsen, particularly when the patient's condition deteriorates. The overall incidence of AIDS dementia was shown to be declining in one large series after the introduction of zidovudine (AZT) (31). Further reductions have been seen since the introduction of multidrug ART.

Early symptoms of dementia may include forgetfulness, inability to concentrate, and confusion and may be accompanied by loss of balance, leg weakness, or difficulty with handwriting and pathologic reflexes (52). Patients often display apathy and social withdrawal or changes in mood. When mild, findings of early AIDS dementia may be misinterpreted as or coexist with symptoms of depression or anxiety. Headaches or seizures occasionally occur.

AIDS dementia typically follows a course marked by steady deterioration over a relatively short period. In advanced cases, psychomotor retardation, mutism, and incontinence may be prominent, and the incidence of ataxia, motor weakness, and tremors increases.

The results of diagnostic studies are nonspecific. Approximately two-thirds of patients are found to have a mildly elevated CSF protein level, and 20% have a mononuclear pleocytosis (35). Viral cultures or tests for viral RNA or other antigen such as p24 may be positive. However, none of these findings, including detection of the virus, is diagnostic of AIDS dementia.

CT typically reveals findings of diffuse cerebral atrophy, including widened cortical sulci and, less commonly, enlargement of the ventricles. Atrophy, however, may also be present without clinical findings of dementia; it was reported in 33% of adult AIDS patients in several early series (53). Diffuse white matter abnormalities with focal areas of demyelination may also be present.

MRI has been demonstrated to be more sensitive than CT in evaluating patients with AIDS dementia (54). In several series (53), MRI detected focal lesions that were missed on CT in 44% of cases.

SYSTEMIC DISORDERS AFFECTING THE CENTRAL NERVOUS SYSTEM

For many reasons HIV-infected patients are prone to systemic disorders that may cause nonfocal CNS abnormalities, particularly at advanced stages of immunodeficiency. Among these are the following:

1. Hypoxemia resulting from diffuse pulmonary infections or malignancies.
2. Anemia resulting from bone marrow involvement by opportunistic infections as a side effect of therapy or as a direct result of HIV infection.
3. Hyponatremia resulting from a variety of causes.
4. Hypoglycemia complicating pentamidine therapy.
5. Uremia complicating HIV nephropathy or caused by nephrotoxic agents such as pentamidine, foscarnet, or amphotericin B.
6. Vitamin B12, folate, or thiamine deficiency.
7. Hepatic encephalopathy complicating viral or alcoholic liver disease.
8. Depression of serum sodium, if severe or sudden, can cause encephalopathy and seizures. Such hyponatremia may be associated with inappropriate secretion of antidiuretic hormone due to medications or pulmonary disorders. Congestive heart failure, which may be otherwise occult, and primary or secondary hypoadrenalism may also present as hyponatremia.
9. Medications commonly used in the treatment of HIV patients may cause alterations in mental status. Common examples include efavirenz and gabapentin. Efavirenz (Sustiva) has been associated with delusions, acute depression, inappropriate behavior, dizziness, abnormal dreams, and insomnia. Gabapentin (Neurontin), used in the treatment of peripheral neuropathy and seizure disorders, can cause somnolence, ataxia, nervousness, depression, and a variety of other central nervous symptoms. For more complete discussion of antiretroviral medication side effects, see chapter 5.

PERIPHERAL NERVOUS SYSTEM

HIV-Related Peripheral Neuropathy

A variety of syndromes involving the peripheral nerves are commonly seen in association with HIV infection. An acute polyneuropathy or cranial nerve palsy may occur shortly after infection (34). Peripheral neuropathy, often in the form of a demyelinating polyneuropathy or mononeuritis multiplex, is seen in 20% of patients with symptomatic HIV infection (34). In more advanced cases, particularly among patients with AIDS, the most common peripheral nervous system complication is a distal, predominantly sensory neuropathy.

Medication-Related Neuropathy

Several medications used to treat HIV infection, specifically didanosine (ddI), zalcitabine (ddC), and zidovudine (AZT), may cause peripheral neuropathy.

OPHTHALMOLOGIC DISORDERS

The eye is a major site of involvement in HIV-related disorders. Opportunistic infections involving various structures within the eye as well as HIV-associated retinopathy and periocular disease such as KS may all produce symptomatic disease. Fortunately, ophthalmologic complications of HIV/AIDS have become significantly less common among patients receiving effective ART. Nonetheless, periodic full ophthalmologic examinations should be performed routinely on all HIV-infected patients, and consultation should be sought promptly for any patient with visual complaints.

Cytomegalovirus Retinitis

Historically, CMV retinitis has been the most commonly diagnosed opportunistic infection of the eye in AIDS. It was seen in 28% of patients in one large series prior to the advent of HAART (55). Without specific therapy, progression to blindness is common, and vision may be threatened at the time the infection is first detected. Bilateral involvement was seen in 35% and 42% of patients in published series (56). Retinal detachment is a common complication (56). Progression of CMV retinitis, despite treatment, is most common with severe immunodeficiency and high HIV viral loads. Coincident with the use of HAART, the incidence of CMV retinitis has declined sharply, and newly diagnosed cases have become a rarity in many centers (57).

Miscellaneous Opportunistic Infections

A variety of other ocular infections have been reported in association with HIV infection. Among these are syphilitic optic neuritis, choroiditis, and optic atrophy associated with cryptococcal meningitis caused either by direct invasion of the optic nerve or by increased intracranial pressure, endophthalmitis caused by *Mycobacterium avium* intracellulare complex (MAC), and keratitis caused by varicella zoster virus.

Kaposi's Sarcoma

Of 100 male homosexuals with KS, 20 were found to have ocular involvement in one series (58). Lesions were present on the eyelid in 16 patients, and on the conjunctiva in 7. Subcutaneous lesions may become evident as spontaneous swelling around the eye or involving the eyelids in the absence of characteristic skin lesions.

Inflammation of the Eye Associated with Immune Recovery

As noted previously, the incidence of CMV retinitis has declined significantly since the advent of highly active ART in the mid-1990s. However, intraocular inflammation, including anterior uveitis, vitritis, cataract formation, cystoid macular edema, and edema of the optic disk, may occur in patients with prior CMV retinitis who manifested immune recovery on ART.

DISORDERS OF THE ORAL CAVITY

The oral cavity may be involved by a variety of opportunistic infections, as well as by KS and lymphoma. In addition, periodontal disease is more common in the setting of HIV infection. For this reason, it is recommended that HIV-infected patients have regular screens for intraoral and dental pathology.

Infections

Candidiasis

Oral candidiasis, which most often appears as white plaques on the buccal mucosa, pharynx, or tongue or as angular cheilitis, may be seen at all stages of HIV infection but is most common and most severe among patients with advanced degrees of cellular immune dysfunction. In such individuals, infection is also most likely to extend into the esophagous and create swallowing and nutritional problems. Candidiasis resistant to oral azole antifungal agents has become increasingly common in recent years and remains a major source of morbidity among patients at advanced stages of disease.

HERPES SIMPLEX INFECTION

In one early series, 10% of AIDS patients were found to have oral herpes simplex infection (59). Lesions are typically painful, progressive ulcerations but may appear as fissures in some cases.

HAIRY LEUKOPLAKIA

Hairy leukoplakia, a white lesion usually found on the sides of the tongue, is commonly seen at all stages of HIV infection, particularly among homosexual men. The appearance of hairy leukoplakia may be predictive of clinical progression. Evidence of an association with EBV has been reported (60).

GINGIVITIS AND PERIODONTAL DISEASE

Necrotizing ulcerative periodontitis occurs in as many as half of patients with symptomatic HIV infection. Severe gingivitis even in the absence of dental plaque is also frequently encountered.

MISCELLANEOUS INFECTIONS

Oral lesions, usually in the form of ulcerations, may be seen in syphilis, tuberculosis, histoplasmosis, cryptococcosis, and anerobic infection.

APHTHOUS STOMATITIS

Oral aphthous ulcers occurred in 3% of HIV-infected patients in one large series (61) and account for the majority of nonhealing mouth ulcers (62).

MISCELLANEOUS DISORDERS

Xerostomia, exfoliative cheilitis, and nonspecific ulcerations were seen in 10%, 9%, and 3%, respectively, in one series (59).

Malignancies

Kaposi's Sarcoma

KS, historically, has been the most common oral malignancy in AIDS, although effective ART has led to a decline in the incidence of KS in recent years. Lesions, which may be mucosal or submucosal or both, typically appear on the palate, gingiva, or buccal mucosa. Oral KS may occur in isolation or with widespread skin or visceral involvement.

LYMPHOMA

AIDS-related lymphoma may become evident as nodular or ulcerating oral lesions.

PULMONARY DISORDERS

Opportunistic Infections

Pneumocystis Pneumonia

Pneumocystis pneumonia in humans is caused by the fungal pathogen *Pneumocystis jirovecii (P. carinii)*. PCP was the commonest of the original infections described in association with AIDS, occurring in 70% to 80% of patients with AIDS before the use of primary propylaxis became widespread (63). PCP remains a common initial opportunistic infection in the United States and other developed countries, although its incidence has declined dramatically among HIV-infected individuals in medical care and receiving specific prophylaxis. PCP is ultimately diagnosed in 80% of patients who do not receive prophylaxis. Almost all cases occur among patients with CD4+ lymphocyte counts below 200 cells/mm^3 (64) who are not receiving preventive therapy.

The clinical manifestations of PCP are nonspecific. The onset of symptoms may be insidious over days to weeks or fulminant. Most patients complain of fever, cough, and dyspnea and have a subacute course. Chills, sputum production, and chest pain are less common. In rare cases, fever or exertional dyspnea may be the only manifestations of disease. The clinical features may be modified and rendered less severe and more slowly progressive in patients receiving prophylaxis.

Bilateral infiltrates are seen on chest radiographs in almost all cases, although unilateral infiltrates, nodules, and cavities occasionally occur. Pleural involvement is extremely unusual. In some cases, the chest radiograph may be completely normal.

PCP is often associated with diffuse, bilateral pulmonary uptake on gallium scanning, which may be apparent before the appearance of radiographic abnormalities. It should be recognized, however, that radiographic and gallium scan findings associated with PCP are nonspecific. Other AIDS-related processes, particularly KS, tuberculosis, histoplasmosis, strongyloidosis, toxoplasmosis, cryptococcosis, cytomegaloviral infection, and lymphocytic interstitial pneumonitis, as well as bacterial pneumonia, may produce identical radiographic patterns. For this reason, histologic or cytologic confirmation of the diagnosis of PCP is necessary in most cases and desirable in all. Examination of induced sputum or specimens obtained at bronchoscopy is almost always effective in confirming the diagnosis.

Occasionally, pneumothorax may complicate PCP. Patients presenting with unexplained pneumothorax who are at risk for PCP should be considered strongly for empiric treatment. Pneumothorax occuring during treatment for PCP confers a worse prognosis. Individuals with recurrent or bilateral pneumothoraces should be evaluated for thoracoscopy, pleurodesis, or surgical repair.

Cryptococcosis

The CNS is the most common site of involvement by *C. neoformans* in AIDS. However, respiratory infection may occur with or without concomitant CNS infection. A variety of radiographic patterns have been associated with pulmonary cryptococcosis. These include interstitial infiltrates and hilar lymphadenopathy, either alone or in combination. Empyema and adult respiratory distress syndrome may also be seen.

Cryptococcal infection may coexist with PCP and other respiratory disorders. The diagnosis is made by lung biopsy or alveolar lavage. Blood cultures and serum cryptococcal antigen assay may also aid in the diagnosis.

Histoplasmosis

Disseminated infection with the fungus *Histoplasma capsulatum* is occasionally seen in AIDS patients from endemic areas such as the Midwestern United States and Central and South America and may be encountered in many regions of the tropics and subtropics. Pulmonary involvement with diffuse, bilateral infiltrates was seen in approximately 40% of cases in one series (65). Hilar lymph node enlargement and extrapulmonary involvement, particularly nodular skin lesions or hepatosplenometaly, may be clues to the diagnosis of pulmonary histoplasmosis. The diagnosis is usually confirmed by lung biopsy or bronchoalveolar lavage.

Coccidioidomycosis

Progressive pulmonary infection caused by the fungal pathogen *Coccidioides immitis* occurs with increased frequency among HIV-infected patients living in endemic areas of the American Southwest and some regions of Central Amercia. Extrapulmonary involvement, particularly skeletal lesions, may also be encountered.

Cytomegalovirus Infection

CMV infection is frequently found at postmortem examination (66) in the lungs of patients who die with AIDS. In clinical series, however, isolated CMV pneumonia is rare, although evidence of CMV infection is often found in association with PCP or other opportunistic respiratory infections.

Toxoplasmosis

Pulmonary toxoplasmosis may mimic PCP on radiographic examination or produce focal infiltrates or nodular densities. Lactate dehydrogenase levels, often elevated in PCP, may be extremely high in pulmonary toxoplasmosis.

Bacterial Pneumonia

Patients with HIV infection are at high risk for infection with *Streptococcus pneumoniae* (67) and *Hemophilus influenzae* (68). Community-acquired pneumonia caused by *Pseudomonas aeruginosa* has been described in patients who had recently been hospitalized (69). Clinical signs and symptoms and radiographic findings may be atypical, particularly among patients at advanced stages of immune deficiency. Diffuse lung involvement and fulminant progression are more common than in non-HIV-infected patients.

Mycobacterial Infection

Tuberculosis

Infection with *M. tuberculosis* is very common among HIV-infected patients at all stages of immune deficiency. The HIV/AIDS epidemic accounted for much of the sudden increase in tuberculosis cases seen in U. S. urban centers in the mid-1980s. The clinical and radiographic manifestations may be atypical in the setting of HIV infection. Lower lobe infiltrates and mediastinal lymph node involvement are common. Tuberculosis is addressed in detail in chapter 8.

ATYPICAL MYCOBACTERIAL INFECTION

Atypical mycobacteria, particularly MAC, are frequently isolated from respiratory secretions from HIV-infected patients, especially those at advanced stages of immune deficiency. Most often, no associated respiratory syndrome or radiographic abnormalities are seen in these patients. On occasion, however, MAC infection may cause lung nodules, focal infiltrates, or cavitary lesions similar to those seen in tuberculosis.

Malignancies

Kaposi's Sarcoma

Bronchopulmonary involvement with Kaposi's sarcoma typically becomes evident as a subacute illness characterized by dyspnea and dry cough occasionally accompanied by hemoptysis or pleuritic chest pain. Fever may be present. Airway involvement may result in wheezing. Clinical progression may be gradual or fulminant, and respiratory failure may occur. Radiographic features are nonspecific and may mimic other disorders, but the presence of diffuse nodular infiltrates, hilar lymphadenopathy, and pleural disease may suggest the diagnosis. In some cases, however, findings may closely resemble those of PCP or other AIDS-related disorders. In contrast to PCP, however, the gallium scan is usually negative in pulmonary KS, and lactate dehydrogenase levels are usually normal or only slightly elevated. Cutaneous KS lesions are usually present but may not be, making the etiology of the lung disease particularly obscure. The diagnosis may be confirmed by lung biopsy, although autopsy data indicate that the sensitivity of this procedure is limited (70). Visualization of characteristic red-purple lesions in the large airways by bronchoscopy may allow a presumptive diagnosis and therapy, even without histologic confirmation.

Lymphoma

Lymphoma is the second most common AIDS-associated malignancy after KS. Although extranodal involvement is seen frequently in AIDS-associated non-Hodgkin's lymphoma (NHL) [occurring in 87% of cases in one large series (71)], the lungs are a relatively unusual site. The reported incidence of pulmonary involvement varies from 0% to 25% (72). Clinical features are nonspecific, and respiratory symptoms are not always present. Chest radiographs may demonstrate abnormalities of the thoracic lymph nodes, lung parenchyma, or pleura. The diagnosis is confirmed by histologic examination.

CARDIOVASCULAR DISORDERS

Cardiovascular disease has long been associated with HIV infection. In the era before effective ART was in use and in regions of the world where large numbers of individuals with advanced infection do not have access to therapy, syndromes described in the first two decades of the epidemic remain significant manifestations of HIV itself or of complicating opportunistic infections. With modern ART and the aging of the population receiving adequate therapy previously unknown or unrecognized, cardiovascular complications of HIV and its treatment have become evident (see chaps. 5 and 9). In this chapter, the discussion of cardiovascular disorders associated with HIV infection will be limited primarily to those to be caused by direct effects of the virus or associated pathogens.

In one early series, 5% of AIDS patients had symptoms of heart disease, usually caused by opportunistic infection or malignancy (73). Male homosexuals and intravenous drug users were equally affected. Opportunistic infections and malignancies may involve the heart, but in many (perhaps most) patients with symptomatic heart disease, the cause is obscure. Myocarditis and pericardial effusion are commonly reported cardiac manifestations (74). Echocardiographic abnormalities are commonly seen in advanced HIV infection. Pericardial effusions and ventricular dysfunction were each noted in 29% of hospitalized AIDS patients (75) and in 26% and 30% of AIDS patients overall (76) in two published series.

The importance of cardiovascular disease has been increasingly recognized over the past two decades and particularly since the advent of modern ART. The dramatically prolonged average survival of effectively patients has underscored the risk of cardiovascular disease as it affects aging populations in general. The aging of the HIV/AIDS population, however, has been accompanied by a growing incidence of symptomatic heart disease associated with traditional risk factors such as hypertension, diabetes, hypercholesterolemia, and tobacco use. Furthermore, the effects of antiretroviral drugs, particularly the protease inhibitors on lipid levels, have long been noted (77).

In addition, however, recent years have witnessed a greater understanding of the direct effects of HIV infection on the cardiovascular system. The following conditions appear to result from these direct effects.

Acute Myocarditis and Dilated Cardiomyopathy

Although the myocardium is frequently affected by HIV infection, the pathogenesis of this phenomenon is not completely understood. Prior to the arrival of modern ART, the incidence of dialated cardiomyopathy among HIV-infected individuals was said to be 15.9/1000 cases (78) and was a poor prognostic sign. Idiopathic cardiomyopathy, possibly directly related to HIV infection, was detected in 44 (15%) of 296 patients in one prospective study. Dilated cardiomyopathy was associated with advanced disease and low CD4+ cell counts and was predictive of poor survival, although spontaneous improvement in heart function has also been described (79).

Prevalence as high as 15% was reported in that era, and cardiomyopathy was highly associated with low CD4 counts. It has been established that direct infection of cardiac myocytes by HIV occurs (80). Nonetheless, it is unclear whether myocardial damage results directly from a cytopathic effect, cytokine release, or coinfection with other agents commonly associated with cardiomyopathy such as enteroviruses and adenoviruses. The full impact of effective ART on the prevalence and ramifications of myocardial involvement by HIV infection has yet to be established.

Pericardial Effusions

Significant but clinically silent pericardial effusions were detected by echocardiography in 7 (26%) of 27 male homosexuals with AIDS (76).

A number of HIV-associated opportunistic infections and malignancies (see the following text) may result in pericardial effusions. As is the case with cardiomyopathy, however, pericardial effusions appear also to be the direct result of HIV infection in some individuals. The majority of such pericardial effusions appear to be idiopathic and appear to be related to capillary leak of serous fluid. They range in severity from small and asymptomatic to large with hemodynamic consequences. The majority of massive effusions and those causing cardiac tamponade are the result of opportunistic infection or malignancy. As in the case of cardiomyopathy, the impact of modern ART on pericardial disease has not yet been fully characterized.

Pulmonary Hypertension

Pulmonary hypertension is estimated to occur in approximately 1 in 200 HIV-infected individuals, and the incidence is roughly 1000 times greater than that in the general population (81) and is a poor prognostic sign. Unlike dilated cardiomyopathy, pulmonary hypertension does not appear to correlate with the degree of immunodeficiency. It may occur in the absence of preexisting lung disease. Another somewhat mysterious entity, pulmonary hypertension, appears to be caused by direct effects of HIV or cytokines released in the setting of HIV infection on the pulmonary arterioles.

Evidence exists that coronary artery disease (82) may also be accelerated in the presence of uncontrolled HIV replication.

As noted above, cardiovascular manifestations of HIV infection, resulting both from the disease and its treatment, have been increasingly recognized in recent years. Although these disorders have received relatively little attention, it has been estimated that 5000 patients per year have heart disease as a result of HIV infection itself or of related disorders. The incidence of significant coronary disease resulting from ART is not yet fully clear. This issue is addressed further in chapter 5.

OPPORTUNISTIC INFECTIONS AND MALIGNANCIES AFFECTING THE CARDIOVASCULAR SYSTEM

Myocardial Disease

A large number of opportunistic pathogens have been associated, in rare instances, with myocarditis in HIV-infected patients. Among these are *P. carinii*, *M. tuberculosis*, MAC, *C. neoformans*, *Aspergillus fumigatus*, *Candida albicans*, *H. capsulatum*, *C. immitis*, *T. gondii*, herpes simplex virus, and CMV. However, myocarditis is not a common manifestation of infection with any of these organisms. With some, myocardial involvement has been reported only in the setting of widespread multisystem infection and has often been first recognized at postmortem examination. The clinical significance of myocardial infection in many such cases is unclear.

Pericardial Disease

Pericardial involvement may complicate tuberculosis, atypical mycobacterial infection, cryptococcosis, nocardiosis, and infection with herpes simplex virus or CMV.

Effusions may be large enough to result in hemodynamic compromise, and both pericarditis and cardiomyopathy should be considered in the evaluation of dyspnea in patients with HIV infection.

Endocarditis

Nonbacterial thrombotic endocarditis, a disorder of unknown origin that may be associated with a variety of wasting diseases, may be seen in association with HIV infection. The condition may be associated with systemic emboli.

HIV-infected injection drug users who continue to use drugs remain at risk for infective endocarditis, which is more likely to be caused by conventional bacteria, particularly *Staphylococcus aureus*, than by opportunistic pathogens otherwise associated with AIDS.

GASTROINTESTINAL AND HEPATIC DISORDERS

Diarrhea

Diarrhea has been recognized as a common manifestation of HIV infection and AIDS since the earliest days of the epidemic. In developing countries, massive diarrhea with profound wasting and ultimate death in association with HIV infection has been seen in association with many infectious agents and as a nonspecific manifestation of immune deficiency. In the United States and other developed countries, a variety of infectious agents, most notably protozoal parasites, have caused great morbidity among patients, especially those at advanced stages of disease. Intestinal involvement by the AIDS-related malignancies, Kaposi's sarcoma, and NHL may be associated with diarrhea. Diarrhea may also be seen as a side effect of therapy, particularly with protease inhibitors (see chap. 5), and colitis due to *Clostridium difficile* toxin in association with an array of antibiotics have achieved great importance. In many instances, however, a specific cause of diarrhea cannot be identified, and the effect of HIV on the bowel mucosa (so-called AIDS enteropathy) or the immune deficiency itself is presumed to be causative. Overall, the incidence of diarrhea associated with identified pathogens has fallen dramatically among patients receiving ART. Specific agents associated with diarrhea are briefly reviewed here. Approaches to therapy are discussed in subsequent chapters.

Bacteria

Agents that frequently produce diarrheal illness in normal hosts, *Salmonella*, *Shigella*, and *Campylobacter*, are commonly encountered in the setting of HIV infection and may produce more refractory symptoms, prone to relapse with discontinuation of therapy. *C. difficile* has become a common cause of diarrhea among patients with advanced degrees of immune deficiency and receive antibiotics, especially those who have been recently hospitalized. In one series, up to 6.4% of patients discharged from this hospital had *C. difficile*–related diarrhea. Clindamycin use, penicillin use, and CD4+ cell count less than 50/mm^3 were found to be risk factors (83).

Parasites

Several protozoal parasites that had not been recognized as human pathogens prior to the AIDS epidemic are frequently identified in the stools of patients with protracted diarrhea. *Cryptosporidium parvum*, the commonest and most difficult to treat of these, is seen almost exclusively among patients with less than 150 CD4+ cells/mm^3 and frequently responds to ART, particularly if there is significant immune reconstitution (84). The diagnosis is made on examination of stool stained with the modified acid-fast technique. Other similar parasites that may be seen include *Isospora belli*, Microsporidia, and *Cyclospora*. Amebiasis and giardiasis may also cause diarrhea but are encountered less frequently than the novel parasites mentioned above.

Mycobacteria

M. tuberculosis may cause infection of the small bowel, which may manifest as persistent diarrhea without other evidence of tuberculosis. MAC may be found in the bowel wall among patients with symptoms of chronic wasting and diarrhea.

Viruses

The enteric viruses that are frequently associated with diarrhea in normal hosts, including rotaviruses, caliciviruses, and others, may be seen in association with HIV infection but do not appear to cause protracted illness. For this reason and because no specific is available for these agents, they are not usually identified outside of a research setting. CMV appears to be the cause of diarrhea in as many as one-quarter of AIDS patients, especially those with the most advanced degrees of immune deficiency. This usually represents infection of the colon and typically presents with small-volume, frequent bowel movements, often containing blood or mucous, and is associated with fever and other systemic signs of infection. Specific antiviral therapy with agents active against CMV may be effective, but ART, when effective, often leads to resolution of symptoms.

Medications

Most, if not all, of the antiretroviral agents currently in use may cause diarrhea. The protease inhibitors, particularly lopinavir, ritonavir and nelfinavir, didanosine, zidovudine, and delavirdine, are all frequently associated with diarrhea, which may make them intolerable (see chap. 5).

Esophagitis

Esophageal involvement with candiasis, cytomegaloviral, or herpesvirus infection or by lymphoma or Kaposi's sarcoma has been described in varying frequency in relation to HIV infection. *Candida* esophagitis is a common initial opportunistic infection.

Diagnosis of esophagitis can often be made on clinical grounds when symptoms of dysphagia and/or odynophagia are present. Oropharyngeal thrush is suggestive of *Candida* esophagitis in the presence of these symptoms. Definitive diagnosis is usually made by endoscopy with biopsy of the esophageal mucosa if necessary.

Pancreatic Disorders

Several medications used in the treatment of HIV infection and its complications may cause pancreatitis. Most common among these are didanosine, pentamidine, zalcitabine, and ritonavir (see chap. 5). Autopsy data indicate that the pancreas may be involved by a number of opportunistic infections, including myco-bacteriosis, toxoplasmosis, pneumocystosis, and a variety of fungi, as well as by HIV itself (85). Pancreatitis resulting from alcohol use, biliary tract disease, trauma, and other medications may also be seen.

Biliary Tract Disease

Several AIDS-related disorders may be associated with biliary obstruction. Both cryptosporidiosis and cytomegaloviral infection may be associated with stenosis of the common bile duct or sclerosing cholangitis or both. CMV may also be seen in association with acalculous cholecystitis. Biliary involvment in HIV infection produces typical symptoms of abdominal pain, nausea, and vomiting. Obstruction may predispose to secondary bacterial infection.

Viral Hepatitis

See chapter 8.

GASTROINTESTINAL MALIGNANCIES

Anal Carcinoma

The risk of anal squamous cell cancer is dramatically increased among HIV-infected men, particularly those with a history of homosexuality.

Lymphoma

The gastrointestinal tract was the most common (24%) extranodal site of involvement by NHL in AIDS patients in one large series. Any segment of the bowel may be involved. Symptoms are typically nonpecific but may include bleeding, perforation, and intestinal obstruction.

MALABSORPTION

Malabsorption may be seen in association with HIV infection. Several infections, particularly cryptosporidiosis and isosporiasis, may cause protracted periods of malabsorption. Lymphoma involving the small bowel is a rare cause.

RENAL DISORDERS

Individuals infected with HIV are prone to a variety of renal disorders. The most common of these is termed HIV-associated nephropathy (HIVAN). Other disorders, particularly diabetes and hypertension, which reflect both the aging of the HIV-infected population and the dyslipidemia associated both with HIV infection and its treatment, have become increasingly common as causes of chronic kidney disease. Antiretroviral medications such as tenofovir and indinavir may have direct renal toxicity. Opportunistic pathogens, particularly CMV, mycobacteria, *C. neoformans*, and *H. capsulatum* may rarely involve the kidneys (86). A number of medications commonly in the treatment of HIV-infected patients may be nephrotoxic in some individuals. These include tenofovir, pentamidine, amphotericin B, foscarnet, and trimethoprim-sulfamethoxazole. Heroin nephropathy may be difficult to distinguish from renal disorders of other etiologies in active users, and renal manifestations of intercurrent infections such as bacterial endocarditis or other disorders may be present.

HIV-Associated Nephropathy

HIV-infected patients have increased susceptibility to a variety of renal disorders, the most important of which is HIVAN. HIVAN is seen disproportionately in males of African descent and injection drug users. It typically presents with proteinuria and progressive renal failure. Kidneys appear normal sized or enlarged on imaging studies, and progression to endstage disease is the rule.

Since the advent of modern ART, the relative incidence of HIVAN among patients with chronic kidney disease and HIV infection has declined (87), the rate of progression of HIVAN is slowed, and disease regression has been described in individuals on treatment (88). Recent guidelines have suggested that HIVAN represents an indication for the intiation of ART regardless of CD4 cell count and viral load (see chap. 5). Survival on dialysis has improved substantially among HIV-infected individuals and is now comparable to the end-stage kidney disease patients without HIV infection. Renal transplantation has been carried out successfully in the setting of HIV infection (89), although the potential complexity of managing ART and immunosuppressive therapy simultaneously following transplantation is daunting and transplant rejection rates have been reported to be higher than in non-HIV-infected patients. Patients with HIVAN who are otherwise candidates for renal transplantation may be considered if their HIV infection is well controlled and they have acceptable CD4 cell counts. Corticosteroids (90) and angiotensin-converting enzyme inhibitors may also produce temporary improvement.

ENDOCRINOLOGICAL DISORDERS

Gonadal Disorders

In one autopsy series (91), 39% of male patients were found to have testicular involvement by opportunistic infections. The most common pathogens were CMV, mycobacteria, and *Toxoplasma*. Functional hypogonadism was documented in 50% of male AIDS patients in one series (92), and significant depression of circulating testosterone levels was seen with the degree of depression correlating with overall clinical status.

Adrenal Disorders

Adrenal cells can be infected with HIV in vitro (93), and the adrenal gland may be a site of involvement of AIDS-related infections and malignancies, including cryptococcosis, mycobacterial infection, and KS (94), although functional hypoadrenalism appears to be rare (95). Symptoms seen in patients with HIV infection are similar to those seen in other settings and may include fatigue, anorexia, weight loss, nausea, abdominal pain, diarrhea, and darkening of the skin. Persistent hyponatremia or hyperkalemia and pronounced orthostatic hypotension should be considered possible indications for adrenal function testing.

MUSCULOSKELETAL DISORDERS

Musculoskeletal complaints are common during the course of HIV infection and may arise at any stage of the disease. In some cases, these symptoms are among the first experienced by the patient. It is worth noting that the initial manifestations of disease in some cases are reminiscent of those of systemic lupus erythematosis and may include arthralgias, cytopenias, butterfly rash, proteinuria, and abnormal urinary sediment.

In one early survey of HIV-positive patients, 72% were found to have rheumatologic manifestations (96), including arthralgias (34.7%), arthritis (11.9%), Reiter's syndrome (9.9%), painful articular syndrome (9.9%), psoriatic arthritis arthritis (1.9%), and polymyositis (1.9%). Arthralgias, which may be mild or severe, most typically involve the knees, shoulders, elbows, or ankles, although the spine or small joints of the hands may also be involved. Features suggestive of sicca complex (97) or Sjogren's syndrome (98) may also occur. The causes of these various conditions are unknown. HIV may play a direct role in the pathogenesis of some of these disorders; others, such as Reiter's syndrome, may sometimes represent reactive states reflecting infection with other organisms commonly seen in HIV-infected individuals.

Myalgias and arthralgias are often a feature of the acute syndrome associated with HIV infection at the time of seroconversion (see chap. 2). Polymyositis has also been associated with HIV infection, as have a variety of autoimmune disorders including thrombocytopenia, circulating rheumatoid factor, and anticardiolipin antibodies, as well as autoantibodies such as antinuclear, antilymphocyte, and antigranulocyte autoantibodies.

Reiter's Syndrome

Reiter's syndrome typically affects young men and appears to be more common in HIV-infected individuals than in the general population. Nearly 10% of patients in various stages of HIV infection had findings consistent with Reiter's syndrome in one prospective series (96).

Several possible reasons for the apparent association between Reiter's syndrome and HIV infection have been proposed (99). Coinfection with organisms such as *Chlamydia* species, known to precipitate Reiter's syndrome, may account for some cases, particularly among patients who test positive for the human lymphocyte antigen B27 (HLA-B27). Bowel infections caused by organisms commonly seen in HIV-infected patients but not previously linked to Reiter's syndrome, such as *Cryptosporidium* organisms or other pathogens not yet characterized, may prove to be important. The stimulation of the immune response that occurs with the onset of Reiter's syndrome may trigger the progression of a preexisting HIV infection. Conversely, the immunodeficiency produced by HIV infection may lead to the development of Reiter's syndrome by an unknown mechanism.

Psoriatic Arthritis

Papulosquamous skin rashes such as seborrheic dermatitis and psoriasis appear to occur more often in HIV-infected patients. In one series (96), 5% of patients had psoriasis and 2% had findings compatible with psoriatic arthritis. Duvic and colleagues (100) described 13 HIV-infected patients with psoriasis, including 9 in whom skin lesions developed after the onset of HIV-related symptoms. Three of these patients had coexistent Reiter's-like symptoms with arthritis, urethritis, and conjunctivitis. Posriasis-associated arthritis may be severe and deforming.

As with Reiter's syndrome, the apparent relationship between HIV and psoriasis and its associated arthritis in some individuals is not well understood. No definite association has been established in these patients between HLA-B27 expression and psoriasis-associated arthritis. In fact, in one series (96), two patients with severe arthritis were HLA-B27 negative. Nonsteroidal anti-inflammatory drugs, sulfasalazine, or gold therapy may be effective in treating psoriatic arthritis. For refractory cases, methotrexate may be considered, although, as noted above, such therapy may result in clinical progression of HIV infection.

HIV-Associated Arthritis

A form of seronegative arthritis not associated with Reiter's syndrome or psoriasis has also been described in some HIV-infected patients (99).

Polymyositis

Polymyositis is the most frequent muscle disorder seen in association with HIV infection. In one large, prospective study (96), 2% of patients were found to have polymyositis on initial evaluation. As with other HIV-related musculoskeletal syndromes, polymyositis may become evident at various stages of HIV infection and may, in fact, be the initial manifestation.

Polymyositis typically becomes evident with proximal muscle weakness, muscle wasting, and elevated creatine kinase levels, often to more than five times normal (99). Electromyographic studies demonstrate abnormalities characteristic of myopathy. In reported cases in which histologic information is available, inflammatory infiltrates of the involved muscles have usually been demonstrated (99).

Sjogren's Syndrome and Sicca Complex

Sicca complex (xerostomia or xerophthalmia) may be seen in association with HIV infection with and without typical features of Sjogren's syndrome. Couderc and colleagues (97) described five HIV-positive patients with progressive generalized lymphadenopathy and sicca complex wit lymphocytic infiltration of salivary glands. Lymphocytic infiltration of one or more extrasalivary sites, including the lungs, liver, kidneys, and bone marrow, was also demonstrated in each of these patients, all of whom had serologic evidence of infection with EBV. In contrast to most cases of classic Sjogren's syndrome, none of these patients were found to have antinuclear antibodies, rheumatoid factor, or other autoantibodies. The relationship between sicca complex, Sjogren's syndrome, and HIV infection remains uncertain, however.

Osteoporosis

Osteopenia and osteoporosis have been recognized, particularly in recent years, to occur with higher prevalence among HIV-infected individuals than in the general population (101), perhaps as a manifestation of what has been postulated to be premature aging in the setting of HIV infection (see chap. 9) (102). Osteoporosis may be seen in association with ART (see chap. 5) (103). Individuals with this condition may develop pathologic fractures.

HEMATOLOGICAL DISORDERS

A remarkable array of hematological disorders may be seen in HIV-infected individuals. These include anemia, leukopenia, thrombocytopenia, coagulopathy, myelofibrosis, hemophagocytosis, plasma cell hyperplasia, and lymphoma.

Some disorders appear to result for the direct effects of HIV on hematopoietic precursor cells; others reflect the production of autoantibodies and perhaps other autoimmune mechanisms. Depletion of CD4+ lymphocytes is, of course, characteristic of HIV infection and at the heart of the immunologic disorders associated with AIDS. Other cell lines, including erythrocytes, granulocytes, and monocytes, may also be directly or indirectly affected by HIV. Refractory anemia, leukopenia, and thrombocytopenia are common in advanced disease. Abnormalities of the peripheral blood smear may include anisocytosis, poikilocytosis, and rouleaux formation. Bone marrow examination, particularly in advanced disease, may reveal dyserythropoiesis, erythroid hypoplasia, megaloblastosis, reticuloendothelial iron block, and a variety of other abnormalities.

Several opportunistic infections associated with AIDS, most notably mycobacteriosis, may involve the bone marrow and lymphoid. Chronic parvovirus infection involving marrow erythroid precursors may occur. A number of therapeutic agents commonly used in HIV infection, especially zidovudine, ganciclovir, acyclovir, and antifolate compounds, often cause significant cytopenias due to bone marrow depression.

In rare cases, hematological manifestations, particularly autoimmune thrombocytopenia, dominate the clinical picture. In patients at advanced stages of immunodeficiency, several disorders, particularly drug toxic effects and involvement of the marrow by opportunistic infections, may coexist.

Autoimmune Thrombocytopenia

Thrombocytopenia is common in HIV-infected individuals. It may be present at any stage of the disease (104) and does not have clear prognostic significance. Mechanisms include both elaboration of antiplatelet antibodies and deposition of immune complexes on the platelet surface.

If possible, the diagnosis of autoimmune thrombocytopenia should be made only after bone marrow examination confirms that platelet production is not depressed. Involvement of the marrow by opportunistic infections and malignancies, or side effects of several commonly used medications, especially ganciclovir, AZT, and antifolate agents such as trimethoprim-sulfamethoxazole or sulfadiazine, may result in thrombocytopenia. Other causes of peripheral consumption of platelets, including hypersplenism, disseminated intravascular coagulation, and drug-induced autoimmune thrombocytopenia, should be excluded.

Other Coagulation Disorders

Patients with HIV infection frequently have anticardiolipin antibodies (105). Clinically significant thrombosis and thromboembolism occur in some of these individuals (106). Lupus-like and heparin-like anticoagulants have also been demonstrated in association with HIV infection (107) as have abnormalities of fibrin polymerization possibly related to high levels of γ-globulins characteristic of HIV infection.

Lymphoproliferative Disorders

Lymphoproliferative disorders have been associated with HIV infection since the earliest days of the AIDS epidemic. The entity of persistent generalized lymphadenopathy (PGL) was recognized as an AIDS-associated phenomenon before the discovery of HIV. Further, generalized lymphadenopathy is a common feature of acute retroviral infection, often occurring a week or two after the onset of other symptoms and persisting for weeks to months. The lymphomas associated with

HIV infection are, to a large extent though not exclusively, associated with EBV infection. The impact of ART on the incidence and prognosis of HIV-associated lymphoma is the subject of some controversy. Some reports suggest a declining incidence and an important role for ART in the management of certain lymphomas, while other data suggest that ART has had little impact on the incidence of lymphoma. It is estimated that approximately 16% of HIV-associated deaths are due to lymphoma in the modern ART era. Unlike many opportunistic infections and KS, lymphoma appears to occur with approximately equal frequency in individuals with both severely and moderately depressed CD4 lymphocyte counts.

LYMPHOMA

The association between HIV infection and lymphoma was recognized in the early days of the HIV/AIDS epidemic, and NHL was considered an AIDS-defining condition by the mid-1980s. It was recognized that most AIDS-related lymphomas were of B-cell origin and frequently presented in extranodal sites, especially the CNS and gastrointestinal tract. It was also clear that lymphoma in the setting of HIV infection carried a particularly poor prognosis and pursued an aggressive course, particularly in the setting of advanced immune deficiency. In the past 20 years, and particularly since the advent of modern ART, knowledge of AIDS-related lymphomas has increased greatly (108). It is now recognized that they represent a heterogeneous group of disorders. The most common histological patterns are noncleaved cell lymphoma, including Burkitt's lymphoma and diffuse large B-cell lymphoma (109). Often several types of histological features are seen within the same lymphoma (110). Further, it appears that Hodgkin's disease (HD) may also be seen with increased frequency in the setting of HIV infection (111). Overall, the majority of AIDS-related B-cell lymphomas have evidence of EBV infection (112), and prior EBV may be a risk factor for the development of lymphoma (113), although the exact link between EBV infection and HIV-related lymphoma remains controversial. HHV-8 has been associated with both Kaposi's sarcoma and a peculiar type of NHL affecting serous body cavities such as the pleural, peritoneal, and pericardial spaces (114).

The clinical presentation of NHL in the setting of HIV infection is remarkably variable but widespread, extranodal involvement is common, and stage IV disease is diagnosed in the majority of cases. Cerebral involvement typically presents with a focal neurological deficit and a mass lesion on cerebral imaging. As discussed above, differentiation between CNS lymphoma and other focal neurological disorders, particularly toxoplasmosis, may be difficult since the radiographic appearance of lesions may be identical. If the clinical situation permits, empiric therapy for toxoplasmosis is generally warranted in patients manifesting cerebral mass lesions with ring enhancement on CT. Patients failing such therapy should be regarded as possibly having lymphoma. Although histological examination is generally required for diagnosis of lymphoma, PET and SPECT, as discussed above, may aid in the distinction between lymphoma and toxoplasmosis. Gastrointestinal lymphoma typically presents with nonspecific abdominal pain, unexplained fever, occult or clinical bleeding, obstruction, ascites, or bowel perforation with peritonitis. The diagnosis is generally suspected on the basis of abdominal imaging, but tissue confirmation is required. Lymphoma at other extranodal sites similarly presents with nonspecific features. Pulmonary involvement may feature nodules, focal or diffuse infiltrates, or pleural effusions, which may mimic pneumonia or tuberculosis. As a rule, the challenge in diagnosing extranodal lymphoma is distinguishing from more common entities that more typically involve the end organ in question.

Similar to NHL, HD, when seen in the setting of HIV infection, tends to present as a multicentric disorder with a high incidence of "B" symptoms at presentation. Extranodal involvement, especially of the liver, spleen, and marrow, is also more common than in non-HIV-related HD, and the disease appears to pursue a more aggressive course (108).

In contrast to the case of Kaposi's sarcoma and many HIV-related opportunistic infections, the incidence of NHL does not appear to be decreasing since the advent of HAART in the mid-1990s (115).

CASTLEMAN'S DISEASE

Castleman's disease (angiofollicular lymphoid hyperplasia) is a lymphoproliferative disorder, which shares some features with lymphoma, including nonspecific respiratory and constitutional symptoms, hepatosplenomegaly, and lymphadenopathy, which may be massive in some cases. Multicentric Castleman's disease may be associated with HIV infection. In some instances, particularly in HIV-infected homosexual men, it may precede the development of Kaposi's sarcoma, and it appears to be associated with HH8 or EBV infection.

GENITAL TRACT DISORDERS

Cervical Neoplasia

It has long been recognized that HIV-infected women have a higher incidence of genital HPV infection, cervical intraepithelial neoplasia, and, very likely, cervical cancer (see chap. 10). This association appears to be true when risk factors for HPV infection other than HIV infection are controlled for and to increase with worsening immune deficiency.

Sexually Transmitted Diseases

Sexually active HIV-infected patients may be at high risk for sexually transmitted diseases, both inflammatory (*gonorrhea*, *Chlamydia*) and ulcerative (syphilis, herpes simplex, chancroid). Vaginal candidiasis, particularly if recurrent and severe, is a common, often overlooked, initial manifestation of HIV infection in women. The approach to diagnosis of these disorders is similar to that taken for non-HIV-infected patients and is outside the scope of this discussion (see chap. 12). In the ambulatory setting, particular attention must be paid to screening for *Chlamydia* and *gonorrhea* as well as forsyphilis with periodic serum tests and for human papillomavirus infection with periodic pelvic examination.

PSYCHIATRIC DISORDERS

Psychiatric disturbances, particularly depression and anxiety, are common among HIV-infected patients. Patients with a history of risk behavior may display denial by avoiding testing. Social isolation, guilt, and uncertainty are common after a diagnosis of AIDS. Stress associated with learning of a positive test result for HIV or being informed that an AIDS-related illness has been diagnosed may precipitate psychiatric crises and feelings of anger, fear, and confusion. Data from the first decade of the epidemic suggested that AIDS was associated with a greatly increased risk of suicide (116).

It may be difficult to distinguish between psychiatric symptoms and those reflecting organic disease, particularly AIDS dementia complex. Opportunistic infections and malignancies as well as medications affecting the CNS may initially cause symptoms suggesting psychiatric disorders.

Cerebral toxoplasmosis, lymphoma, cryptococcosis, tuberculosis, listeriosis, and neurosyphilis may all present with a clinical picture of toxic psychosis. It is especially important that these conditions be excluded with appropriate diagnostic studies in patients presenting with the new onset of psychotic symptoms. Reactions to medications may also be confused with psychiatric disorders. For example, hypoglycemia resulting from pentamidine therapy may manifest as delerium. Efavirenz may cause confusion and vivid nightmares (see chap. 5).

REFERENCES

1. Daher EF, Silva GB, Barros FA, et al. Clinical and laboratory features of disseminated histoplasmosis in HIV patients from Brazil. Trop Med Int Health 2007; 12(9):1108–1115.
2. Skinner-Adams TS, McCarthy JS, Gardiner DL, et al. HIV and malaria coinfection: interactions and consequences of chemotherapy. Trends Parasitol 2008; 24(6):264–271.
3. Ustianowski AP, Lawn SD, Lockwood DN. Interactions between HIV infection and leprosy: a paradox. Lancet Infect Dis 2006; 6(6):350–360.
4. Batista MD, Porro AM, Maeda SM, et al. Leprosy reversal reaction as immune reconstitution inflammatory syndrome in patients with AIDS. Clin Infect Dis 2008; 46(6):e56–e60.
5. Kaplan JE, Benson CB, Holmes KK, et al. Guidelines for prevention and treatment of opportunistic infections in HIV-infected adults and adolescents. Recommendations from CDC, the National Institutes of Healt and the HIV Medicine Associaion of the Infectious Diseases Society of America. Morbid Mortal Weekly Rep 2009; 58(RR04):1–198.

6. Zolopa A, Andersen J, Komarow L, et al. Immediate versus deferred ART in the setting of actue-related OI: final results of a randomized strategy, ACTG A5164. 15th CROI, 2008, Boston, MA, Abstract 142.

7. Khan FA, Minion J, Pai M, et al. Treatment of active tuberculosis in HIV-coinfected patients: a systematic review and meta-analysis. Clin Infect Dis 2010; 50(9):1288–1299.

8. Tantisiriwat W, Tebas P, Clifford DB, et al. Progressive multifocal leukoence-phalopathy in patients with AIDS receiving highly active antiretroviral therapy. Clin Infect Dis 1999; 28:1152–1154.

9. Carr A, Marriott D, Field A, et al. Treatment of HIV-1-associated microsporidiosis and cryptosporidiosis with combination antiretroviral therapy. Lancet 1998; 351:256–261.

10. Murdaca G, Campelli A, Setti M, et al. Complete remission of AIDS/Kaposi's sarcoma after treatment with a combination of two nucleoside reverse transcriptase inhibitors and one non-nucleoside reverse transcriptase inhibitor [letter]. AIDS 2002; 16:304–305.

11. Lawn SD, Torok ME, Wood R. Optimum time to start antiretroviral therapy during HIV-associated opportunistic infection. Curr Opin Infect Dis 2011; 24(1):34–42.

12. Mofenson LM, Brady MT, Danner SP, et al. Guidelines for the prevention and treatment of opportunistic infections among HIV-exposed and HIV-infected children: recommendations from CDC, the National Institutes of Health, the HIV Medicine Association of the Infectious Diseases Society of America, the Pediatric Infectious Diseases Society, and the American Academy of Pediatrics. Morbid Mortal Weekly Rep Recomm Rep 2009; 58(RR11):1–248.

13. Valle SL. Dermatologic finding related to human immunodeficiency virus infection in high-risk individuals. J Am Acad Dermatol 1987; 17:951.

14. Goodman DS, Teplitz ED, Wishner A, et al. Prevalence of cutaneous disease in patients with acquired immunodeficiency syndrome (AIDS) or AIDS-related complex. J Am Acad Dermatol 1987; 17:210.

15. Melbye M, Grossman RJ, Goedert JJ, et al. Risk of AIDS after herpes zoster. Lancet 1987; 1(8535):728–731.

16. Koehler JE, Quinn FD, Berger TG, et al. Isolation of *Rochalimaea* species from cutaneous and osseous lesions of bacillary angiomatosis. N Engl J Med 1992; 327:1625–1631.

17. Cockerell CJ, Leboit PE. Bacillary angiomatosis: a newly characterized pseudo-neoplastic, infectious cutaneous vascular disorder. J Am Acad Dermatol 1990; 22:501.

18. Perkocha LA, Geaghan SM, Yen TS, et al. Clinical and pathological features of bacillary peliosis hepatis in association with human immunodeficiency virus infection. N Engl J Med 1990; 323(23):1581–1586.

19. Rico MJ, Penneys NS. Cutaneous cryptococcosis resembling molluscum contagiosum in a patient with AIDS. Arch Dermatol 1985; 121:901.

20. Beyt BE, Ortbals DW, Santa Cruz DJ, et al. Cutaneous mycobacteriosis: analysis of 34 cases with a new classification of the disease. Medicine 1981; 60:95.

21. Beral V, Peterman TA, Berkelman RL, et al. Kaposi's sarcoma among persons with AIDS: a sexually-transmitted infection? Lancet 1990; 335(8682):123–128.

22. Mesri EA, Cesarman E, Boshoff C. Kaposi's sarcoma and its associated herpes-virus. Nat Rev Cancer 2010; 10(10):707–719.

23. Jacobson LP, Jenkins FJ, Springer G, et al. Interaction of human immunodeficiency virus type1 and human herpesvirus type 8 infection on the incidence of Kaposi's sarcoma. J Infect Dis 2000; 181:1940.

24. Friedman-Kien A, Laubenstein LJ, Rubinstein P, et al. Disseminated Kaposi's sarcoma in homosexual men. Ann Intern Med 1982; 96:693–700.

25. Gnepp DR, Chandler W, Hyams V. Primary Kaposi's sarcoma of the head and neck. Ann Intern Med 1984; 100:107–114.

26. Hasan FA, Jeffers LJ, Welsh SW, et al. Hepatic involvement as the primary manifestation of Kaposi's sarcoma in the acquired immunodeficiency syndrome. Am J Gastroenterol 1989; 84:1449–1451.

27. Silver MA, Macher AM, Reichert CM, et al. Cardiac involvement by Kaposi's sarcoma in acquired immune deficiency syndrome (AIDS). Am J Cardiol 1984; 53:983.

28. Rasokat H, Steigleder GK, Bendick C, et al. Malignant menaloma and HIV infection. Z Hautdr 1989; 64:581–582.

29. Wilkins K, Turner R, Delov JC, et al. Cutaneous and human immunodeficiency virus disease. J Am Acad Dermatol 2006; 54(2):189–206.

30. Gabuzda DH, Hirsch MS. Neurologic manifestations of infection with human immunodeficiency virus: clinical features and pathogenesis. Ann Intern Med 1987; 107:383.

31. Portegies P, de Gans J, Lange JM, et al. Declining incidence of AIDS dementia complex after introduction of zidovudine treatment. BMJ 1989; 299:819–821.

32. Hollander H, Stringari S. Human immunodeficiency virus-associated meningitis: clinical course and correlations. Am J Med 1987; 83:813.

33. Goldstick L, Mandybur TI, Bode R. Spinal cord degeneration in AIDS. Nerulogy 1985; 35:103.

34. Parry GJ. Peripheral neuropathies associated with human immunodeficiency virus infection. Ann Neruol 1988; 23(suppl):S49.

35. Navia BA, Jordan BD, Price RW. The AIDS dementia complex. I. Clinical features. Ann Neurol 1986; 19:517–524.

36. Israelski DM, Remington JS. Toxoplasmic encephalitis in patients with AIDS. Infect Dis Clin North Am 1988; 2:429.

37. Elkin CM, Leon E, Grenell SL, et al. Intracranial lesions in the acquired immunodeficiency syndrome: radiological (computed tomography) features. JAMA 1985; 253:393–396.

38. Hoffman JM, Washkin HA, Schifter T, et al. FDG-PET iin differentiating lymphoma from nonmalignant central nervous system lesions in patients with AIDS. J Nucl Med 1993; 34:567.

39. Cohen JA, McMeeking A, Cohen W, et al. Evaluation of the policy of empiric treatment of suspected *Toxoplasma* encephalitis in patients with the acquired immunodeficiency syndrome. Am J Med 1989; 86:521.

40. Ambinder RF, Bhatia K, Martinez-Maza O, et al. Cancer biomarkers in HIV patients. Curr Opin HIV AIDS 2010; 5(6):531–537.

41. Utsuki S, Oca H, Abe K, et al. Primary central nervous system lymphoma in acquired immune deficiency syndrome mimicking toxoplasmosis. Brain Tumor Pathol 2011; [Epub ahead of print].

42. Levy RM, Bredesen DE, Rosenblum ML, et al. Neurological manifestations of the acquired immunodeficiency syndrome (AIDS): experience of UCSF and review of the literature. J Neruosurg 1985; 62:475–495.

43. Cinque P, Koralnik LJ, Gerevini S, et al. Progressive multifocal leukoencephalopathy in HIV-1 infection. Lancet Infect Dis 2009; 9(10):625–636.

44. Centers for Disease Control and Prevention, Update: acquired immunodeficiency syndrome: United States. Morbid Mortal Weekly Rep 1986; 35:17.

45. Page KR, Chaisson R, Sande M. Cryptococcosis and other fungal infections (histoplasmosis and coccidioidomycosis) in HIV-infected patients. In: Volberding PA, Sande MA, Lange J, et al., eds. Global HIV/AIDS Medicine. Philadelphia: Saunders Elsevier, 2008.

46. Zuger A, Louie E, Holzman RS, et al. Cryptococcal disease in patients with the acquired immunodeficiency syndrome: diagnostic features and outcome of treatment. Ann Intern Med 1986; 104:234–240.

47. Fiala M, Cone LA, Cohen N, et al. Responses of neurologic complications of AIDS to 3′azido3′deoxythymidine and 9-(1,3-dihydroxy-2-propoxylmethyl) guanine. I. Clinical features. Rev Infect Dis 1988; 10:250–256.

48. Holland NR, Power C, Mathews VP, et al. Cytomegalovirus encephalitis in acquired immunodeficiency syndrome (AIDS). Neurology 1994; 44:507–514.

49. Kalayjian RC, Cohen ML, Bonomo RA, et al. Cytomegalovirus ventriculoencephalitis in AIDS: a syndrome with distinct clinical and pathologic features. Medicine (Baltimore) 1993; 72:67–77.

50. Cohen BA, et al. Neurological prognosis of cytomegalovirus polyradiculomyelopathy in AIDS. Neurology 1993; 43:493.

51. Musiani M, Zerbini M, Venturoli S, et al. Rapid diagnosis of cytomegalovirus encephalitis in patients with AIDS using in situ hybridization. J Clin Pathol 1994; 47:886–891.

52. Lipton SA, Genderlman HE. Dementia associated with acquired immunodeficiency syndrome. N Engl J Med 1995; 332:934.

53. De La Paz R, Enzmann D. Neuroradiology of acquired immunodeficiency syndrome. In: Rosunblum ML, Levy RM, Bredesen DE, eds. AIDS and the Nervous System. New York: Raven, 1988:121–154.

54. Post MJ, Tate LG, Quencer RM, et al. CT, MR and pathology in HIV encephalitis and meningitis. AJR Am J Roentgenol 1988; 151(2):373–380.

55. Jabs DA, Green WR, Fox R, et al. Ocular manifestations of acquired immunodeficiency syndrome. Opthalmology 1989; 96:1092–1099.

56. Jabs DA, Enger C, Bartlett JG. Cytomegalovirus retinitis and acquired immunodeficiency syndrome. Arch Opthtalmolol 1989; 107:75.

57. Whitcup SM. Cytomegalovirus retinitis in the era of highly active antiretroviral therapy. JAMA 2000; 283:653.

58. Shuler JD, Holland GN, Miles SA, et al. Kaposi sarcoma of the conjunctiva and eyelids associed with the acquired immunodeficiency syndrome. Arch Opthalmol 1989; 107:858.

59. Phelan JA, Saltzman BR, Friedland GH, et al. Oral findings in patients with acquired immunodeficiency syndrome. Oral Surg Oral Med Oral Pathol 1987; 64:50–56.

60. Greenspan JS, Greenspan D, Lennette ET, et al. Replication of Epstein-Barr virus within the epithelial cells of "hairy: leukoplakia, and AIDS-associated lesion. N Engl J Med 1985; 313:1564–1571.

61. Muzyka BC, Glick M. Major aphthous ulcers in patients with HIV disease. Oral Surg Oral Med Oral Pathol 1994; 77:116.

62. Friedman M, Brenski A, Taylor L. Treatment of aphthous ulcers in AIDS patients. Laryngocscope 1994; 104(5 pt 1):566.
63. Phair J, Munoz A, Detels R, et al. The risk of *Pneumocystis carinii* pneumonia among men infected with human immunodeficiency virus type 1. Multicenter AIDS Cohort Study Group. N Engl J Med 1990; 322:161–165.
64. Masur H, Ognibene FP, Yarchoan R, et al. CD4 counts as predictors of opportunistic pneumonias in human immunodeficiency virus (HIV) infection. Ann Intern Med 1989; 111:223–231.
65. Wheat LJ, Slama TG, Zeckel ML. Histoplasmosis in the acquired immune deficiency syndrome. Am J Med 1985; 78:203–210.
66. Welch K, Finkbeiner W, Alpers CE, et al. Autopsy finding in the acquired immune deficiency syndrome. JAMA 1984; 252:1152–1159.
67. Selwyn PA, Feingold AR, Hartel D, et al. Increased risk of bacterial pneumonia in HIV-infected intravenous drug without AIDS. AIDS 1988; 2:267–272.
68. Farley MM, Stephens DS, Brachman PS Jr., et al. Invasive *Haemophilus influenza* disease in adults: a prospective, population-based surveillance. Ann Intern Med 1992; 116:806–812.
69. Mendelson MH, Gurtman A, Szabo S, et al. *Pseudomonas aeruginosa* bacteremia in patients with AIDS. Clin Infect Dis 1994; 18:886–895.
70. Meduri GU, Stover DE, Lee M, et al. Pulmonary Kaposi's sarcoma in the acquired immune syndrome: clinical, radiographic and pathologic manifestations. Am J Med 1988; 81:11–18.
71. Knowles DM, Chamulak GA, Subar M, et al. Lymphoid neoplasia associated with the acquired immunodeficiency syndrome (AIDS): the New York University Medical Center experience with 105 patients (1981-1986). Ann Intern Med 1988; 108:744–753.
72. White DA, Matthay RA. Noninfectious pulmonary complications of infection with the human immunodeficiency virus. Am Rev Respir Dis 1989; 140:1763.
73. Monsuez J, Kinney EL, Vittecoq D, et al. Comparison among acquired immune deficiency syndrome patients with and without clinical evidence of crdiac disease. Am J Cardiol 1988; 62:1311.
74. Yunis NA, Stone VE. Cardiac manifestations of HIV/ADS: a review of disese spectrum and clinical management. J Acquir Immune Defic Syndr Hum Retrovirol 1998; 18:145.
75. Himelman RB, Chung WS, Chernoff DN, et al. Cardiac manifestations of human immunodeficiency virus infection: a two-dimensional echocardiographic study. J Am Coll Cardiol 1989; 13:1030–1036.
76. Hecht SR, Berger M, Van Tosh A, et al. Unsuspected cardiac abnormalities in the acquired immune deficiency syndrome: an echocardiographic study. Chest 1989; 96:805–808.
77. The DAD Study Group. Class of antiretroviral drugs and the risk of myocardial infarction. N Engl J Med 2007; 356(17):1723–1735.
78. Barbaro G. Cardiovascular manifestations of HIV infection. Circulation 2002; 106:1420–1425.
79. Hakas JF, Geralovich T. Spontaneous regression of cardiomyopathy in a patient with the acquired immunodeficiency syndrome. Chest 1991; 99:770.
80. Barbaro G, Di Lorenzo G, Grisorio B, et al. Cardiac involvement in the acquired immunodeficiency syndrome: a multicenter clinical-pathological study. Gruppo

Italiano per lo Studio Cardiologico dei pazienti affetti da AIDS Investigators. AIDS Res Hum Retroviruses 1998; 14:1071–1077.

81. Mesa RA, Edell ES, Dunn WF, et al. Human immunodeficiency virus infection and pulmonary hypertension: two new cases and a review of 86 reported cases. Mayo Clin Proc 1998; 73:37–45.

82. Currier JS, Baden LR. Getting smarter—the toxicity of undertreated HIV infection. N Engl J Med 2006; 355(22):2359–2361.

83. Barbul F, Meynard JL, Guiguet M, et al. *Clostridium difficile* associated diarrhea in HIV-infected patients: epidemiology and risk factors. J Acquir Immune Defic Syndr Hum Retroviral 1997; 16:176–181.

84. Flanigan T, Whalen C, Turner J, et al. *Cryptosporidium* infection and CD4 cell counts. Ann Intern Med 1992; 116:840.

85. Chehter EZ, Longo MA, Laudanna AA, et al. Involvement of the pancreas in AIDS: a propectively study of 109 post-mortems. AIDS 2000; 14:1879–1886.

86. Glassrock RJ, Cohen AH, Danovitch G, et al. Human immunodeficiency (HIV) infection and the kidney. Ann Intern Med 1990; 112:35–49.

87. Wyatt CM, Klotman PE. HIV-associated nephropathy in the era of antiretroviral therapy. Am J Med 2007; 120(6):488–492.

88. Chemlal K, Nochy D, Kenouch S, et al. Dramatic improvement of renal dysfunction in a human immunodeficiency virus-infected woman treated with high active antiretroviral therapy. Clin Infect Dis 2000; 31:805.

89. Trulas TC, Mocroft A, Cofan F, et al. Dialysis and renal transplantation in HIV-infected patients: a European study. J Acquir Immune Def Syndr 2010; [Epub ahead of print].

90. Smith MC, Austen JL, Carey JT, et al. Prednisone improves renal function and proteinuria in human immunodeficiency virus-associated nephropathy. Am J Med 1996; 101:41.

91. De Paepe ME, Guerrieri C, Waxman M. Opportunistic infections of the testis in the acquired immunodeficiency syndrome. Mt Sinai J Med 1990; 57:25.

92. Dobs AS, Dempsey MA, Ladenson PW, et al. Endocrine disorders in men infected with human immunodeficiency virus. Am J Med 1988; 84(3 pt 2):6111–6116.

93. Barboza A, Castro BA, Whalen M, et al. Infection of cultured human adrenal cells by different strains of HIV. AIDS 1992; 6(12):1437–1443.

94. Glasgow BJ, Steinsapir KD, Anders K, et al. Adrenal pathology in the acquired immune deficiency syndrome. Am J Clin Pathol 1985; 84(5):594–597.

95. Gripshover B, Kalayjian R. Adrenal insufficiency in AIDS; prevalence and clinical characteristics. Int Conf AIDS (1993): 465 (abstract no. PO-B25 1980).

96. Berman A, Espinoza LR, Diaz JD, et al. Rheumatic manifestations of human immunodeficiency virus infection. Am J Med 1988; 85:59–64.

97. Couderc L, D'Agay MF, Danon F, et al. Sicca complex and infection with human immunodeficiency virus. Arch Intern Med 1987; 147:898.

98. DeClerck LS, Couttenye MM, de Broe ME, et al. Acquired immunodeficiency syndrome mimicking Sjogren's syndrome and systemic lupus erythematosus. Arthritis Rheum 1988; 31:272.

99. Kaye BR. Rheumatologic manifestations of infection with human immunodeficiency virus (HIV). Ann Intern Med 1989; 111:158.

100. Duvic M, Johnson TM, Rapini RP, et al. Acquired immunodeficiency syndrome-assoicated psoriasis and Reiter's syndrome. Arch Dermatol 1987; 123:1622–1632.

101. Bonjoch A, Figueras M, Estany C, et al. High prevalence of and progression to low bone mineral density in HIV-infected patients: a longitudinal cohort study. AIDS 2010; 24(18):2827–2833.

102. Onen NF, Overton ET. A review of premature frailty in HIV-infected persons; another manifestation of HIV-related accelerated aging. Curr Aging Sci 2010; [Epub ahead of print].

103. Ofotokun I, Weitzmann MN. HIV-1 infection and antiretroviral therapies: risk factors for osteoporosis and bone fracture. Curr Opin endocrinol Diabetes Obes 2010; 17(6):523–529.

104. Ratner L. Human immunodeficiency virus-associated autoimmune thrombocytopenic purpura: a review. Am J Med 1989; 86:194.

105. Stimmler MM, Quismorio FP Jr, McGehee WG, et al. Anticardiolipin antibodies in acquired immunodeficiency syndrome. Arch Intern Med 1989; 149:1833–1835.

106. Cappell MS, Simon T, Tiku M. Splenic infarction associated with anticardiolipin antibodies in a patient with acquired immunodeficiency syndrome. Dig Dis Sci 1993; 38(6):1152.

107. Guez T, Toulon P, Sienczewska M, et al. Fibrin polymerization defect in patients with AIDS. In Conf AIDS 1991; 7:261.

108. Tirelli U, Spina M, Gaidano G, et al. Epidemiological, biological and clinical features of HIV-related lymphomas in the era of highly active antiretroviral therapy. AIDS 2000; 14:1675–1688.

109. Carbone A, Tirelli U, Vaccher E, et al. A clinicopathologic study of lymphoid neoplasias associated with human immunodeficiency virus infection in Italy. Cancer 1991; 68:842–852.

110. Raphael M, Gentilhomme O, Tulliez M, et al. Histopathologic features of high-grade non-Hodgkin's lymphomas in acquired immunodeficiency syndrome. Arch Pathol Lab Med 1991; 115:15–20.

111. Tirelli U, Errante D, Dolcetti R, et al. Hodgkin's disease and human immunodeficiency virus infection: clinicopatholgic and virologic features of 114 patients from the Italian Cooperative Group on AIDS and Tumors. J Clin Oncol 1995; 13:1758–1767.

112. Ballerinii P, Gaidano G, Gong JZ, et al. Multiple genetic lesions in acquired immmunodeficiency syndrome-related non-Hodgkin's lymphoma. Blood 1993; 81:166–176.

113. Shibata D, Weiss LM, Nathwani BN, et al. Epstein-Barr virus in benign lymph node biopsies from individuals infected with the human immunodeficiency virus is associagted with concurrent or subsequent development of non-Hodgkin's lymphoma. Blood 1991; 77:1527.

114. Nador RG. Primary effusion lymphoma: a distinct clinicopathologic entity associated with Kaposi's sarcoma-associagted herpes virus. Blood 1996; 88:6465.

115. Jacobson LP, Yamashita TE, Detels R, et al. Impact of potent antiretroviral therapy on the incidence of Kaposi's sarcoma among HIV-1-infected individuals. J Acquir Immune Defic Syndr 1999; 21(suppl:S34):S34–S41.

116. Marzuk PM, Tierney H, Tardiff K, et al. Increased risk of suicide in persons with AIDS. JAMA 1988; 259:1333–1337.

4

Symptom-oriented evaluation and management

INTRODUCTION

A variety of medical complaints are commonly voiced by HIV-infected individuals, especially those at advanced stages of immune deficiency. A challenge for the clinician is to recognize how the presence of HIV infection may change the significance and implications of a specific complaint or physical finding. Among patients with advanced HIV infection, relatively minor complaints such as a headache, fever, or cough may signify life-threatening opportunistic infections or malignancies, which would not be considerations in the normal host. Even at earlier stages in the natural history of HIV infection, such common problems as diarrhea, chest pain, and fatigue must be viewed from the unique perspective of the complex, multisystem disorder that the virus causes. Furthermore, antiretroviral therapy (ART) has brought with it new disorders, such as the lipodystrophy syndrome, lactic acidosis/hepatic steatosis associated with several of the nucleoside reverse transcriptase inhibitors, severe hypersensitivity reactions to abacavir, acute hepatitis associated with nevirapine, and renal disorders associated with tenofovir among others. Finally, of course, the presence of HIV infection does not preclude other unrelated disorders.

This chapter presents an approach to the differential diagnosis and diagnostic evaluation of symptoms commonly encountered with HIV infection. Although minor complaints are common among HIV-infected patients, this chapter emphasizes the presenting manifestations of serious, debilitating, and life-threatening complications of HIV infection.

RECOGNIZING HIV INFECTION

Acute HIV Infection

Acute HIV infection is accompanied by a symptomatic illness in the majority of individuals. After an incubation period between one and six weeks, this illness is characterized by sore throat, skin rash, and, later, lymphadenopathy. Aseptic meningitis and other neurologic abnormalities may also manifest in association with acute HIV infection. Despite its apparently high incidence, the acute retroviral syndrome is seldom diagnosed largely because it shares features with many other disorders and because the risk of HIV infection in an individual may not be recognized either by themselves or by providers evaluating their complaints. What often marks the syndrome and may permit its recognition is its relative chronicity, often weeks to a month or more, while other similar illnesses, largely viral respiratory or enteroviral infections, typically last a week or less. Generalized lymphadenopathy and the diffuse rash that accompany the syndrome are also rare in other viral infections among adult patients. Despite these potential clues, however, the provider evaluating unexplained aseptic meningitis or other "viral syndromes" should carefully question the patient about potential HIV exposure, particularly within the preceding month or two. A similar illness may occur in individuals with chronic HIV infection during periods of rising viral load because of treatment failure or poor adherence to ART.

Chronic HIV Infection

Because of the multisystem nature of HIV infection and the remarkable variety of associated clinical disorders (see chap. 3), recognizing the nonspecific signs and symptoms of chronic HIV infection may be difficult, even among patients known to be at risk. When there is no clinical suspicion of HIV infection, this task may be impossible. The true significance of such nonspecific HIV-related symptoms as lymph node enlargement, diarrhea, and weight loss may not be initially recognized. Diagnostic confusion is particularly likely when the patient is not known to be at high risk for HIV infection and in geographic areas where prevalence rates are low. Even disorders associated with advanced stages of immune deficiency, such as invasive herpes simplex infection and lymphoma, may not initially be appreciated as being related to HIV infection. Therefore, evaluating disorders that result from HIV infection requires familiarity with the commonly seen syndromes, an ability to assess the likelihood of HIV infection, and a high level of awareness.

The likelihood that HIV-related signs or symptoms will be recognized as such can be increased by routinely and systematically questioning all patients about risk behavior during the course of the initial medical evaluation and, as discussed in chapter 1, offering HIV testing to everyone aged 13 to 64. Even after meticulous risk factor assessment, directed testing may fail to identify a substantial proportion of HIV-infected patients because they are unaware of potential exposure or are reticent to discuss risk behaviors.

Although some disorders, such as Kaposi's sarcoma (KS), may be virtually diagnostic of HIV infection, all the symptoms and many of the specific disorders discussed in this chapter are encountered frequently in patients not infected with HIV. The new appearance of certain signs or symptoms, such as unexplained weight loss, fever, and persistent diarrhea, in a patient not known to be HIV infected should prompt careful assessment or reassessment of potential risk factors. It should be kept in mind that many patients first come to medical attention with manifestations of advanced HIV infection, including AIDS, without any history of earlier HIV-related complaints.

What follows is an overview of the differential diagnosis and suggested diagnostic evaluation of several of the most common symptoms and signs seen in HIV-infected individuals. As with all patients, the evaluation of symptoms and signs of disease in HIV-infected patients must be individualized. The morbidity and cost of diagnostic studies must be taken into account, and the extent of the diagnostic workup should reflect the likelihood that a treatable cause of the disorder can be identified.

As noted above, the recent availability of a large number of new medications for the treatment of HIV infection and its complications has complicated the interpretation of symptoms. Side effects affecting the central nervous, skin, or gastrointestinal tracts may cause diagnostic confusion with some of the entities discussed here. The reader is referred to chapter 5 for discussions of interpretation and management of medication side effects.

FEVER OF UNKNOWN ORIGIN

Incidence

Unexplained persistent fever, that is, fever of several weeks' duration for which no cause can be identified after a routine diagnostic evaluation, is a common phenomenon in HIV infection and may be encountered at any stage of disease (1,2).

Differential Diagnosis

The differential diagnosis of persistent fever varies, depending on the stage of disease and degree of immunodeficiency. Self-limited fever is a common feature of acute HIV infection, but it is typically accompanied by other signs, including rash, headache, and oral ulcerations. Persistent fever may be seen in early symptomatic patients, especially in association with generalized lymphadenopathy; along with other constitutional signs, it was formerly termed lymphadenopathy syndrome or AIDS-related complex (ARC).

In patients with more advanced HIV infection, particularly those with CD4+ lymphocyte counts below 200 cells/mm^3 or with a previous diagnosis of AIDS, opportunistic infections may give rise to fever before the onset of more specific symptoms. A number of studies have demonstrated that mycobacterial infection is a relatively frequent cause of fever of unknown origin in this setting (Fig. 4.1) (4,5). A variety of other pathogens, including *Mycobacterium tuberculosis*, *Pneumocystis carinii* pneumonia (PCP), cytomegalovirus (CMV), and, in endemic areas, histoplasmosis, coccidioidomycosis, and leishmaniasis may

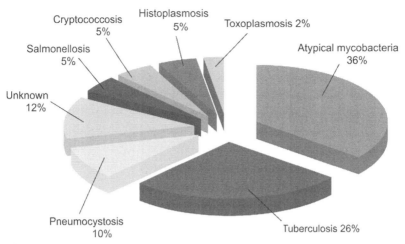

Figure 4.1 Causes of persistent fever in 42 AIDS patients. *Source*: Adapted from Ref. 3.

also become apparent in this fashion. Visceral KS and lymphoma may also cause nonspecific fever. Bacterial and fungal superinfections are particularly common among patients with indwelling intravenous catheters. Sinusitis, as well as periodontal and perirectal infections, all common in HIV-infected patients, occasionally become evident as undifferentiated fever. Endocarditis should be considered a potential cause of fever of unknown origin, especially among active injection drug users. Drug hypersensitivity is strikingly common in HIV-infected patient and may manifest as fever without any specific signs of allergy. This entity should be considered carefully in any patient with fever of obscure etiology, common in HIV-infected patients, should also be considered when appropriate. For the purposes of this discussion, patients with specific end organ syndromes, for example, headache, cough, diarrhea, rash, etc., are excluded, and the approach to diagnosis presumes that fever is persistent (>2 weeks) and origin is obscure.

Diagnostic Evaluation

The approach to a patient with persistent fever of unknown origin should be individualized, taking into account prior history, travel, exposure to other individuals who may have infection, animal exposure, and food history. Most importantly, the nature of prophylactic therapy the patient is receiving and the degree of immune impairment as indicated by the CD4+ lymphocyte count provide invaluable information to aid the clinician in determining the range of possible disorders to which the patient is susceptible (Fig. 4.2). If routine X rays and laboratory studies, including cultures of blood, urine, and stool repeatedly

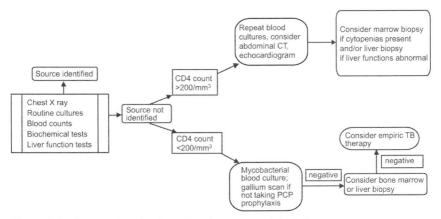

Figure 4.2 Suggested evaluation of persistent, unexplained fever.

fail to provide a clue to the source of the fever, radionuclide scans, biopsy of the liver or bone marrow, or both may reveal the diagnosis.

Differential Diagnosis by CD4+ Cell Count

The opportunistic infections classically associated with AIDS (PCP, cerebral toxoplasmosis, cryptococcal meningitis, disseminated mycobacterium avium complex (MAC) infection, and locally invasive Herpes simplex) occur exclusively in the setting of profound cellular immune dysfunction. In general, these disorders can be excluded in patients with stable CD4+ cell counts above $200/mm^3$. Patients receiving and complying with trimethoprim-sulfamethoxazole prophylaxis are almost completely protected from both PCP and toxoplasmosis, and those receiving prophylaxis directed at MAC are at considerably lower risk of developing symptomatic infection with this organism. Much of the published data on evaluation of fever has come from studies of patients with advanced immune deficiency. Fever at earlier stages of HIV infection, particularly among patients with CD4+ cell counts above $500/mm^3$, should generally be evaluated as it would in non-HIV-infected hosts. It should be noted, however, that tuberculosis and infections due to *Streptococcus pneumoniae* and varicella zoster virus occur at increased frequency even at early stages of HIV infection before the onset of significant, measurable cellular immune dysfunction.

The Use of Radionuclide Studies

Gallium-67 and indium-111 scanning may identify localized infections in some patients. In a study by Fineman and colleagues (6) of 36 AIDS patients with unexplained fever, 21 (78%) and 12 (44%) of 27 documented localized infections were identified by indium and gallium scanning, respectively. Although less sensitive overall, gallium studies were particularly effective in detecting early PCP and infections involving the lymph nodes in this series. Other recent reports have indicated that gallium scanning leads to a diagnosis in a substantial proportion of AIDS patients with fever of unknown origin (7). More recently, fluorodeoxyglucose-positron emission tomography (FDG-PET) scanning (8) as well as FDG-PET combined with anatomical imaging with computed tomography (CT) have proven to be sensitive means of detecting occult inflammatory disorders.

Liver Biopsy

Because of the high incidence of liver involvement by opportunistic infections in AIDS, the efficacy of liver biopsy in evaluating unexplained fever in HIV-infected patients (particularly those with a history of AIDS-related infections) appears to be substantially higher than in non-HIV-infected patients. In one series, liver biopsy provided a specific diagnosis in most patients at various stages of HIV infection referred to for evaluation of fever, but the diagnostic yield was more than twice as high in patients with a history of AIDS-defining infections than in those with no history of AIDS (9). In this series, liver biopsy was substantially more effective than bone marrow biopsy in detecting mycobacterial infection. The sensitivity of liver biopsy is particularly high in the presence of abnormalities of serum alkaline phosphatase and liver function tests (10). The yield of liver biopsy in the diagnosis of MAC infection was greater than that of bone marrow biopsy or blood culture in one comparative study (11). The role of liver biopsy, however, has been controversial. Advocates point to the high diagnostic accuracy for mycobacterial infection, whereas others believe that most treatable infections diagnosed by liver biopsy may be identified by less invasive means.

Bone Marrow Aspirate/Biopsy

Examination and culture of bone marrow may identify the cause of unexplained fever in approximately one-quarter of cases of patients with AIDS (11). Disseminated infection with mycobacteria and *Histoplasma capsulatum* is commonly identified in this manner, particularly among patients at advanced stages of immune deficiency. ART, although characteristic histologic abnormalities were not present in the bone marrow and culture in the evaluation of unexplained fever, is probably most valuable when the CD+ lymphocyte count is below 200 cells/mm^3. Hematologic indications for bone marrow examination, such as thrombocytopenia and anemia, may arise at earlier stages of HIV infection.

Special Culture Techniques

Blood and tissue specimens, particularly of bone marrow and liver, should be stained specifically for the presence of mycobacteria and fungi. Because mycobacteria do not grow on routine culture media, pathology and microbiology laboratories should be informed when these organisms are suspected so that the specimen can be preserved properly and specific culture media can be used.

Disseminated histoplasmosis may be diagnosed by appropriate culture of blood or tissue specimens, although results of these tests are often negative or require several weeks of incubation. Serologic studies for histoplasmosis are relatively insensitive in immunocompromised patients.

Infection with CMV may be diagnosed by specific viral culture of blood or urine.

LYMPHADENOPATHY

Incidence

Nonspecific lymph node enlargement was recognized as a common finding in HIV-infected patients early in the history of the HIV/AIDS epidemic. In one early study, 71% of HIV-infected homosexual men at various stages of disease were found to have significant lymphadenopathy (12). The syndrome of persistent generalized lymphadenopathy, defined as unexplained palpable lymph node enlargement of more than 1 cm in two or more extrainguinal sites for at least three months, represents an exaggerated reaction to HIV infection in most cases.

Nonspecific lymphadenopathy in early HIV infection often regresses with time, although the incidence of lymph node enlargement in AIDS and other advanced stages of HIV infection is less clear. Perhaps because hyperplastic lymph nodes tend to regress with progression to AIDS, autopsy series have shown low rates of significant lymphadenopathy. However, involvement of the lymph nodes by opportunistic infections or malignancies becomes increasingly common as HIV infection progresses. Since the era of highly active antiretroviral therapy (HAART) began in the mid-1990s, a syndrome associated with immune reconstitution in which latent opportunistic infections are activated has been described (see chap. 6), often in association with significant lymphadenopathy.

Intraabdominal lymphadenopathy was found in 48% of HIV-infected patients, primarily intravenous drug users, in one series (13) and correlated poorly with the presence of peripheral lymph node enlargement. Such lymphadenopathy has implications similar to those of generalized node enlargement and may represent nonspecific hyperplasia, infection, or malignancy.

Differential Diagnosis

The diagnostic significance of lymph node enlargement varies with the stage of HIV infection. As noted previously, a nonspecific generalized lymphadenopathy may be present at any point in the disease but is most common before the onset of profound immune deficiency and AIDS-related infections or malignancies. Histologic examination of lymph nodes from patients with persistent generalized lymphadenopathy typically reveals nonspecific hyperplasia. The challenge to the clinician is to distinguish persistent generalized lymphadenopathy, which requires no specific therapy, from opportunistic infection or neoplasm. Among the HIV-related infections that cause lymph node enlargement, mycobacterial infection, particularly tuberculosis, has been the most common in a number of published clinical series. In a retrospective chart review of lymph node biopsies in injection drug users in New York, 65% of biopsies from HIV-infected individuals revealed significant histologic findings, compared with 30% of specimens from non-HIV-infected patients (14). Tuberculosis was the most common diagnosis in both groups in this study.

Bacillary angiomatosis, as well as infection with *Cryptococcus neoformans*, *H. capsulatum*, *Toxoplasma gondii*, and a variety of other organisms, may also involve the lymph nodes. Lymphoma may cause generalized or localized lymph node enlargement. Metastatic involvement of the lymph nodes was found in 44% of patients with cutaneous KS in one autopsy series.

Diagnostic evaluation. Lymph node biopsy should be performed in all cases in which a reasonable working diagnosis cannot be established on other grounds. Nonetheless, the decision to perform a biopsy must be individualized (Fig. 4.3). Patients with CD4 lymphocyte counts above 500/mm^3 who have symmetric, generalized lymph node enlargement may not require immediate biopsy because of the relatively small chance of opportunistic infection or malignancy. It should be noted, however, that lymphoma or lymphadenopathic KS may occasionally occur before the onset of severe immune deficiency. While the incidence of KS has declined since the advent of current ART, the incidence of lymphoma has not, and, in fact, may be rising (see chap. 4).

Patients at all stages with new, asymmetrical lymph node enlargement of uncertain etiology, particularly if it is rapidly enlarging, should generally undergo prompt biopsy. Those with lymphadenopathy confined to the inguinal

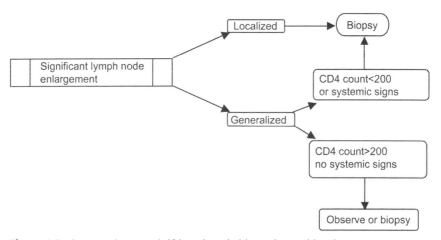

Figure 4.3 Suggested approach if lymph node biopsy is considered.

region should be evaluated for syphilis and other sexually transmitted diseases (e.g., chancroid and lymphogranuloma venereum) before being considered for biopsy.

In skilled hands, fine-needle lymph node aspiration and cytologic examination may provide as much information as excisional biopsy and represents a less invasive alternative.

If lymph node tissue is obtained, specific stains and cultures for mycobacteria and fungi should be performed on all specimens because histopathologic studies alone may be misleading (e.g., granulomata may be absent in some cases of disseminated mycobacterial infection). With possible cryptococcal or *T. gondii* infection of the lymph nodes, serologic studies may be helpful in confirming the diagnosis.

Evaluation of deep intraabdominal or intrathoracic node, where biopsy may be difficult, is especially challenging. If percutaneous biopsy is not feasible, bone marrow examination should be considered as a safe, intermediate diagnostic step. Open biopsy of lymph nodes in such cases is occasionally necessary, however, especially in the setting of unexplained fever or other systemic signs or when the lymph nodes are enlarging. If the decision is made to defer biopsy, the patient should have frequent (monthly) reassessments. If additional lymphadenopathy develops or the nodes under observation undergo significant further enlargement, or if systemic signs such as fever, weight loss, and respiratory, gastrointestinal, or neurologic symptoms occur, biopsy should be reconsidered.

It should be remembered that the cause of lymph node enlargement can only be definitively established by tissue examination and culture.

HEADACHE

Incidence

Headache is a common complaint among HIV-infected patients in all stages of disease. Nearly 3% of patients who were admitted to an AIDS unit, as compared with 0.2% of those who were admitted to a neurology service, complained of headache in one series (15). As the presence and severity of pain are subjective, it is important to recognize that pain at any site may be easily underestimated and HIV care providers often have an inadequate appreciation of pain and other complaints (16).

Differential Diagnosis

The central nervous system (CNS) is a common site of involvement by HIV and AIDS-related infections and malignancies. Cryptococcal meningitis and toxoplasmosis, the most common infections, and lymphoma are life-threatening disorders that are often accompanied by headache. Because headaches in HIV-infected patients often have such organic causes but are more often caused by non-life-threatening conditions, evaluation of this symptom may pose a difficult challenge to the primary care physician.

As with other clinical syndromes associated with HIV infection, the differential diagnosis is extensive and varies with the degree of immune deficiency. In general, headache is most likely due to a benign, noninfectious cause (migraine, tension headache, depression) early in the course of HIV infection, prior to the onset of significant immunologic impairment (17).

HIV itself may cause meningitis at the time of acute infection or later in the course of disease. HIV meningitis may become evident as a self-limited process marked by fever, headache, and neck stiffness or as a chronic headache not associated with meningeal signs. This syndrome is seldom associated with signs of encephalopathy of focal neurologic deficits, which often accompany opportunistic infections involving the CNS. Syphilis with CNS involvement may present with headache. In endemic regions, malaria and typhoid fever may present with headache, typically accompanied by high fever.

When the CD4+ lymphocyte count falls below 200 cells/mm^3, opportunistic infections and CNS lymphoma become increasingly important causes of headache. Cryptococcal meningitis typically becomes evident as a subacute illness marked by fever and headache and, occasionally, focal neurologic signs. In a significant minority of cases, the course may be more fulminant with rapid progression to coma and death. Cerebral toxoplasmosis is typically associated with headache, a depressed level of consciousness, or focal neurologic abnormalities of recent onset, or a combination of these.

Sinusitis has been increasingly recognized as a complication of HIV infection at all stages of disease and may become evident as acute or chronic headache with or without clear evidence of sinus tenderness or nasal congestion. Periodontal disease, also common regardless of degree immune deficiency, may also become evident as referred pain and headache. Localized varicella zoster infection frequently involves the head in HIV-infected patients and may present as obscure, unilateral headache prior to the eruption of characteristic vesicles.

Several medications commonly prescribed for the HIV-infected may also cause headaches. A syndrome of fever, malaise, nausea, and headache may be encountered in patients receiving trimethoprim-sulfamethoxazole, and headache is a common side effect of several antiretroviral agents: the nucleoside reverse transcriptase inhibitors zidovudine (AZT), zalcitabine (DDC), and the non-nucleoside reverse transcriptase inhibitors delavardine and efavirenz, as well as the chemokine blocker maraviroc among others (see chap. 5).

Diagnostic Evaluation

Because of the potentially life-threatening nature of the opportunistic infections and malignancies that may cause headache in HIV-infected patients, this symptom must always be regarded with concern and evaluated carefully

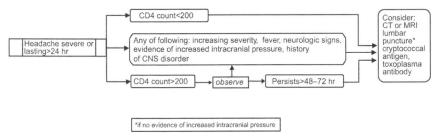

Figure 4.4 Suggested evaluation of persistent headache.

and promptly, particularly in patients with CD4+ lymphocyte counts below 200 cells/mm^3 (Fig. 4.4).

In the patient with advanced immune deficiency, the evaluation of headache that lasts longer than several days or progressively worsens or is accompanied by fever, neurologic abnormalities or evidence of increased intracranial pressure should include CT or magnetic resonance imaging (MRI) and, if necessary, neurologic consultation. Serum cryptococcal antigen is almost always positive in cryptococcal meningitis. A lumbar puncture should be performed unless there is reason to suspect an intracranial mass lesion. Sinus radiographs or CT and dental evaluation should be considered for more subacute syndromes or if the workup is unrevealing.

SEIZURE

Incidence

Because CNS involvement by opportunistic infections and malignancies and HIV itself is common, seizures are a relatively common manifestation of HIV

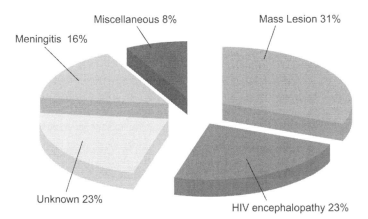

Figure 4.5 Etiologies of new-onset seizures. *Source*: Adapted from Ref. 18.

infection (Fig. 4.5). In a retrospective review of more than 600 hospitalized patients at all stages of immune deficiency, 12% were noted to have new-onset seizures (19). Of these patients, 46% had single and 54% had recurrent seizures. Seizures were generalized in 94%.

Differential Diagnosis

Approximately one-third of HIV-infected patients with new-onset seizures are found to have an intracerebral mass lesion, 10% to 16% have meningitis, and 3% to 11% have metabolic causes (18,19).

Seizures have been reported to complicate 4% to 8% of cases of cyrptococcal meningitis (20,21), 14% to 23% of cerebral toxoplasmosis (22,23), and 17% of cases of primary CNS lymphoma (24). Less common HIV-related disorders such as CNS tuberculosis, progressive multifocal leukoencephalopathy (PML), and herpes simplex encephalitis may also become evident as seizures, as may metabolic disturbances such as hyponatremia, uremia, and hypoglycemia.

The role of direct infection of the CNS by HIV is suggested by the observation that 7% to 44% of patients with AIDS dementia complex have seizures (25). Early studies have indicated that 24% to 46% of new-onset seizures may be attributed to HIV encephalopathy (18,19).

Diagnostic Evaluation

HIV-infected patients with new-onset seizures or focal neurologic deficits or both should undergo a thorough evaluation for CNS infection, malignancy, and metabolic derangements. Intracerebral mass lesions should be promptly excluded by CT or MRI. Serologic studies for toxoplasmosis and cryptococcosis may also provide helpful information.

PERSISTENT COUGH OR DYSPNEA

Incidence

The lung is a target organ for many HIV-related disorders. Bacterial pneumonia and tuberculosis are seen more commonly among HIV-infected individuals than in the general population, even prior to or during the early stages of immune deficiency. True opportunistic respiratory infections, particularly PCP, are among the commonest complications of advanced immune deficiency. In addition, sinusitis and bronchitis and other viral respiratory infection, including influenza, may be seen more frequently and cause more severe illness. Pulmonary hypertension may be seen, especially, but not exclusively, among patients with a history of injection drug use. Extrapulmonary disorders such as cardiomyopathy and hypercoagulable states with thromboembolic disease are also more likely in the presence of HIV infection. For all of these reasons, cough and dyspnea are frequent complaints among patients at all stages of immune deficiency.

Differential Diagnosis

The differential diagnosis of persistent cough or dyspnea in HIV-infected patients varies greatly with the stage of disease. In patients with CD4+ lymphocyte counts below 200 cells/mm^3 or with a history of AIDS opportunistic respiratory infections such as PCP are of primary concern, particularly, but not exclusively, when fever or other systemic signs of infection are present. In contrast, bacterial pneumonia and pulmonary tuberculosis are common at all stages of HIV infection.

Diagnostic Evaluation

The evaluation of HIV-infected patients with a new or persistent cough should be guided, if time and the clinical situation permit, by the results of immunologic staging. New respiratory complaints in patients with CD4+ lymphocyte counts below 200 cells/mm^3 should be promptly evaluated with a chest radiograph and sputum analysis, including stain for acid-fast bacilli as well as routine, fungal, and mycobacterial culture. It should be recalled that PCP may present with a completely normal chest X ray (see chap. 4). If expectorated sputum is unrevealing or if PCP is suspected, sputum induction with immunofluorescent stain for *Pneumocystis* should be performed. Properly performed, this procedure has a sensitivity in excess of 90%. In cases where sputum cannot be obtained by induction, bronchoscopy with bronchoalveolar lavage (BAL) may be required to exclude the diagnosis of PCP. Blood cultures should be performed in febrile patients. The patient should be quickly assessed for evidence of opportunistic malignancy or infection, particularly KS and tuberculosis. Measurement of arterial blood gas levels and immediate hospitalization may be necessary, particularly for patients with progressive dyspnea accompanying a cough. If the chest radiograph is normal and there is no evidence of systemic bacterial infection, pulmonary gallium scanning may be useful in detecting early PCP among patients with advanced immune deficiency.

If radiographic examination and gallium scanning provide no insight into the cause of cough, echocardiogram may identify patients with occult cardiomyopathy causing congestive heart failure as well as pulmonary hypertension or pericardial disease. The possibility of bacterial endocarditis should be considered carefully, especially in patients who are active injection drug users. Pulmonary function tests may be very useful in establishing the presence of airways disease. High-resolution CT of the chest may identify interstitial disease not apparent on routine X rays.

Evaluation of cough in patients with CD4+ lymphocyte counts above 200 cells/mm^3 should also include an early chest radiograph and assessment for systemic infection, in particular, infection caused by *S. pneumoniae*,

Hemophilus influenzae, *Legionella* species, or tuberculosis. In these patients, particularly the CD4+ lymphocyte counts above 500 cells/mm^3, the diagnostic workup should also be directed at respiratory disorders unrelated or indirectly related to HIV infection, such as asthma, chronic bronchitis, lung cancer, emphysema, and chronic interstitial disease.

CHEST PAIN

Incidence

Chest pain is an uncommon symptom in HIV-infected patients, although the exact incidence is unknown. As survival is prolonged by advances in therapy and the population of HIV-infected individuals ages, cardiovascular disease is likely to become an increasingly common cause of chest pain. Perhaps accelerating this trend is the hyperlipidemia syndrome associated with ART, which has been associated with progression of coronary artery disease in some individuals (see chaps. 5 and 9).

Differential Diagnosis

All HIV-infected patients with chest pain should be evaluated promptly with chest radiograph and electrocardiogram. If the pain is substernal, esophageal and cardiac causes are most likely. Patients with esophagitis usually note exacerbation of pain with swallowing. The evaluation of such patients is outlined in the following discussion of dysphagia.

The evaluating of chest pain in the setting of HIV infection should generally proceed along the same lines as indicated for other patients. Individuals with traditional risk factors for coronary artery disease (e.g., diabetes, smoking, hypertension, hyperlipidemia, family history) should be evaluated for acute ischemia, especially if they are taking ART. It should be borne in mind that HIV infection itself appears to represent a possible independent risk factor for coronary artery disease (see chap. 9) and that certain antiretroviral drugs (e.g., lopinavir/ritonavir; abacavir) may be specifically associated with cardiovascular disease (see chap. 5). Cocaine use, which is disproportionately common among HIV-infected individuals, has also been associated with acceleration of coronary artery disease as well as with acute coronary spasm.

Pulmonary causes of chest pain to be considered, especially if pain is accompanied by dyspnea at rest or with exertion, include pneumothorax resulting from active or past PCP, pulmonary embolism associated with hypercoagulability or immobility, and pulmonary hypertension related to prior injection drug use.

Substernal pain related to esophageal disorders (see below) is typically made worse by eating but may, in some individuals, mimic acute myocardial ischemia.

Diagnostic Evaluation

The evaluation of chest pain in the setting of HIV infection should proceed along the same lines as in other patients. The nature and pattern of the pain, the likelihood of significant coronary artery disease, and, if warranted, evaluation by electrocardiogram and cardiac enzymes should dictate whether additional evaluation should be directed at the exclusion of coronary artery disease or other syndromes.

DYSPHAGIA AND ODYNOPHAGIA

Incidence

Difficulty swallowing (dysphagia) and pain on swallowing (odynophagia) are common complaints in HIV-infected patients, particularly among those at advanced stages of immune deficiency.

Differential Diagnosis

Esophageal candidiasis is the most common cause of dysphagia and odynophagia in patients with advanced immune deficiency (26). Other common esophageal disorders that may produce these symptoms include infection herpes simplex virus, CMV, and, in rare instances, other opportunistic pathogens. Esophageal ulcers directly related to HIV infection may also present in this fashion.

Other HIV-related disorders that may result in pain or discomfort on swallowing include painful oral lesions and noninfectious disorders involving the pharynx or esophagus, including apththous ulcers, KS, squamous cell carcinoma, and lymphoma. Disruption of esophageal motility may complicate HIV-related esophageal disorders and contribute to the severity of symptoms.

The presence of oral candidiasis in patients with symptoms of esophagitis indicates a high likelihood of *Candida* esophagitis. However, either oral or esophageal candidiasis may occur alone. Pain on swallowing may be a clue to the presence of invasive infection.

Diagnostic Evaluation

Uncertainty may exist regarding the optimum diagnostic workup for an HIV-infected patient with symptoms of dysphagia or odynophagia, specifically on the need for and timing of upper gastrointestinal tract endoscopy. Potential strategies include endoscopy with biopsy as the initial diagnostic study, blind brushing of the esophagus through a nasogastric tube, barium radiography followed by endoscopy if the diagnosis is uncertain, and therapeutic trial of an antifungal agent such as fluconazole with radiographic or endoscopic investigation or both for patients who do not respond to empiric therapy (Fig. 4.6).

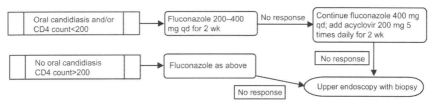

Figure 4.6 Therapeutic trial for patients with odynophagia.

In one large series in which double-contrast barium radiography was compared prospectively with endoscopy in HIV-infected patients who had a variety of upper gastrointestinal tract complaints, radiography had an overall sensitivity of only 31.1% and was particularly ineffective in detecting esophageal candidiasis (27). In contrast, endoscopy was found to have a sensitivity of 97.5% in cases in which a diagnosis was confirmed by histopathologic examination. These data indicate that negative results of barium radiography cannot always exclude active esophagitis. In another prospective study, blind brushing of the esophagus through a nasogastric tube was found to have a sensitivity similar to endoscopy in the diagnosis of esophageal candidiasis in patients complaining of dysphagia or odynophagia (28).

Despite the excellent diagnostic results that endoscopy provides, it may not be necessary that all patients be subjected to the discomfort, inconvenience, and potential morbidity and cost of this procedure. Because of the high degree of correlation between oral and esophageal candidiasis, a therapeutic trial of fluconazole can be considered in patients with oral candidiasis and esophageal symptoms, reserving endoscopy for those whose symptoms do not respond. Blind esophageal brushing, which could potentially be performed by the primary health care provider, might provide a relatively safe, inexpensive alternative to endoscopy in selected cases (28), although the diagnostic sensitivity of the procedure compared with endoscopy has not been thoroughly evaluated.

When therapy for candidal esophagitis is initiated without histologic confirmation of the diagnosis, it should be recalled that other HIV-related disorders may produce identical symptoms.

NAUSEA/VOMITING

Incidence

Nausea and vomiting are common complaints among patients with advanced disease as well as patients taking a variety of commonly used medications.

Differential Diagnosis

Disorders such as viral hepatitis, pancreatitis, biliary disease, and intestinal obstruction due to lymphoma, KS, or other mass lesions may present in this fashion. Many commonly used medications, including trimethoprim/

sulfamethoxazole, protease inhibitors, nucleoside reverse transcriptase inhibitors, nonnucleoside reverse transcriptase inhibitors (especially nevirapine), hydroxyurea and macrolide antibiotics, isoniazid, and pyrazinamide may cause nausea and vomiting on the basis of hepatic inflammation or pancreatic inflammation or as idiopathic side effects. Persistent vomiting should also be considered a possible manifestation of increased intracranial pressure caused by cerebral mass lesions associated with toxoplasmosis, lymphoma, or other disorders.

Diagnostic Evaluation

Intestinal obstruction should be excluded with appropriate radiographic studies in any patient with persistent vomiting. Liver function tests and amylase and lipase determinations should be obtained. Abdominal imaging studies may be necessary to exclude cholelithiasis or mass lesions resulting in partial bowel obstruction. A careful neurologic examination should be performed. If papilledema, focal neurologic deficits, or headache are present or if no other etiology of persistent vomiting can be established, CT or MRI of the brain should be performed.

ABDOMINAL PAIN

Incidence

Abdominal pain is a frequent complaint among patients at advanced stages of HIV infection and may reflect disease of the bowel, spleen, pancreas, peritoneum, liver, or biliary system as well as medication side effects. Bowel perforation and other surgical emergencies occur in HIV patients, perhaps more frequently than in the general patient population. The challenge to the clinician is distinguishing among the large number of causes or origins of abdominal pain that do not require immediate intervention and the occasional intraabdominal catastrophe or life-threatening medication effect.

Published studies of patients who seek medical attention with abdominal pain or intraabdominal disease have focused on those with advanced HIV infection. Less is known about the incidence of abdominal pain in earlier stages of disease. In one series of more than 200 hospitalized AIDS patients, 12.3% reported abdominal pain for two or more days during their hospitalization (29). In another study, 4.2% of more than 900 consecutive hospitalized AIDS patients required abdominal surgical procedures, including cholecystectomy, appendectomy, and exploratory (30).

Differential Diagnosis

Pain associated with diarrhea or vomiting suggests infectious enteritis such as that caused by cryptosporidiosis, microsporidiosis, isosporiasis, salmonellosis, and infection with *Clostridium difficile* and other pathogens. Cryptosporidiosis was the most common intestinal infection in one large early series of AIDS patients with abdominal pain, being seen in 31% of cases (29). Infections with *Campylobacter* species and *Giardia lamblia* were also seen. The pain associated with intestinal infections in these patients was most often diffuse. Diarrhea and hypoalbuminemia were evident in the majority of cases, and more than 40% of patients complained of nausea and vomiting.

Pain localized to the right upper quadrant or more generalized throughout the abdomen may indicate biliary tract disease or hepatitis.

Generalized intraabdominal infection with CMV, *Cryptococcus*, or MAC may be associated with abdominal pain. Diffuse pain with peritoneal signs should raise the possibility of peritonitis resulting from (*i*) bowel perforation caused by invasive infections or malignancies, including tuberculosis, histoplasmosis, CMV, aspergillosis, lymphoma, and Kaposi's sarcoma, or (*ii*) direct involvement of the peritoneum by HIV-related infections such as tuberculosis, toxoplasmosis, histoplasmosis, or cryptococcosis. HIV-infected patients undergoing chronic ambulatory peritoneal dialysis appear to be at higher risk for bacterial and fungal peritonitis than other such patients (31).

Midepigastric or left upper-quadrant pain may signify pancreatits related to biliary tract disease or to drug therapy, particularly with pentamidine, didanosine, DDC, lopinavir, or foscarnet. Appendicitis with typical right-sided abdominal pain may occur in association with CMV infection and aspergillosis.

An important, and potentially life-threatening, cause of abdominal pain is the syndrome of lactic acidosis, hepatomegaly, and hepatic steatosis associated with nucleoside therapy (see chap. 5).

GASTROINTESTINAL BLEEDING

Incidence

Although incidence data are sparse, significant bleeding appears to be an uncommon manifestation of HIV-related gastrointestinal tract disorders but is included in this discussion because it may rapidly become life threatening and has a broad differential diagnosis.

Differential Diagnosis

Causes of bleeding not related to HIV infection should be sought in HIV-infected individuals with significant gastrointestinal blood loss. Potential HIV-associated causes include esophagitis, invasive infection of the small or large bowel (e.g., with CMV, *Salmonella* or *Aspergillus* species), and Kaposi's sarcoma or lymphoma involving any region of the intestinal tract.

Diagnostic Evaluation

Evaluation should proceed as in non-HIV-infected patients. Confirmed or suspected bleeding should be investigated with barium studies and endoscopic procedures when indicated.

SPLENOMEGALY

Incidence

Splenomegaly is a common nonspecific manifestation of HIV infection at advanced stages of disease. More than 70% of AIDS were found at autopsy to have enlarged spleens in one early series (32). A comparably high incidence of splenomegaly has been detected by CT (33). The incidence of splenomegaly in earlier stages of HIV infection is less clear.

Differential Diagnosis

The cause of splenomegaly in HIV-infected patients is often obscure. The diagnostic evaluation should serve to exclude treatable diseases.

OPPORTUNISTIC INFECTIONS

Opportunistic infections directly involving the spleen are most likely to occur in patients at advanced stages of immune deficiency. Infection with MAC, *Salmonella*, and CMV as well as involvement with Kaposi's sarcoma was seen in one series of patients undergoing splenectomy (34). Cryptococcosis and histoplasmosis with splenic involvement as well as tuberculosis may also be seen as variety of less common infections. In tropical areas of South America, Asia, and Africa, visceral leishmaniasis, malaria, and schistosomiasis should be considered.

MALIGNANCIES

The spleen is a common site of involvement by metastatic Kaposi's sarcoma (34) and lymphoma (35).

Diagnostic Evaluation

The best diagnostic approach to splenomegaly in the setting of HIV infection is unknown. Large clinical series focusing on the causes of splenomegaly at various stages of HIV infection and the yield of various diagnostic tests are not available to guide the clinician. Because of this lack of clear data, it is probably prudent to attempt to identify a specific cause in all patients when feasible. The wide variety of disorders that may involve the spleen and the frequency with which splenomegaly is seen in HIV-infected patients may present obstacles to designing an efficient workup. Patients with splenomegaly and unexplained fever, weight loss, or other signs or symptoms that may represent a disseminated infection or malignancy should probably be evaluated more extensively than those without these.

Even in other asymptomatic patients, a careful effort should be made by means of the history, physical examination, routine laboratory data, and other diagnostic studies to establish a working diagnosis (e.g., nonspecific splenic enlargement caused by HIV infection itself or by a specific disorder unrelated to HIV infection, such as cirrhosis with portal hypertension).

Diagnostic studies of potential value include abdominal imaging studies to evaluate for mass lesions or abscesses within the spleen and to identify other organ involvement, such as hepatomegaly and lymphadenopathy, that might provide a clue to the cause of the splenic enlargement. A thorough evaluation of other common sites of involvement by opportunistic infections and malignancies is important, including the respiratory and gastrointestinal tracts, the skin, the lymphatics, and the CNS. Blood cultures for pathogens known to disseminate to the spleen, particularly MAC, *Cryptococcus*, *Histoplasma*, and CMV, as well as routine bacteria, may be necessary. Biopsy of the liver or bone marrow, if feasible, may aid in excluding disseminated infection (mycobacterial or fungal) or malignancy involving the spleen. Exploratory laparotomy may be necessary in rare instances of symptomatic patients in whom a definitive or reasonable working diagnosis cannot be made.

DIARRHEA

Diarrhea, defined as at least two watery bowel movements per day, is a common complaint among HIV-infected patients at all stages of disease. In chapter 3, specific etiologic agents and, in chapter 6, the approach to diagnosis and management of serious intestinal disorders presenting as diarrhea are addressed. Diarrhea is a common side effect of several antiretroviral agents (see chap. 5).

PERIPHERAL NEUROPATHY

Symmetrical, distal sensory neuropathy is a common manifestation of HIV infection, particularly among patients with severe immune deficiency with an annual incidence of approximately 8% when the CD4 cell count is below $100/mm^3$ (36). Other causes, particularly diabetes mellitus, vitamin deficiencies, and side effects from several nucleoside antiretroviral agents (see chap. 5) may produce similar findings. The diagnosis is usually made on clinical grounds, although myelopathy must be excluded if the diagnosis is in doubt. Therapy with analgesics is often inadequate. Other medications that may be effective include amitriptyline, gabapentin, carbamazepine, dilantin, and valproate.

REFERENCES

1. Sepkowitz KA, Telzak EE, Carrow M, et al. Fever among outpatients with advanced human immunodeficiency virus infection. Arch Intern Med 1993; 153:1909–1912.
2. Bissuel F, Leport C, Perronne C, et al. Fever of unknown origin in HIV-infected patients: a critical analysis of a retrospective series of 57 cases. J Intern Med 1994; 236:529–535.

3. Pierone G, Lin J, Masci J, et al. Fever of unknown origin in AIDS. Int Conf AIDS 1990; 6(1):257 (abstract no. Th.B.540).
4. Hot A, Schmulewitz L, Viard JP, et al. Fever of unknown origin in HIV/AIDS patients. Infect Dis Clin North Am 2007; 21(4):1013–1032.
5. Miralles P, Moreno S, Pérez-Tascón M, et al. Fever of uncertain origin in patients infected with the human immunodeficiency virus. Clin Infect Dis 1995; 20:872–875.
6. Fineman DS, Palestro CJ, Kim CK, et al. Detection of abnormalities in febrile AIDS patients with In-111-labeled leukocyte and Ga-67 scintigraphy. Radiology 1989; 170 (3 pt 1):677–680.
7. Knockaert DC, Mortelmans LA, De Roo MC, et al. Clinical value of gallium-67 scintigraphy in evaluation of fever of unknown origin. Clin Infect Dis 1994; 18:601–605.
8. Zhuang H, Yu JQ, Alavi A. Applications of fluorodeoxyglucose-PET scanning in the detection of infection and inflammation and other benign disorders. Radiol Clin North Am 2005; 43:121–134.
9. Cappell MS, Schwartz MS, Biempica L. Clinical utility of liver biopsy in patients with serum antibodies to the human immunodeficiency virus. Am J Med 1990; 88:123.
10. Rogeaux O, Priqueler L, Hoang C, et al. Diagnostic usefulness of liver biopsy for unexplained fever in HIV patients. Int Conf AIDS 1993; 9:446.
11. Nichols L, Florentine B, Lewis W, et al. Bone marrow examination for the diagnosis of mycobacterial and fungal infections in the acquired immunodeficiency syndrome. Arch Pathol Lab Med 1991; 115:1125–1132.
12. Lang W, Anderson RE, Perkins H, et al. Clinical, immunologic and serologic findings I men at risk for acquired immunodeficiency syndrome: the San Francisco Men's Heath Study. JAMA 1987; 252:1152.
13. Cassani F, Costigliola P, Zoli M, et al. Abdominal lymphadenopathy detected by ultrasonography in HIV-1 infection: prevalence and significance. Scand J Infect Dis 1993; 25:221–225.
14. Albu E, Abeebe L, Beniwal JS, et al. Lymph node biopsy in intravenous-drug abusers and patients with HIV infection. Infect Med 1995; 137:125.
15. Brew BJ, Miller J. Human immunodeficiency virus-rrelated hadache. Neurology 1993; 43:1098.
16. Justice AC, Rabeneck L, Hays RD, et al. Sensitivity, specificity, reliability, and clinical validity of provider-reported symptoms: a comparison with self-reported symptoms. Outcomes Committee of the AIDS Clinical Trials Group. J Acquir Immune Defic Syndr 1999; 12:126–133.
17. Holloway RG, Kieburtz KD. Headache and the human immunodeficiency virus type 1 infection. Heacache 1995; 35:245.
18. Holtzman DM, Kaku DA, So YT. New-onset seizures associated with human immunodeficiency virus infection: causation and clinical features in 100 cases. Am J Med 1989; 87:173.
19. Wong MC, Suite ND, Labar DR. Seizures in human immunodeficiency virus infection. Arch Neurol 1990; 47:640.
20. Chuck SL, Sande MA. Infections with *Cryptococcus neoformans* in the acquired immunodeficiency syndrome. N Engl J Med 1989; 321:794.

21. Zuger A, Louie E, Holzman RS, et al. Cryptococcal disease in patients with the acquired immunodeficiency syndrome: diagnostic features and outcome of treatment. Ann Intern Med 1986; 104:234.

22. Cohn JA, McMeeking A, Cohen W, et al. Evaluation of the policy of empiric treatment of suspected *Toxoplasma* encephalitis in patients with the acquired immunodeficiency syndrome. Am J Med 1989; 86:521–527.

23. Wong B, Gold JW, Brown AE, et al. Central nervous system toxoplasmosis in homosexual men and parenteral drug abusers. Ann Intern Med 1984; 100:36–42.

24. Gill PS, Levine AM, Meyer PR, et al. Primary central nervous system lymphoma in homosexual men: clinical, immunologic, and pathologic features. Am J Med 1985; 78:742–748.

25. Navia BA, Jordan BD, Price RW. The ADIS dementia complex. I Clinical features. Ann Neurol 1986; 19:517.

26. Raufman JP. Odynophagia/dysphagia in AIDS. Gastroenterol Clin North Am 1988; 17:599.

27. Connolly GM, Forbes A, Gleeson JA, et al. Investigation of upper gastrointestinal symptoms in patients with AIDS. AIDS 1989; 3:453–456.

28. Bonacini M, Laine L, Gal AA, et al. Prospective evaluation of blind brushing of the esophagus for *Candida* esophagitis in patients with human immunodeficiency virus infection. Am J Gastroenterol 1990; 85:385–389.

29. Barone JE, Gingold BS, Arvanitis ML, et al. Abdominal pain in patients with acquired immune deficiency syndrome. Ann Surg 1986; 204:619–623.

30. LaRaja RD, Rothenberg RE, Odom JW, et al. The incidence of intra-abdominal surgery in acquired immunodeficiency syndrome: a statistical review of 904 patients. Surgery 1989; 105(2 pt 1):175–179.

31. Dressler R, Peters AT, Lynn RI. Pseudomonal and candidal peritonitis as a complication of continuous ambulatory peritoneal dialysis in human immunodeficiency virus-infected patients. Am J Med 1989; 86:787.

32. Wheeler AP, Gregg CR. *Campylobacter* bacteremia, chholecystitis and the acquired immunodeficiency syndrome. Ann Intern Med 1986; 105:804.

33. Arrive L, Frija J, Couderc LJ, et al. Results of abdominal x-ray computed tomography in 25 patients with the acquired immunodeficiency syndrome. J Radiol 1986; 67:219–223.

34. Mathew A, Raviglione MC, Niranjan U, et al. Splenectomy in patients with AIDS. Am J Hematol 1989; 32:184–189.

35. Levine AM, Meyer PR, Begandy MK, et al. Development of B-cell lymphoma in homosexual men: clinical and immunologic findings. Ann Intern Med 1984; 100:7–13.

36. Moyle GJ, Sadler M. Peripharal neuropathy with nucleoside antiretrovirals. Risk factors, incidence and management. Drug Safety 1998; 19:481.

5

Antiretroviral therapy

INTRODUCTION

The remarkable advances in the therapy of HIV infection, which began in the mid-1990s, have continued and accelerated in recent years. Additional anti-retroviral agents have been developed in each of the initial therapeutic classes: drugs that blocked either reverse transcriptase or viral protease. These newer agents have proven to have higher barriers to resistance and to be, by and large, more simple to take and less prone to significant side effects. In addition, several new categories have of drugs have now become available to expand the treatment options for patients who have failed initial therapy. Two specific novel agents have recently been added to the antiretroviral armamentarium: maraviroc, a chemokine (CCR5) receptor antagonist, and raltegravir, an integrase strand transfer inhibitor. These drugs, when used in combination with older agents, have greatly expanded the options for patients failing long-term therapy.

The evolution of antiretroviral therapy (ART) represents one of the most remarkable examples of new drug development that modern medicine has seen. Monotherapy with zidovudine (AZT) gave way, sequentially, to combinations of related nucleoside reverse transcriptase inhibitors (NRTIs). This was followed in the mid-1990s by the advent of nonnucleoside reverse transcriptase inhibitors (NNRTIs), protease inhibitors (PIs), and three-, four-, and five- drug regimens. The newer agents were developed in each of these categories during the late 1990s and early 2000s to reduce pill burden, enhance antiviral activity, and limit side effects. Much work was done to establish optimal treatment regimens based on these drug classes. The last few years have witnessed new breakthroughs with the arrival of the newer agents noted above. Since 2003, nine new drugs and three new drug classes have been approved (1). As clinical trials proceed to establish the proper place of each of these new agents in therapy, newer agents and drug classes are on the horizon. These developments have served to transform symptomatic HIV infection from a rapidly fatal disorder to a treatable chronic condition. Vast numbers of patients, particularly in resource-rich settings, have seen their health and quality of life improve. In addition, increasing numbers of asymptomatic patients can now avoid profound immune deficiency and its consequences for decades. There is new hope for patients who have developed resistance to multiple classes of agents, and the goal of achieving complete suppression of viral replication is often achievable even in the most treatment-experienced patient.

Treatment strategies have also undergone substantial evolution. An initial emphasis on early, aggressive treatment gave way to more cautious approaches as the significant side effects of early generation antiretroviral agents were more fully appreciated and adherence to the often complex regimens was difficult for many. In recent years, however, taking into account current less toxic and more convenient drug formulations, some data has suggested that early treatment may have clear advantages for many patients, especially when viral load is significantly elevated. The long-term effects of viremia itself and the chronic inflammatory state and endorgan disease with which it is associated have come into sharper focus (see chap. 9) and have also influenced treatment guidelines.

As new classes of drugs continue to be developed and new agents within the older classes of drugs become easier to tolerate, the prospects for continued improvement in life expectancy and quality of life appear strong in regions of the world where access to therapeutic advances is readily available. Unfortunately, in much of the world, including regions where prevalence of HIV infection is highest, new agents and the technology to direct therapy effectively continue to disseminate slowly.

With the advances in therapy, however, have come a variety of new challenges. Viral resistance has been reported to each of the classes of drugs, and many individuals who have received various forms of highly active antiretroviral therapy (HAART) therapy for the past several years may still have very limited options for effective therapy. Although newer agents and new formulations and combinations of older agents have resulted in much more simple treatment regimens and reduced pill burden as an obstacle to adherence, second- and third-line regimens still often call for patients to take many pills on confusing schedules. A host of drug interactions continue to hamper the use of some effective agents. Finally, ART does not always lead to significant restoration of immune function even when viral suppression is achieved, especially in individuals at advanced stages of immune deficiency.

In addition, reconstitution of the immune response itself, particularly when it occurs rapidly after the initiation of effective ART, has brought with it the peculiar entities dubbed the immune reconstitution inflammatory syndrome (IRIS) and immune reconstitution disease. These disorders, which are discussed in association with specific infections in chapter 6, represent either recrudescence of the inflammatory response to previously controlled opportunistic infections or the clinical appearance of infections that had been latent and not manifest in the absence of a strong cellular immune response.

On balance, though improvements in therapy have been dramatic and undeniable and have triggered intense research into the development of newer antiretroviral agents, new classes of compounds have been developed and attempts to change pharmacokinetic parameters of older agents to improve the effectiveness and tolerability of therapy have been largely successful (2).

Therapeutic strategies in the management of HIV infection are in constant evolution. Indications for initiating therapy and for changing therapy as well as recommended dosing regimens are all subject to change as new data is accumulated. Nonetheless, a general consensus has emerged at the time of this writing on each of these issues and will be presented in this chapter. In view of the rapid advances that have been seen over a very few years, however, the reader is urged to consult updated treatment guidelines and the results of new clinical trials.

As is the case for all of the topics discussed in this text, the material and guidelines presented here apply to care of the adult patient.

RESOURCE-LIMITED SETTINGS

As discussed in chapter 13 and elsewhere in this book, resource-limited settings continue to face great challenges in providing adequate ART to the vast numbers of individuals for whom it is indicated. Lack of sufficient and predictable supplies of drugs, interruptions in therapy due to difficulty with adherence and maintenance in care and the inability to measure either effectiveness or toxicity of antiretroviral agents plague the poorest countries and even some middle-income regions.

THE IMPACT OF ANTIRETROVIRAL THERAPY

Survival

Evidence abounds that effective ART has dramatically improved the prognosis of HIV infection for many individuals since the introduction of PIs in 1996 (3).

Opportunistic Infections, Malignancies

Effective ART has had a major impact on the incidence of HIV-related opportunistic infections and malignancies. Although the relative frequency of such disorders as mucosal candidiasis, cytomegaloviral retinitis, disseminated *Mycobacterium avium* intracellulare complex (MAC), *Pneumocystis carinii* pneumonia (PCP), and Kaposi's sarcoma have remained constant, their overall incidence has dropped markedly (4).

Transmission

The impact of effective ART on transmission of HIV infection has been somewhat more difficult to assess. Although suppression of viremia reduces the risk of perinatal and, possibly, sexual transmission (5), concern exists that improvements in therapy carry the risk of complacency, potentially leading some to resume or increase high-risk behavior. There is no plasma viral load below which transmission of HIV is known to be impossible.

GOALS OF ANTIRETROVIRAL THERAPY

On the basis of the correlation between viral load, immune function, and overall prognosis, the goals of ART can be viewed as follows:

> Durable suppression of viral replication
> Stabilization or improvement in immune function as measured by CD4 cell count
> Improvement in quality of life by reduction of HIV-related complications
> Improvement in survival
> Likely reduction in transmission of HIV

Specific antiviral regimens should be selected with the goal of maximizing viral suppression, minimizing side effects, and preventing or delaying the emergence of viral resistance to preserve future treatment options. These goals are attainable only with nearly complete adherence to the therapeutic regimen. For this reason, regimens should be designed for maximum convenience. It should be borne in mind, however, that complete viral suppression may be unachievable, especially in the patient who has received combined ART previously and thus accumulated multiple resistance genes. However, even in such individuals, clinical improvement may be seen with partial suppression. Similarly, the CD4 lymphocyte count may not rise in some patients who achieve complete viral suppression and/or clinical improvement.

The risks of ART, however, must also be taken into account. These include the following:

> Medication side effects, hypersensitivity reactions, and interactions with other drugs
> Emergence of resistance with resultant reduction in future therapeutic options and potential transmission of resistant viral strains

Given the complexity of ART and the high failure rate among patients who are not strictly adherent to their treatment regimens under almost all circumstances, it is crucial that the decision to begin therapy be made jointly by the provider and patient only after thorough discussion of effectiveness, side effects, and adherence issues.

Antiretroviral Drugs

At the time of this writing, five classes of drugs comprising over two dozen compounds have been licensed for the treatment of HIV infection (Boxes 5.1–5.4), and several more are anticipated within the next few years. Some are available in fixed-drug combination formulations designed to improve convenience. What follows is a general discussion of available agents, focused primarily on evidence of effectiveness and current clinical role for each agent.

Box 5.1 Nucleoside and Nucleotide Reverse Transcriptase Inhibitors

1. Abacavir (Ziagen)
2. Didanosine (ddI; Videx, Videx EC)
3. Lamivudine (3TC; Epivir)
4. Stavudine (d4T; Zerit)
5. Zalcitabine (ddC; Hivid)
6. Zidovudine (ZDV; Retrovir)
7. Emtricitabine (FTC, Emtriva)
8. Tenofovir DF (TDF, Viread)
9. A fixed combination of zidovudine and lamivudine (Combivir)
10. A fixed combination of zidovudine, lamivudine, and abacavir (Trizivir)
11. A fixed combination of Abacavir and Lamivudine (Epzicom, Kivexa)
12. A fixed combination of tenofovir DF and emtricitabine (Truvada)

Box 5.2 Nonnucleotide Reverse Transcriptase Inhibitors

1. Delavirdine (Rescriptor)
2. Efavirenz (Sustiva)
3. Nevirapine (Viramune)
4. Etravirine (Intelence)

Box 5.3 Protease Inhibitors

1. Fosamprenavir (FPV, Lexiva)
2. Indinavir (IDV, Crixivan)
3. Nelfinavir (NFV, Viracept)
4. Ritonavir (RTV, Norvir)
5. Saquinavir (SQV, Invirase)
6. Lopinavir/ritonavir (LPV/r, Kaletra)
7. Atazanavir (Reyataz)
8. Darunavir (DRV, Prezista)
9. Tipranavir (TPV, Aptivus)

Box 5.4 Other Agents

1. Fusion inhibitor: Enfuvirtide (ENF or T-20, Fuzeon)
2. Entry inhibitor: Maraviroc (Selzentry)
3. Integrase inhibitor: (Isentress)
4. Three-agent combination: Efavirenz/Emtricitabine/Tenofovir (Atripla)

As will be noted, not all agents can be used in combination with all other agents. Treatment regimens are typically constructed on a "backbone" of two NRTI agents or a nucleotide reverse transciptase inhibitor (NtRTI) agent combined with a nucleoside agent. Additional agents, either an NNRTI or a PI complete the regimen. In most PI-based regimens, one PI is combined with a low dose of the PI ritonavir to enhance drug levels. This strategy of combining PIs is termed boosting. Some of the agents described below have fallen out of favor for reasons of toxicity or rapid emergence of resistance. These agents and data supporting their early roles in therapy are provided since they remain commonly used agents in some resource-limited areas. Current treatment guidelines are provided in the final section of this chapter.

All drugs except Fuzeon, which is given as a twice-daily injection, are available in oral form, some also as liquids or powders. Zidovudine, which is normally taken by mouth, is available for intravenous infusion for use in the peripartum period to reduce the risk of vertical transmission of HIV. Although clinical efficacy has been established for each drug individually, one- or two-drug regimens with current agents with the possible exception of certain boosted PIs (see below) are felt to be inadequate at this time.

NUCLEOSIDE REVERSE TRANSCRIPTASE INHIBITORS
Mode of Action

NRTIs inhibit viral reverse transciptase, thereby slowing or preventing replication within infected cells.

Evidence of Efficacy

Although antiretroviral agents should not be used in single-drug regimens outside of the setting of pregnancy, clinical evidence of efficacy for individual drugs will be briefly reviewed here in part to clarify the evolution of current therapy and to provide the reader with a basis for understanding the role of each drug in current and future therapeutic regimens.

Zidovudine (AZT, Retrovir)

Therapeutic benefit was established in early studies (ACTG 016, ACTG 019) (6,7), demonstrating a delay in disease progression for individuals with CD4+ lymphocyte counts between 200 and 500 cells/mm^3. Benefit was not established for asymptomatic patients in other studies. The most compelling evidence of clinically significant antiviral effect came when zidovudine has been shown to reduce the incidence of perinatal transmission of HIV (see chap. 10).

Didanosine (ddl, Videx)

Prior to the advent of modern combined antiretroviral regimens, no consistent differences in outcome were found between patients with little or no prior therapy receiving either zidovudine or didanosine. For symptomatic patients with CD4+ lymphocyte counts below 300 cells/mm^3 or asymptomatic patients with counts below 200 cells/mm^3 who had received prolonged (four months or more) prior to therapy with zidovudine, didanosine (500 mg daily) was superior to zidovudine in delaying progression to AIDS, although it did not confer a survival advantage (8). Largely because of the significant incidence of side effects, particularly peripheral neuropathy and pancreatitis, the use of didanosine has declined in recent years in favor of other NRTIs when feasible.

Lamivudine (3TC, Epivir)

The clinical efficacy of lamivudine has been demonstrated primarily in combination therapy. Significant decreases in viral load have been demonstrated with zidovudine and lamivudine together when compared with either agent alone (9).

Stavudine (D4T, Zerit)

Although early studies demonstrated in vitro activity of stavudine and it has represented a potential alternative to zidovudine (10), stavudine, like didanosine, has largely given way to other NRTIs because of its general high level of toxicity and its relatively strong association with the development of lactic acidosis (11).

Zalcitabine (ddC, Hivid)

Zalcitabine was initially approved for use only in combination with zidovudine. Although it was subsequently approved as monotherapy, it is not used in this fashion and is considered an adjunct to therapy with other nucleoside agents.

As is the case with didanosine and stavudine, zalcitabine is seldom used when alternatives are available because of toxicities.

Abacavir (Ziagen)

Abacavir is available as a single agent or in combination with lamivudine (Epzicom, Kivexa) or in combination with lamivudine and zidovudine (Trizivir). In a study of treatment-naïve patients, combination therapy with abacavir, lamivudine, and zidovudine resulted in a significantly higher rate of complete viral suppression (75% vs. 37%) compared with lamivudine, zidovudine, and placebo (12). In treatment-experienced patients, results have been mixed. Abacavir has also been shown to result in significantly greater viral suppression at 48 weeks when added to stable combination regimens after week 16, so called intensification therapy (13). When substituted for PIs or used in regimens containing PIs or NNRTIs, abacavir has been comparable to other nucleoside agents (14).

Tenofovir (Viread)

Tenofovir disoproxil fumarate (tenofovir; Viread) was the first nucleotide reverse transcriptase inhibitor approved for the treatment of HIV infection. Because of its long (12–14 hour) half-life (15) and sustained intracellular levels (16), it has the advantage of once-daily dosing and, in combination with emtricitabine, (17) has become one of the favored "backbone" agents for therapy of treatment naïve patients (see below). Other advantages include a relatively high barrier to resistance (18) and a lack of association with lipid abnormalities seen with other antiretroviral agents (19). Unfortunately, tenofovir can cause renal injury with loss of renal function (20) and Fanconi syndrome (21), although the risk and severity of renal toxicity may not preclude its use in resource-deprived regions (20).

Patterns of use. Two NRTIs or a combination of one NRTI and one NtRTI are typically prescribed together either a ritonavir-boosted PI (PIr) or a NNRTI in initial treatment regimens for retroviral naïve patients. Certain NRTI pairings are appropriate, and others are not. For example, zidovudine and stavudine should not be combined because of clinically significant drug antagonism, while didanosine and zalcitabine may produce additive toxicities of pancreatitis or peripheral neuropathy. Appropriate combinations include tenofovir/emtricitabine, abacavir/lamivudine, zidovudine/lamivudine; zidovudine/didanosine; stavudine/lamivudine; stavudine/didanosine; and zidovudine and zalcitabine, although zalcitabine is less potent than the other agents and has fallen out of widespread use and, as mentioned above, didanosine and stavudine are associated with significant side effects and have been largely replaced, when possible, by other drugs of this class.

Recent data indicate that regimens combining three NRTI agents (specifically, zidovudine, lamivudine, and abacavir) may be almost as effective as those employing two NRTIs (zidovudine and lamivudine) and a PI (indinavir) (22), but superiority of dual NRTI regimens or NRTI NtRTI regimens combined with NNRTI or ritonavir-boosted PIs has been demonstrated, and at present, three-drug NRTI combinations are not considered optimal in initial therapy in current guidelines (see below). However, further study is needed to establish the validity of these preliminary data and the full potential of regimens, which do not employ either a PI or an NNRTI at the time of this writing. Hypersensitivity reactions to abacavir, which may be severe or even life threatening, have been associated with the presence of the HLA-B*5701 allele. Prospective screening for this genetic marker can dramatically reduce the risk of such reactions (23).

Resistance. Resistance to each NRTI has been documented, and patterns of cross resistance have been established.

NONNUCLEOSIDE REVERSE TRANSCRIPTASE INHIBITORS

Mode of Action

NNRTIs also inhibit viral reverse transcriptase by different mechanisms than the NRTI drugs.

Evidence of Efficacy

Many studies have demonstrated that NNRTIs have clinically significant anti-retroviral activity and, when used in combination regimens, can provide additive activity to other agents to significantly lower viral load and raise CD4 counts. Regimens employing two NRTIs and either delavirdine or nevirapine appear to lead to less durable viral suppression than PI-containing regimens, especially in individuals with high pretreatment viral loads (24).

However, data comparing an efavirenz-containing regimen with a PI-containing regimen suggest that the efavirenz regimen was more effective (25). Analysis comparing nevirapine and efavirenz in combination with two nucleosides indicates that they are approximately equal in effectiveness (26). On the basis of these and other data, the use of NNRTIs has become increasingly common, especially in treatment-naïve patients when there is a desire to avoid PIs or in patients intolerant of PI therapy.

Etravirine is the newest approved drug in this class and has been shown to be highly active against sensitive viral strains (27). In addition, it may play a role in combination salvage regimens for patients who have failed first-line therapy (28).

Patterns of Use

In standard treatment guidelines, efavirenz is currently considered acceptable and possibly superior to a PI in combination with two NRTI agents (see below), and as indicated above, nevirapine may be equally effective in such combinations especially for individuals with pretreatment viral loads of less than 100,000 copies/mm^3. Because of their convenient dosing schedules (once daily and twice daily, respectively), efavirenz and nevirapine are generally favored, although delavirdine may significantly raise PI levels and may eventually have an important role in salvage regimens incorporating PIs.

Resistance

One important problem in the use of NNRTIs is that resistance to any of the agents is indicative of resistance to all of them.

PROTEASE INHIBITORS

Mode of Action

They prevent cleavage of viral protein precursors required for HIV replication and entry into cells.

Evidence of Efficacy

Most agents in this class are potent inhibitors of HIV replication. A number of PIs typically combined (boosted) with low-dose ritonavir (PIr) inhibitors, in combination regimens with nucleoside drugs, have been shown to lead to significant clinical improvement and prolonged survival.

The central role of PI-containing regimens has been reinforced by a number of clinical trials.

Patterns of Use

PIs should be used as components of multidrug regimens. Although limited data suggest that the fixed combination of lopinavir and ritonavir (Kaletra) or darunavir and ritonavir without other agents (so-called boosted PI monotherapy) may be effective in some patients (29), controversy exists concerning the effectiveness of this strategy, and European guidelines include this treatment option for selected patients, but U.S. guidelines do not.

PIs, with the exception of nelfinavir, are typically given in combination with ritonavir, while ritonavir itself, because of its relatively high incidence of side effects, is administered in a subtherapeutic dose with other PIs to increase serum concentrations of the other PIs. When combined with ritonavir, darunavir (30,31) has a higher resistance threshold, is as effective as lopinavir/ritonavir, and is often effective in patients with virus resistant to earlier agents. They also have the advantage of lower rates of lipid disorders than earlier agents (31,32).

Resistance

Resistance to one PI is often predictive of resistance to one or more other drugs in this class. Resistance testing may not fully reveal such cross-resistance among PIs.

REGIMENS CONTAINING A PI AND NNRTI OR PI, NNRTI, AND NRTI

Combining PI and NNRTI agents, although theoretically appealing, raises practical considerations because of interactions between drugs of these classes and difficult dosing schedules. Regimens that combine agents of all three classes may also be quite potent but may leave no proven options if resistance develops. For these reasons, such regimens are generally not advisable for initial therapy, unless primary multiclass viral resistance is documented. At present, the use of these combinations is typically reserved for salvage therapy in cases of virologic failure.

INTEGRASE STRAND INHIBITOR

Mode of Action

Raltegravir, the first and currently only approved drug in this class, inhibits strand transfer, the final step in integration of the HIV provirus into host DNA.

Evidence of Efficacy

Raltegravir, the first marketed agent in this category, was approved for use in treatment-experienced patients in 2007 (33,34). Its effectiveness has been evaluated in the Blocking Integrase in Treatment Experienced Patients with a Novel Compound Against HIV (BENCHMRK-1 and BENCHMRK-2) studies (35). In a randomized trial of treatment-naïve patients comparing several dosing regimens of raltegravir with efavirenz, each combined with tenofovir and lamivudine, complete viral suppression was comparable at 48 weeks (36). In treatment-experienced patients with resistance to at least one PI, NNRTI, and NRTI, raltegravir was found to be superior to placebo when combined with optimized additional therapy (35).

Patterns of Use

On the basis of data available at the time of this writing, raltegravir can be used in initial regimen (see below) or reserved for use in treatment-experienced patients without other reasonable treatment options due to viral resistance. It must be used in combination with other active agents because of its apparent low barrier to resistance (see below).

Resistance

Current data suggests that raltegravir has a relatively low barrier to resistance related to at least two mutations in the integrase enzyme (37). For this reason, its clinical utility may be limited, unless it is used in combination with multiple effective agents. Nonetheless, raltegravir was found to be superior to placebo when combined with an optimized background even among patients with high viral loads ($>$100,000) and low CD4 counts ($<$50 cells/mm^3) and broad resistance to other agents (38).

CHEMOKINE CCR5 RECEPTOR ANTAGONIST

Mode of Action

Maraviroc, the first chemokine receptor antagonist to receive approval, blocks the CCR5 coreceptor. Binding to this receptor is necessary for entry into cells by certain HIV-1 cells with specific CCR5 tropism (so-called R5 viruses). Since not all HIV-1 strains are R5, CCR5 tropism assays must be performed and tropism demonstrated before maraviroc can be reliably used.

Evidence of Efficacy

Maraviroc was equivalent to efavirenz when each was combined with zidovudine and lamivudine at achieving complete viral suppression at 48 weeks in treatment-naïve patients (39). Effectiveness of maraviroc has also been demonstrated in treatment-experienced patients with CCR5 tropic virus when it is combined with other active agents (40).

Patterns of Use

Maraviroc is not currently recommended for use in initial therapeutic regimens (41). Because it is effective only against R5 strains of the virus and patients may be infected with R5-tropic and nontropic strains, overuse of maraviroc may lead to increasing emergence of non-R5 tropic virus and further limit its usefulness in the future. To prevent this phenomenon, maraviroc should be used only with an otherwise optimized regimen and only when CCR5 tropism has been demonstrated.

Resistance

Resistance to this agent is manifest both as a shift away from R5-tropic virus to strains using the CXCR4 coreceptor as well as to specific mutations in gp120 of the virus (42).

The Patient on Antiretroviral Therapy with Incomplete Viral Suppression

Although there is no uniform standard of virologic failure, a one-log reduction in viral load by eight weeks of therapy is recommended as an indication of therapeutic success in published treatment guidelines. Failure to achieve this milestone or, ultimately, failure to achieve complete viral suppression within six months is a common phenomenon in clinical practice. For patients achieving a partial response, several options exist. One approach is so-called treatment intensification. In this strategy, a single additional agent is added to a regimen that has produced partial, but not complete, improvement in viral load. It is prudent to reserve this option for patients with almost complete suppression (e.g., less than 1000 copies/mm^3) to avoid sequential drug resistance. Recent data regarding intensification in various settings and with several agents, including raltegravir and abacavir, has been discouraging (43,44). However, the strategy may be effective in the setting of the reverse transcriptase mutation K65R using zidovudine for intensification (45), and it may hold promise in other situations. Other options include continuation of the initial regimen if CD4 cell counts are rising or stabilizing or completely revising the treatment regimen.

Virologic Failure

Sequencing of ART in patients who have not responded to their initial or subsequent regimens is a complicated process. Little controlled data are currently available to guide the clinician in choosing subsequent regimens, but certain factors must be taken into account.

Cross-resistance to other agents within a class (NRTI, PI, NNRTI) is likely and, in the case of NNRTI failure, should be assumed to be present.

Resistance testing may fail to identify subpopulations of resistant virus.

Discordant responses to therapy (see below) in which a significant rise in CD4 cell count occurs despite failure to achieve complete viral suppression may be adequate under some circumstances when safe and effective options are very limited or nonexistent.

Discordant Responses

Patients who remain on ART often remain clinically stable with stable or, rarely, rising CD4+ lymphocyte counts despite virologic failure. This phenomenon, which may reflect reduced fitness of viral strains with resistance mutations, provides a rationale for continuing a suboptimal but well-tolerated regimen when no alternatives exist. In a prospective comparative study from France, it was found that the likelihood of an AIDS-defining complication after six months of HAART was equal among patients manifesting a significant immunologic response, regardless of virologic response (46). Patients with a virologic but not immunologic response had significantly worse outcomes. Complete non-responders had the worst prognosis. Observations such as this support the continued importance of CD4 cell count monitoring (47) and serve as an indicator that immune reconstitution itself should be a primary goal of therapy.

Interestingly, and perhaps relevant to the phenomenon of discordant responses to therapy, multidrug-resistant viral strains often manifest diminished infectivity and rate of replication (48).

MONITORING ANTIRETROVIRAL THERAPY

The measurement of plasma viral RNA and of CD4+ lymphocyte counts, along with clinical assessment, can provide an accurate picture of disease activity and progression for most patients. It has been observed that blood levels of antiretroviral agents are variable among individuals, and treatment failure may indicate subtherapeutic levels. In the future, monitoring of drug levels may become a standard practice; however, at this time, access to such assays is limited.

MONITORING FOR EFFECTIVENESS

Viral Load

Despite the data mentioned above regarding the importance of immunologic improvement, plasma levels of viral RNA have been shown to correlate closely with clinical outcome. Over a dozen clinical trials, which included thousands of patients, have demonstrated this correlation in patients at various stages of disease and with a wide variety of prior treatment histories (49–51). In addition, the level of viremia (viral load) measured in this way provides the most precise means of establishing whether or not a response to antiviral therapy has occurred. In the untreated patient or in individuals on stable therapeutic regimens, viral load should generally be measured every three to four months.

In patients beginning therapy or those changing therapy for virologic failure, viral load should be measured immediately prior to initiation and two to eight weeks later, by which time it typically falls by at least 1 log in the presence of effective therapy. In most of such patients, the viral load becomes undetectable (less than 50 copies/mL) by four to five months. An absent or incomplete response of the viral load to ART should raise concerns about viral resistance or poor patient compliance with therapy.

At the time of this writing, only the polymerase chain reaction (PCR) measure of viral RNA has been approved by the U.S. Food and Drug Administration for clinical staging and assessment of therapy of HIV infection.

Lymphocyte Subsets

CD4+ lymphocyte count, expressed as cells/mm^3 of blood, is a somewhat less precise indicator of clinical stage and response than viral load but is a valuable adjunctive study and can permit immunologic staging and decisions regarding prophylaxis against opportunistic infections. CD4+ cells counts should be measured at the time of diagnosis of HIV infection and every three to six months thereafter. The CD4+ response to ART can be unpredictable, and although a significant rise often occurs among patients treated with effective ART, the absence of such a rise should not be taken to mean viral resistance or poor patient compliance if the viral load declines appropriately. This lack of correlation between viral load and CD4+ cell response is particularly common among patients with extremely low initial CD4 cell count (e.g., less than 50 cells/mm^3).

Clinical Signs and Symptoms

The appearance of signs and symptoms of acute HIV infection (see chap. 4) in a previously asymptomatic patient should be regarded as a poor prognostic indicator. As mentioned above, symptomatic HIV infection is considered an independent indication for the initiation of ART regardless of viral load and immune parameters. The appearance of symptoms in a patient receiving ART should prompt a reassessment of the treatment regimen and patient compliance.

MONITORING FOR SIDE EFFECTS

Bone Marrow Depression

Bone marrow depression is most often associated with zidovudine therapy. Significant cytopenias become more common in the later stages of symptomatic HIV infection.

Lipodystrophy/Hyperlipidemia

In patients receiving PIs or efavirenz, serum triglyceride levels and routine biochemical tests, including liver function assays, should be determined prior to beginning therapy and periodically thereafter.

Glucose Intolerance

Blood glucose levels should be monitored periodically among patients receiving PIs. Patients at high risk of glucose intolerance (e.g., obesity, hyperlipidemia, pancreatitis, family history of diabetes) may also be monitored with periodic determination of glycosylated hemoglobin (hemoglobin A1C) or glucose tolerance test to identify intermittent periods of hyperglycemia.

Peripheral Neuropathy

Patients taking nucleoside drugs, particularly didanosine, zalcitabine, or stavudine, should be monitored for clinical signs and symptoms of peripheral neuropathy including numbness, tingling, or pain in the hands or feet. These symptoms are seen more commonly in patients with advanced HIV infection or prior history of neuropathy. Discontinuation of these agents usually results in gradual improvement.

Pancreatitis

Serum amylase levels should be monitored periodically among patients receiving zalcitabine who have a history of pancreatitis or ethanol abuse or who are at high risk for pancreatitis on the basis of hyperalimentation or underlying medical conditions. Didanosine should be avoided in patients at high risk of pancreatitis if possible. If such patients are receiving didanosine, amylase levels should be monitored periodically.

Lactic Acidosis/Hepatic Steatosis

The syndrome of lactic acidosis/hepatic steatosis (see above) has most often been associated with nucleoside therapy. Manufacturers of individual NRTIs recommend the following:

Stavudine, abacavir, didanosine, lamivudine, and zalcitabine should be used with caution in patients at risk for liver toxicity, although cases of the syndrome have occurred in the absence of definite hepatotoxicity. These agents should be discontinued in any patient developing signs consistent with lactic acidosis (including unexplained decrease in serum bicarbonate level) or liver toxicity.

Hepatoxicity

Hepatotoxicity, which may be fulminant, has most often been associated with nevirapine therapy. The manufacturer strongly recommends monitoring of transaminases, particularly during the first six months of therapy and discontinuing the drug if moderate or severe abnormalities occur. The drug should be avoided if liver function abnormalities recur upon rechallenge. The manufacturer of efavirenz recommends periodic monitoring of liver function tests in patients having a history of hepatitis B or C.

Miscellaneous Side Effects

Diarrhea. Diarrhea is a frequent complication of PI therapy.

Central nervous system effects. Both efavirenz and zidovudine can cause insomnia and mood alterations.

Drug interactions. Numerous interactions between antiretroviral drugs, particularly PIs and other medications, have been described. Some interactions may cause serious morbidity or mortality.

INTERPRETING VIROLOGIC FAILURE

Confirmation

In general, virologic failure should not be based on the result of one viral load determination. Repeat testing is warranted, especially if a change in ART is contemplated.

Measuring Drug Levels

Drug levels have been shown to correlate with clinical success for several agents. At the present time, however, these assays are not widely available.

ISSUES IN COMPLIANCE WITH THERAPY

Compliance with ART and adherence to complex treatment regimens are essential for achieving durable suppression of viral load. Even patients who only occasionally miss doses of their antiviral drugs run an increased risk of early emergence of resistance, viral breakthrough, and clinical progression. The practical impact of treatment adherence is seen in the contrast between rates of viral suppression seen in clinical trials, often greater than 95% (52), and those reported from clinical settings, often less than 50% (53,54). Many factors may represent obstacles to full compliance with therapy, however.

Denial

Failure to accept the reality of HIV infection frequently leads patients, particularly those who are asymptomatic, to doubt the need for ART or to be less than meticulous in taking their prescribed medications.

Lack of Acceptance of Therapy

Side effects of therapy, concerns about safety, whether real or imagined, or skepticism about traditional medicine may lead some individuals to openly decline appropriate retroviral therapy or to adhere poorly.

Number of Pills

Such practical issues as the large number of pills, the fact that some antiretroviral medications must be taken either with meals or on an empty stomach, and lack of privacy at home or in the workplace may lead even highly motivated patients to miss doses frequently.

Depression

Depression, more frequent among HIV-infected patients at all stages of disease, may be accompanied by feelings of hopelessness so intense that therapy and visits to the provider may seem pointless.

Physical Obstacles

A large proportion of HIV-infected individuals live in marginal housing or are homeless. Lack of a stable living situation can be a significant impediment to treatment adherence.

In general, in most cases, interruption of HAART therapy is followed by rebound of viremia and decline in CD4 cell count. For this reason, such an interruption should occur only under controlled circumstances.

STRUCTURED TREATMENT INTERRUPTION

Because of the limited number of antiretroviral agents available and the problem of cross resistance between agents, some patients may have exhausted all feasible drug combinations. In addition, a substantial number of individuals have achieved sustained viral suppression and immune reconstitution over a period of years. Because of these scenarios, efforts have been made to establish whether treatment interruption may be appropriate either to allow the overgrowth of more sensitive viral strains in those patients with limited treatment options or to reduce the long-term side effects of ART in those who have well-controlled viremia and high CD4 lymphocyte counts. Recent data, primarily from the Strategies for Management of Anti-retroivral Therapy (SMART) study, have indicated that interruption of therapy may not be appropriate and may have a negative impact on long-term outcomes. (55–60).

ACHIEVING THE GOALS OF ANTIRETROVIRAL THERAPY

With current therapeutic strategies, durable suppression of viral replication as indicated by viral load is achieved in approximately 50% of individuals beginning therapy for the first time. Treatment failure appears to represent either viral resistance or poor patient compliance in most cases. As noted above, adherence to ART can be difficult, especially when treatment regimens are complex and confusing. It is the responsibility of the provider to specifically address adherence by fostering a close relationship with the patient. In this way, the patient will be more likely to be frank about compliance issues, and the provider will be able to help formulate specific strategies for improvement. Treatment regimens should be as simple as possible, and unnecessary medications should be eliminated. Reminders such as alarms, printed schedules, and, when helpful, periodic telephone discussions should be considered even for apparently compliant patients. The support of family and friends should be enlisted when confidentiality permits. An intentional or unintentional interruption of therapy with any of the agents in the regimen should be reported to and discussed with the provider. In general, if therapy must be stopped for reasons of logistics, side effects, or lifestyle, all agents should be stopped and ultimately resumed simultaneously. Patients should be provided with an updated list of their medications and instructed to contact the provider promptly if they are hospitalized so that unnecessary interruption of therapy is avoided.

Among symptomatic patients with advanced immune deficiency, treatment regimens must be constantly reconsidered as the need for other, potentially interacting drugs may arise. Interruption of ART, although not desirable, may be inevitable in some of these patients.

Above all else, treatment adherence must be regarded as a likely constant struggle for all patients receiving ART, and time should be set aside at each patient contact to discuss this vital issue.

DRUG RESISTANCE TESTING

Several factors have made antiretroviral drug resistance testing increasingly important and necessary for effective management of HIV infection. The widespread use of combination therapy for nearly two decades has resulted in a large number of individuals who have experienced virologic failure of their initial regimen. In addition, the availability of new agents PIs and reverse transcriptase inhibitors has necessitated resistance testing to determine their utility in new combinations and to avoid the development of resistance to these drugs. Finally, the advent of entry inhibitors, such as maraviroc, has mandated the need for CCR5 coreceptor tropism assays to identify patients for whom this agent is appropriate. Recently updated guidelines by the International AIDS Society-USA Panel include the recommendation that resistance testing be conducted, whenever possible, before the initiation of any ART and that their importance be reinforced in identifying appropriate agents to be used when therapy is changed (61). Unfortunately, although resistance testing is widely available in developed countries, it is typically unavailable in the developing world. Transmission of resistance virus is a well-established phenomenon (62–64). The negative impact of empiric therapy not guided by viral load monitoring and thus by resistance testing has been demonstrated in recent data from South Africa (65,66).

Drug Resistance Assays

Two types of resistance assays are available in clinical practice. Genotypic assays employ gene sequencing to detect mutations associated with specific drug resistance. Phenotypic assays utilize cell culture techniques to measure viral replication in the presence and absence of specific drugs. Both techniques pose technical challenges to proper interpretation. Genotypic assays can be difficult to interpret in treatment-experienced patients in the presence of blends of viral strains with different resistance mutations (67) and in patients with relatively low viral loads (68).

Genotypic Assays

These tests employ predetermined panels of drug resistance mutations for each antiviral agent (69). The correlation between the presence of resistance mutations and clinical failure has improved in recent years for the majority of antiviral agents in each of the oldest three classes: PIs, NRTIs, and NNRTIs. Combinations of resistance mutations have resulted in the development of algorithms used to predict the likelihood of resistance to a variety of agents (69). A "virtual phenotype" can be characterized on the basis of mutational patterns determined by genotypic assays combined with corresponding phenotypic assays (70), although this technique has not been demonstrated to be superior to genotypic assays alone in predicting the likelihood of viral suppression (71).

Phenotypic Assays

This technique employs amplification of HIV-1 protease and a component of reverse transcriptase genes. These are then combined with other standardized laboratory HIV-1 genes. Susceptibility of the resultant recombinant "pseudovirus" is then determined by exposure to antiretroviral drugs (72).

TREATMENT SCENARIOS

U.S. and international expert panels have issued and revised antiretroviral treatment guidelines periodically. What follows represents 2010 updates to recommendations addressing situations in which therapeutic decisions should be made. In initiating lifelong therapy, issues regarding patient acceptance, obstacles to adherence, and potential for negative consequences of treating or not treating as discussed above and elsewhere in this text must be taken into account. These guidelines presume that these issues have been fully considered.

When Should Antiretroviral Treatment Be Started in the Treatment-Naïve HIV-Positive Patient?

The International AIDS Society USA (IAS-USA) Panel (41) recommends therapy for adults.

> All patients with symptomatic disease, including primary infection (highest-rated recommendations according to available evidence)
> All patients with CD4 cell count <500 cells/mm^3
> All patients with CD4 cell count <350 cells/mm^3 (highest-rated recommendations according to available evidence)
> All pregnant women (highest-rated recommendations according to available evidence)
> Patients with HIV viral RNA levels above 100,000 copies/mL
> All patients whose CD4 count falls at a rate of 100 cells/mm^3 or greater

Patients with active hepatitis B or hepatitis C infection

Patients with active cardiovascular disease or those at high risk

Patients with HIV-associated nephropathy

When the risk of transmission to others is considered high, as in discordant sexual partners

Patients with CD4 count above 500/mm^3 unless HIV viral load is less than 50 copies/mL ("elete controller") or CD4 count is stable and viremia is at low levels

Guidelines issued by an expert panel of the World Health Organization (73) were also updated in 2010 and include the following:

All patients, including HIV-pregnant women, with CD4 cell count below 350 cells/mm^3

All patients with severe or advanced disease (WHO clinical stage 3 or 4)

All patients with active tuberculosis

All patients with hepatitis B infection requiring treatment

What Drugs Should Be Used as Initial Therapy?

The IAS-USA (41) and WHO (73) panels both recommend combination regimens consisting of a "backbone" consisting of two NRTIs (tenofovir/emtricitabine by IAS-US and a regimen containing either zidovudine or tenofovir by the WHO) combined with an NNRTI (WHO), specifically efavirenz (IAS-USA). Boosted PI agents (atazanavir/ritonavir or darunavir/ritonavir) or raltegravir are endorsed as third agents by the IAS-USA panel (Table 5.1).

The IAS-USA panel considers abacavir/lamivudine as an alternative dual NRTI backbone (assuming patient negative for HLA-B*57-1) and lopinavir/ritonavir, foasamprenavir/ritonavir, or maraviroc (assuming viral tropism for CCR5 studies indicates susceptibility) as alternative third agents (41).

It should be noted that efavirenz is teratogenic and, if possible, should be avoided in pregnancy, particularly during the first trimester.

What Drugs Should Be Used as Second- or Third-Line (Salvage) Therapy?

Ideally, therapy for patients who have failed initial therapy should be guided by viral resistance studies. Efforts should be made to confirm treatment adherence and to address and treat specific side effects among patients with apparent treatment failure. For those with proven or suspected virologic failure, it is prudent to assume that NNRTI-containing regimens will have to be replaced with regimens not containing this class of drug because of the high rate of cross-resistance. All drugs within a failing regimen should be replaced. The complexities of identifying the optimal salvage regimen are of course magnified in resource-deprived regions lacking access to viral susceptibility testing. Ideal alternate regimens in any setting have not been clearly defined, although recommendations have been made to help guide the clinician (41).

Table 5.1 Antiretroviral Therapy for Chronic HIV Infection in Adults

Preferred initial regimen: general recommendations

Dual nucleoside/nucleotide reverse transcriptase (NRTI) component

    Tenofovir/emtricitabine

       Or

    Abacavir/lamivudine

Plus

    Efavirenz

       Or

    Atazanavir/ritonavir *or*

    Darunavir/ritonavir *or*

    Raltegravir

Alternative agents

    Lopinavir/ritonavir

    Fosamprenavir/ritonavir

    Maraviroc (if CCR5 viral tropism documented)

Note: See Appendix I for recommended adult dosing and side effects.
Source: From Ref. 41

ANTIRETROVIRAL THERAPY IN PREGNANCY

The role of ART as well as other strategies for the prevention of maternal-to-child transmission (PMTCT) is addressed in chapter 10. As indicated above, HIV infection in the setting of pregnancy is considered an indication for treatment with combination therapy in both the IAS-USA and WHO guidelines. To minimize the likeliness of maternal-to-child transmission, therapy antepartum, intrapartum, and prophylaxis of the infant postpartum are recommended (74) (Table 5.2). If antepartum therapy has not been given to the mother, intrapartum therapy and prophylaxis to the infant should be provided. If neither antepartum nor intrapartum therapy has been administered, it is recommended that the infant receives zidovudine for the first six weeks of life (74).

POSTEXPOSURE PROPHYLAXIS

Postexposure prophylaxis is intended to prevent transmission of HIV infection from an infected index case to an uninfected contact. Guidelines for preventive therapy in both occupational (health care) settings (75) and nonoccupational settings (76) have been developed and frequently re-evaluated. The reader is referred to these guidelines and their periodic updates for detailed recommendations.

Table 5.2 Antiretroviral Therapy in Pregnancy

First-trimester women known to be HIV-infected at the beginning of pregnancy
If already receiving ART:
> Continue therapy if full viral suppression has been achieved. Efavirenz (teratogenic) and combination therapy with stavudine and didanosine (lactic acidosis) should be avoided. Substitute PI-based regimen if possible.

If not receiving ART:
> *Obtain resistance assays if possible*
> *Optimal regimen:* Zidovudine/lamivudine plus nevirapine or PI/ritonavir. Nevirapine should be avoided if possible if CD4 count is above 250 cells/mm^3 because of the risk of fulminant hepatitis.

Women receiving ART during pregnancy but failing to achieve complete viral suppression:
> *Ceasarian section if viral load exceeds 1000 copies/mm^3 at term.*

Women with no prior ART presenting in labor:
> Intravenous zidovudine during labor and delivery. Oral zidovudine for infant for 4-6 wk.
> A large number of other options have been studied, which may be particularly appropriate in resource-limited settings (74).

Note: See Appendix I for recommended adult dosing and side effects.

PREEXPOSURE PROPHYLAXIS

The potential to reduce transmission by administering antiretroviral medications to uninfected individuals engaging in high-risk behavior has received increased attention in recent years. In a multinational study published in 2010 (77), it was found that the risk risk of HIV infection was reduced by 73% among sexually active men who have sex with men (MSM) who were at least 90% compliant with once-daily therapy with the combination drug tenofovir-emtricitabine (FTC-TDF). Concerns have been raised regarding this strategy including potential toxicity, incomplete adherence, and the possibility of the emergence of viral resistance, which was observed in this study (78). Additional studies designed to further examine this strategy of reducing transmission are under way.

REFERENCES

1. Havlir DV. HIV integrase inhibitors—out of th epipeline and into the clinic. N Engl J Med 2008; 359:416–418.
2. Hirschel B, Calmy A. Initial treatment for HIV infection—an embarrassment of riches. N Engl J Med 2008; 358:2170–2172.
3. Department of Health and Human Services Centers for Disease Control and Prevention. HIV/AIDS among persons aged 50 and older, 2008. Available at: http://www.cdc.gov/hiv.

4. Forrest DM, Seminari E, Hogg RS, et al. The incidence and spectrum of AIDS-defining illnesses in persons treated with antiretroviral drugs. Clin Infect Dis 2000; 27:1379–1385.

5. Quinn TC, Wawer MJ, Sewankambo N, et al. Viral load and heterosexual transmission of human immunodeficiency virus type 1. Rakai Project Study Group. N Engl J Med 2000; 342:921–929.

6. Fischl MA, Richman DD, Hansen N, et al. The safety and efficacy of zidovudine (AZT) in the treatment of patients with mildly symptomatic human immunodeficiency virus type 1 (HIV) infection. A double-blind, placebo-controlled trial. Ann Intern Med 1990; 112:727.

7. Volberding P, Lagakos SW, Grimes JM, et al. The duration of zidovudine benefit in persons with asymptomatic HIV infection. JAMA 1994; 272:437–442.

8. Kahn JO, Lagakos SW, Richman DD, et al. A controlled trial comparing continued zidovudine with didanosine in human immunodeficiency virus infection. N Engl J Med 1992; 327:581–587.

9. Eron JJ, Benoit SL, Jemsek J, et al. Treatment with lamivudine, zidovudine or both in HIV positive patients with 200 to 500 CD4 cells per cubic millimeter. N Engl J Med 1995; 327:581.

10. Spruance S, Pavia AT, Mellors JW, et al. Clinical efficacy of monotherapy with stavudine compared with zidovudine in HIV infected, zidovudine-experienced patients. A randomized, double-blind, controlled trial. Ann Intern Med 1997; 126:355–363.

11. Dragovic GJ, Smith CJ, Jevtovic DJ, et al. Comparison of nucleoside reverse transcriptase inhibitor use as part of first-line therapy in a Serbian and a UK HIV clinic. HIV Clin Trials 2009; 10(5):306–313.

12. Fischl M, Greenberg S, Clumeck N, et al. Ziagen (abacavir, aBC, 1592) combined with 3TC and ZDV is highly effective and durable through 48 weeks in HIV-1 infected antiretroviral-therapy naïve subjects. 6th Conference on Retroviruses and Opportunistic Infections, Chacago, 1999.

13. Vernazza P, Katlama C, Clotet B, et al. Intensification of stable background therapy with abacavir: preliminary 48 weeks data. Seventh European Conference on Clinical Aspects and Treatment of HIV Infection, 1999; Lisbon, Portugal.

14. Hammer S, Squires K, Degrutolla V, et al. Randomized trial of abacivr (ABC) and nelfinavir (NFV) in combination with efavirenz (EFV) and adefovir dipivoxil (ADV) as salvage therapy in patients with virologic failure receiving indinavir (IDV), 6 the Conference on Retroviruses and Opportunistic Infections, 1999; Chicago.

15. Fung HB, Stone EA, Piacenti FJ. Tenofovir disoproxil fumarate: a nucleotide reverse transcriptase inhibitor for the treatment of HIV infection. Clin Ther 2002; 24(10):1515–1548.

16. Pham PA, Gallant JE. Tenofovir disoproxil fumarate for the treatment of HIV infection. Expert Opin Drug Metab Toxicol 2006; 2(3):459–469.

17. Chowers M, Gottesman BS, Leibovici L, et al. Nucleoside reverse transcriptase inhibitors in combination therapy for HIV patients: systematic review and meta-analysis. Eur J Clin Microbiol Infect Dis 2010; 29(7):779–786.

18. Antoniou T, Park-Wyllie LY, Tseng AL. Tenofovir: a nucleotide analog for the management of human immunodeficiency virus infection. Pharmacotherapy 2003; 23(1):29–43.

19. Pozniak A. Tenofovir: what have over 1 million years of patient experience taught us? Int J Clin Pract 2008; 62(8):1285–1293.

20. Cooper RD, Wiebe N, Smith N, et al. Systematic review and meta-analysis: renal safety of tenofovir disoproxil fumarate in HIV-infected patients. Clin Infect Dis 2010; 51(5):496–505.

21. Quimby D, Trito MO. Fanconi syndrome associated with use of fenofovir in HIV-infected patients: a case report and review of the literature. AIDS Read 2005; 15 (7):357–364.

22. Shey M, Kongnyuy EJ, Shang J, et al. A combination of abacavir-lamivudine-zidovudine (Trizivir) for treating HIV infection and AIDS. Cochrane Database Syst Rev 2009; 8(3):CD005481.

23. Mallal S, Phillips, E, Carosi G, et al. HLA-B*5701 screening for hypersensitivity to abacavir. N Engl J Med 2008; 358:568–579.

24. Raboud J, Montaner JS, Rae S, et al. Patients with higher baseline pVL are less likely to have a virologic response in a meta-analysis of two trials of ADV/ddI vs. ZDV/ddI/NVP (abstr II236I), 12 International Conference on AIDS, 2000, Geneva.

25. Stazewski S, Morales-Ramirez J, Tashima KT, et al. Efavirenz plus zidovudine and lamivudine, efavirenz plus indinavir and indinavir plus zidovudine and lamivudine in the treatment of HIV-1 infection in adults. N Engl J Med 1999; 341:1865–1873.

26. Nunez M, Soriano V, Martin-Barbonero L, et al. SENC (Spanish efavirenz vs. nevirapine comparison) trial: a randomized, open-label study in HIV-infected anive individuals. HIV Clin Trials 2002; 3(3):186–194.

27. Clumek N, Cahn P, Molina JM, et al. Virological response with fully active etravirine: pooled results from the DUET-1 and DUET-2 trials. Int J STD AIDS 2010; 21(11):738–740.

28. Santos JR, Librfe JM, Domingo P, et al. High effectiveness of etravirine in routine clinical practice in tgreatment-experienced HIV type 1-infected patients. AIDS Res Hum Retroviruses 2011 Jan 15 (Epub ahead of print).

29. Pulido F, Matarranz M, Rodriguez-Rivera V, et al. Boosted protease inhibitor monotherapy. What have we learnt after seven years of research? AIDS Rev 2010; 12(3):127–134.

30. Madruga JV, Berger D, McMurchie M, et al. Efficacy and safety ofdarunavir-ritonavir copared with that of lopinavir-ritonavir at 48 weeks in treatment-experienced, HIV-infected patients in TITAN: a randomized controlled phase III trial. Lancet 2007; 370(9581):49–58.

31. Curran A, Ribera Pascuet E. Darunavir as first-line therapy. The TITAN study. Enferm Infecc Microbiol Clin 2008; 26(suppl 10):14–22.

32. Molina JM, Andrade-Villanueva J, Echevarria J, et al. Once-daily atazanavir/ritonavir compared with twice-daily lopinavir/ritonavir each in combination with tenofovir and embricitabine, for management of antiretroviral-naïve HIV-1-infected patients: 96 week efficacy and safety results of the CASTLE study. J Acquir Immune Defic Syndr 2010; 53(3):323–332.

33. Steigbigel R, Kumar P, Eron J, et al. Results of BENCHMRK-2, a phase III study evaluating the efficacy and safety of MK-0518, a novel HIV-1 integrase inhibitor, in patients with triple-class resistant virus. 14th Conference on Retroviruses and Opportunistic Infections; February 25-28, 2007; Los Angeles, CA. Abstract 105bLB.

34. Cooper D, Gatell J, Rockstroh J, et al. Results of BENCHMRK-1, a phase III studey evaluating the efficacy and safety of MK-0518, a novel HIV-1 integrase inhibitor, in

patients with triple-class resistant virus. 14th Conference on Retroviruses and Opportunistic Infections; February 25-28, 2007; Los Angeles, CA. Abstract 105aLB.

35. Steigbigel RT, Cooper DA, Kumar PN, et al. Rategravir with optimized background therapy for resistant HIV-1 infection. N Engl J Med 2008; 359:339–354.

36. Markowitz M, Nguyen BY, Gotuzzo E, et al. Rapid and durable antiretroviral effect of the HIV-1 integrase inhibitor raltegravir as part of combination therapy in treatment-naïve patients with HIV-1 infection: result of a 48-week controlled study. J Acquir Immune Defic Syndr 2007; 46(2):125–133.

37. Hazuda DJ, Miller MD, Nguyen BY, et al. P005 Study Team. Resistance to the HIV-integrase inhibitor raltegravir: analysis of protocol 005, a phase II study in patients with triple-class resistant HIV-1 infection. Antivir Ther 2007; 12(suppl):S10.

38. Cooper DA, Stigbigel RT, Gatell JM, et al. Subgroup and resistance analyses of raltegravir for resistant HIV-1 infection. N Engl J Med 2008; 359:355–365.

39. Saag M, Ive P, Heera J, et al. A multicenter, randomized, double-blind, comparative trial of a novel CCR5 antagonist, maraviro versus efavirenz, both in combination with combivir (zidovudine [ZDV]/lamivudine [3tc], for the treatment of anti-retroviral naïve subjects infected with R5 HIV-1: week 48 results of the MERIT study. 4th International AIDS Society Conference on HIV Pathogenesis, Treatment and Prevention; July 22-25, 2007; Sydney, Australia, Abstract WESS104.

40. Haardy D, Reynes J, Konourina I, et al. Efficacy and safety of maraviroc plus optimized background therapy in treatment-experienced patients infected with CCR5-tropic HIV-1: 48-week combined analysis of the MOTIVATE studies. 15th Conference on Retroviruses and Opportunistic Infections; February 3-6, 2008; Boston, MA. Abstract 792.

41. Thompson MA, Aberg JA, Cahn P, et al. Antiretroviral treatment of adult HIV infection: 2010 recommendations of the International AIDS Society USA Panel. JAMA 2010; 304(3):321–333.

42. Hammer SM, Eron JJ, Reiss P, et al. Antiretroviral treatment of adult HIV infection. 2008 recommendations of the International AIDS Society-USA Panel. JAMA 2008; 300(5):555–570.

43. Gandhi RT, Zheng L, Bosch RJ, et al. The effect of raltegravir intensification on low-level residual viremia in HIV-infected patients on antiretroviral therapy: a randomized controlled trial. PloS Med 2010; 7(8). Pii:e1000321.

44. Hammer SM, Ribaudo H, Bassett R, et al. A randomized, placebo-controlled trial of abacavir intensification in HIV-1-infected adults with virologic suppression on a protease inhibitor-containing regimen. HIV Clin Trials 2010; 11(6):312–324.

45. Stephan C, Dauer B, Bickel M, et al. Intensification of a failing regimen with zidovudine may cause sustained virologic suppression in the presence of resensitising mutations including K65R. J Infect 2010; 61(4):346–350.

46. Grabar S, Le Moing V, Goujard C, et al. Clinical outcome of patients with HIV-1 infection according to immunologic and virologic response after 6 months of highly active antiretroviral therapy. Ann Intern Med 2000; 133:401–410.

47. Gulick RM, Mellors JW, Havlir D, et al. 3-year suppression of HIV viremia with indinavir, zidovudine, and lamivudine. Ann Intern Med 2000; 133:35–39.

48. Kaufman D, Muñoz M, Bleiber G, et al. Virological and immunological characteristics of HIV treatment failure. AIDS 2000; 14:1767–1774.

49. Mellors JW, Rinaldo CR Jr, Gupta P, et al. Prognosis in HIV-1 infection predicted by the quantity of virus in plasma. Science 1996; 272:1167–1170.

50. Mellors JW, Muñoz A, Giorgi JV, et al. Plasma viral load and CD4+ lymphocytes as prognostic markers of HIV-1 infectino. Ann Intern Med 1997; 126:946–954.

51. Powderly WG, Saag MS, Chapman S, et al. Predictors of optimal virological response to potent antiretroviral therapy. AIDS 1999; 13:1873–1880.

52. Gulick RM, Mellors JW, Havlir D, et al. Treatment with indinavir, zidovudine and lamivudine in adults with human immunodeficiency virus infection and prior anti-retroviral therapy. N Engl J Med 1997; 337:734–739.

53. Valdez H, Lederman MM, Woolley I, et al. Human immunodeficiency virus 1 protease inhibitors in clinical practice: predictors of virological outcome. Arch Intern Med 1999; 159:1771–1776.

54. Bozzette SA, Berry SH, Duan N, et al. The care of HIV-infected adults in the United States. HIV cost and services utilization study consortium. N Engl J Med 1998; 339:1897.

55. Strategies for Management of Antiretroviral Therapy (SMART) Study Group. CD4+ count-guided interruption of antiretroviral treatment. N Engl J Med 2006; 355:2283–2296.

56. The SMART Study Group. Risk for opportunistic disease and death after reinitiating continuous antiretroviral therapy in patients wit HIV previously receiving episodic therapy. A randomized trial. Ann Intern Med 2008; 149:289–299.

57. Silverberg MJ, Neuhaus J, Bower M, et al. Risk of cancers during interrupted antiretroviral therapy in the SMART study. AIDS 2007; 21:1957063.

58. Phillips AN, Carr A, Neuhaus J, et al. Interruption of antiretroviral therapy and risk of cardiovascular disease in persons with HIV-1 infection: exploratory analyses from the SMART trial. Antivir Ther 2008; 13:177–187.

59. Burman WJ, Grund B, Roediger MP, et al. SMART Study Group. The impact of episodic CD4 cell count-guided antiretroviral therapy on quality of life. J Acquir Immune Defic Syndr 2008; 47:185–193.

60. Strategies for Management of Antiretroviral Therapy (SMART) Study Group. Inferior clinical outcome of the CD4+ cell count-guided antiretroviral treatment interruption strategy in the SMART study: role of CD4+ cell counts and HIV RNA levels during followup-up. J Infect Dis 2008; 197:1145–1155.

61. Hirsch MS, Gunthard HF, Schapiro JM, et al. Antiretroviral drug resistance testing in adult HIV-1 infection: 2008 recommendations of an International AIDS Society-USA panal. Clin Infect Dis 2008; 47:266–285.

62. Brenner B, Wainberg MA, Salomon H, et al. Resistance to antiretroviral drugs in patients with primary HIV-1 infection. Investigators of the Quebec Primary Infection Study. Int J Antimicrob Agents 2000; 16:429–434.

63. Chaix ML, Descamps D, Harzic M, et al. Stable prevalence of genotypic drug resistance mutatons but increase in non-B virus among patients with primary HIV-1 infection in France. AIDS 2003; 17:2635–2643.

64. Yerly S, Von Wyl V, Ledergerber B, et al. Transmission of HIV-1 drug resistance in Switzerland: a 10-year molecular epidemiology survey. AIDS 2007; 21:2223–2229.

65. Marconi VC, Sunpath H, Lu Z, et al. Prevelence of HIV-1 durg resistance after failure of a first highly active antiretroviral therapy regien in KwaZulu Natal, South Africa. Clin Infect Dis 2008; 46(15 May):1589–1597.

66. Smith DM, Schooley RT. Running with scissors: using antiretroviral therapy without monitoring viral load. Clin Infect Dis 2008; 46:1598–1600.

67. Ross L, Boulme R, Fisher R, et al. A direct comparison of drug susceptibility to HIV type 1 from antiretroviral experienced subjects as a ssessed by the antivirograqm and PhenoSense assays and by seven resistance algorithms. AIDS Res Hum Retroviruses 2005; 21:933–939.

68. Descamps D, Dalaugerre C, Masquelier B, et al. Repeated HIV-1 resistance genotyping external quality assessments improve virology laboratory performance. J Med Virol 2006; 78:153–160.

69. MacArthur RD. An updated guide to go tenotype interpretation. AIDS Read 2004; 14:256–258, 261–261, 266.

70. Mazzotta F, Lo Caputo S, Torti C, et al. Real versus virtual phenotype to guide treatment in heavily pretreated patients: 48-week follow-up of the Genotipo-Fenotipo di Resistenza (GenPheRex) trial. J Acquir Immune Defic Syndr 2003; 32:268–280.

71. Torti C, Quiros-Roldan E, Regazzi M, et al. A randomized controlled trial to evaluate antiretroviral salvage therapy guided by rules-based or phenotype-driven HIV-1 genotypic drug-resistance interpretation with our without concentration-controlled intervention: the Resistance and Dosage Adapted Reimens (RADAR) study. Clin Infect Dis 2005; 40:1828–1836.

72. Walter H, Schmidt B, Korn K, et al. Rapid, phenotypic HIV-1 drug sensitivity assay for protease and reverse transcriptase inhibitors. J Clin Virol 1999; 13:71–80.

73. World Health Organization. Antiretroviral therapy for HIV infection in adults and adolescents. Recommendations for a public health approach. 2010 revision. World Health Organization, 2010.

74. Panel on Treatment of HIV-Infected Pregnant Women and Prevention of Perinatal Transmission. Recommendations for use of antiretroviral drugs in pregnant HIV-1-infected women for maternal health and interventions to reduce perinatal HIV transmission in the United States, May 24, 2010; pp1–117.

75. Panlilio AL, Cardo dM, Grohskopf LA, et al. Updated U.S. Public Health Service guidelines for the management of occupational exposures to HIV and recommendations for postexposure prophylaxis. Centers for disease control and prevention. MMWR Recomm Rep 2005:54(RR-9):1–17.

76. Smith DK, Grohskopf LA, Black RJ, et al. Antiretroviral postexposure prophylaxis after sexual, injection-drug use, or other nonoccupational exposure to HIV in the United States. Recommendations from the U.S. Department of Health and Human Services. MMWR Recomm Rep.2005; 54(RR02):1–20.

77. Grant RM, Lama JR, Anderson PL, et al. Preexposure chemoprophylaxis for HIV prevention in men who have sex with men. N Engl J Med 2010; 363(27):2587–2599.

78. Michael NL. Oral preexposure prophylaxis for HIV—another arrow in the quiver. N Engl J Med 2010; 363(27):2587–2599.

6

Therapy of selected serious HIV-related disorders and the immune reconstitution syndrome

INTRODUCTION

Modern antiretroviral therapy (ART) has resulted in a dramatic reduction in the incidence of severe and life-threatening opportunistic infections associated with HIV infection. Such disorders as *Pneumocystis carinii* pneumonia (PCP), *Toxoplasma* encephalitis, and cryptococcal meningitis, which cost many lives, and *Cytomegalovirus* (CMV) retinitis, a frequent cause of blindness, during the first 15 years of the AIDS epidemic have become unusual among patients receiving effective ART. In fact, many such patients have experienced such significant increases in CD4+ lymphocyte counts that preventive therapy for such previously common disorders as CMV retinitis, PCP, and toxoplasmosis infection has been withdrawn. Nonetheless, many patients continue to suffer and die from HIV-related opportunistic infections, particularly in the resource-limited settings that exist in most of the areas of the world most impacted by HIV/AIDS. There are several reasons for this. Many individuals enter care late and present with opportunistic infections as their initial manifestation of AIDS before ART is instituted. In addition, many have failed multiple antiretroviral regimens and have not seen significant immune reconstitution. Finally, prophylaxis directed against some opportunistic pathogens is not universally prescribed and taken.

The clinical manifestations and approach to diagnosis and prevention of the disorders discussed in this chapter are presented in chapters 2, 3, and 8 [tuberculosis (TB) and viral hepatitis]. The focus of this discussion is on therapy of these conditions including the approach to related manifestations of the immune reconstitution syndrome (IRIS), an inflammatory disorder, occasionally serious, which often accompanies the initiation of effective therapy of HIV.

PNEUMOCYSTIS PNEUMONIA

Therapy

Trimethoprim/sulfamethoxazole (TMP-SMX) is the preferred treatment for confirmed or suspected PCP (1,2) and should be continued for 21 days. Oral therapy with TMP-SMX was effective in 90% of patients with initial episodes of mild-to-moderate PCP (partial pressure of oxygen >60 mmHg) (3) and can be considered for compliant patients without gastrointestinal tract disease who can be closely monitored for respiratory symptoms.

Combination therapy with clindamycin and primaquine or with pentamidine (4,5) represents alternatives for patients with moderate-to-severe disease. Confirmed or suspected PCP may be treated with either TMP-SMX (20 mg/kg daily TMP and 100 mg/kg daily SMX in a fixed combination given in four divided doses) or pentamidine (4 mg/kg in a single daily dose). Reported response rates have been in the range of 70% to 95% depending on the severity of disease (6).

Side effects with either TMP-SMX or pentamidine are common. Rash and anemia were each encountered in approximately 40% of patients receiving TMP-SMX, whereas more than 60% of patients receiving pentamidine had nephrotoxic effects, and approximately one-fourth had hypotension or hypoglycemia in one controlled study (7). TMP-SMX is generally favored by clinicians, with pentamidine held in reserve for patients failing or intolerant of therapy.

Combination therapy with clindamycin (600 mg four times daily or 900 mg three times daily intravenously or 300–450 mg four times daily by mouth) and primaquine (15 mg base once daily by mouth) may be effective in some patients unresponsive to or intolerant of conventional therapy (8) and represents a third parenteral option in patients unable to take oral medications.

The oral agent atovaquone is approved for the therapy of mild-to-moderate PCP for patients intolerant of TMP-SMX. In a dose of 750 mg three times daily, atovaquone is somewhat less effective than conventional therapy with TMP-SMX (1).

Combined therapy with oral dapsone (100 mg/day) and TMP (20 mg/kg daily) has been shown to be as effective as conventional therapy for mild-to-moderate PCP (3). As noted previously, oral therapy is appropriate only in selected cases.

Prognostic Indicators

Several factors have prognostic significance in HIV-related PCP. The overall condition of the patient as indicated by degree of wasting and serum albumen level and the degree of gas exchange abnormality is indicated by arterial blood gas determination (9).

Adjunctive Therapy with Corticosteroids

Corticosteroids, when initiated within the first 72 hours, have improved the survival of patients with $PO_2 < 70$ mmHg or arterial-alveolar O_2 gradient > 35 mmHg (10). In 1990, a consensus panel of the National Institute of Allergy and Infectious Disease recommended that patients with PCP whose oxygen pressure is below 70 mmHg or whose arterial-alveolar oxygen pressure difference is greater than 35 mmHg receive adjunctive corticosteroids within 72 hours of starting anti-PCP therapy. The panel recommended the following regimen: prednisone 40 mg twice daily, days 1 through 5; 20 mg twice daily, days 6 through 10; and 20 mg once daily, days 11 through 21.

Concerns have been expressed that other, undiagnosed, opportunistic infections may accelerate because of further immunosuppression caused by corticosteroids. Although this risk must be considered, it appears to be small, and the impact on survival of moderate-to-severe PCP of corticosteroid therapy has been substantial.

Prophylaxis of PCP represents cornerstones in HIV care. These topics are reviewed in chapter 2. The approach to secondary prophylaxis is comparable to that for primary prophylaxis. Secondary prophylaxis can usually be safely discontinued after the CD4 cell count has risen above 200 cells/mm^3 for at least three months (11) unless the episode of PCP occurred at counts above this level.

The Immune Reconstitution Syndrome and PCP

The IRIS (12) with recrudescence of symptomatic disease following treatment has been described after the initiation of ART. It is unclear at this time what the optimal timing of ART after PCP should be (11).

CEREBRAL TOXOPLASMOSIS

Therapy

The initial treatment of choice for cerebral toxoplasmosis is the combination of sulfadiazine (1–2 g qid) and pyrimethamine (100–200 mg daily). This regimen is continued for four to eight weeks after which sulfadiazine may be reduced to 2 to 4 g in four divided doses daily and pyrimethamine to 25 to 50 mg daily. Leucovorin (5–50 mg daily) should be administered simultaneously. Clindamycin (600 mg qid) may be substituted for sulfadiazine and has been shown to be equally effective in initial therapy (13) although not as effective in maintenance. Radiographic and clinical signs of improvement are usually apparent after two weeks of therapy. If no improvement occurs in this time period, other disorders, particularly lymphoma and TB, should be considered strongly.

In patients responding, suppressive therapy may be continued indefinitely, although consideration can be given to discontinuing this in cases where there is sustained immune reconstitution with CD4+ cell counts maintained over 200/ mm^3 for three to six months.

Evidence has accumulated that several alternative agents may be effective in some patients not responding to or unable to tolerate either sulfadiazine- or clindamycin-based regimens.

Azithromycin

Conflicting data regarding the potential role of azithromycin have been published. While progression of cerebral toxoplasmosis was seen in two patients treated with azithromycin alone in one study, cases of response to combination therapy with azithromycin and pyrimethamine have been reported (14).

Atovaquone

Following initial therapy with sulfadiazine/pyrimethamine, atovaquone was effective in long-term suppressive therapy in one study of 65 patients (15). Although 26% of individuals in this study suffered relapses of cerebral toxoplasmosis, only the duration of initial therapy correlated with risk of relapse. Another study indicated that atovaquone may be effective in salvage therapy (16). The dose of atovaquone used in both studies was 750 mg by mouth four times daily.

The Immune Reconstitution Syndrome and Toxoplasmosis

There have been few reports of recurrence or progression of toxoplasmosis attributed to immune reconstitution (11).

CRYPTOCOCCAL INFECTION

Therapy

Extraneural Infection

Patients presenting with infection in the lungs or other extraneural sites should undergo lumbar puncture to evaluate for CNS involvement (17). Little information is available on outcomes of various treatment strategies for extraneural infection in HIV-infected patients. There is a consensus that all such patients should receive systemic antifungal therapy and that surgical resection should be considered for refractory pulmonary or skeletal lesions. Therapy with oral azole agents, particularly fluconazole with or without flucytosine, can be considered for patients with mild-to-moderately severe extraneural disease. Amphotericin B is most appropriate for individuals with severe disease.

Meningitis

Both amphotericin B and fluconazole are effective in the therapy of cryptococcal meningitis. However, mortality rates within the first two weeks of therapy are lower among patients receiving amphotericin B than among those receiving fluconazole (8% and 15%, respectively) (18). Combination therapy with amphotericin B (0.7–1.0 mg/kg intravenously daily) and flucytosine 100 mg/kg in four divided doses orally continued for at least two weeks is considered the treatment of choice for HIV-associated cryptococcal meningitis (11). Patients intolerant of flucytosine may be treated with amphotericin B alone. Lipid-based amphotericin B preparations may offer a lower risk of nephrotoxicity, although dosing regimens are not as well established as they are for conventional amphotericin B. Less desirable initial regimens include fluconazole (400–800 mg/day) and flucytosine 100 mg/kg/day for six weeks or fluconazole or itraconazole alone.

After successful induction therapy with clinical improvement and sterilization of the cerebrospinal fluid, fluconazole 400 mg/day or itraconazole should be administered for at least eight weeks (11).

Relapse rates after the completion of therapy may exceed 50% (19). For this reason, following the completion of consolidation therapy, maintenance therapy with fluconazole (200–400 mg daily) should be instituted and continued until sustained immune reconstitution has been achieved. Itraconazole, used for maintenance, was associated with a significantly higher relapse rate than fluconazole in one series (20). Amphotericin B (1 mg/kg intravenously 1–3 times weekly) should be reserved for patients intolerant of or resistant to azole compounds.

Increased Intracranial Pressure

Neurologic deficits, particularly hearing loss, can be more pronounced among patients with cryptococcal meningitis complicated by increased intracranial pressure. For this reason, it is recommended that patients with intracranial pressure greater than 250 mm H_2O undergo large-volume CSF drainage (17).

The Immune Reconstitution Syndrome and Cryptococcal Infection

The IRIS has been reported to be relatively frequent following initiation of ART, occurring in approximately 30% of individuals (21). It is particularly common among patients who are ART naïve or who have high HIV RNA levels load (22). It may be advisable to delay initiation of ART until the completion of the initial two-week phase of therapy has been successfully completed (22). In addition to continuation of antifungal therapy and ART, a brief course of glucocorticoid therapy is recommended by some for severe IRIS.

PROGRESSIVE MULTIFOCAL LEUKOENCEPHALOPATHY

Therapy

Therapy of progressive multifocal leukoencephalopathy (PML) has been frustrating. No antiviral agent has demonstrated consistent efficacy. Potent ART has resulted in clinical and radiographic improvement (23) in some individuals, as well as improved survival (24). Antiretroviral drugs may reduce central nervous system replication of the JC virus, the causative agent of PML (25).

The Immune Reconstitution Syndrome and PML

The potential for robust immune reconstitution after initiation of ART in patients with PML presents a unique challenge. Since improvement in immunologic function appears to be beneficial in treatment of PML and, in contrast to the other opportunistic infections described in this chapter, there is no other effective therapy for PML, IRIS may result in an abrupt, severe, and even fatal degree of cerebral edema after the initiation of ART. Short courses of corticosteroids may be considered in this situation (11). Discontinuation of ART is not currently recommended (11).

MYCOBACTERIUM AVIUM COMPLEX INFECTION

Therapy

Treatment strategies for *Mycobacterium avium* complex (MAC) infection in the setting of HIV infection have focused on those patients with disseminated MAC, defined as documented bacteremia. Significant progress has been made in the treatment of this condition, primarily reflecting the effectiveness of the macrolide antibiotics azithromycin and clarithromycin, although current guidelines include both a macrolide and a second agent, typically ethambutol (11). Of the macrolides, clarithromycin has been the most studied and appears to eradicate the organism from the blood more rapidly (26) than azithromycin. Mycobacteremia was eradicated or significantly reduced in two to four weeks among patients receiving clarithromycin in one large series (27). As in other mycobacterial infections, therapy of disseminated MAC infection with a single agent is associated with emergence of secondary resistance (46%) to clarithromycin in the study cited above.

Standard treatment regimens for MAC include at least two agents, one of which should be either azithromycin (1200 mg weekly) or clarithromycin (500 mg twice daily). Ethambutol (15 mg/kg daily) is most often used as the second drug and is most effective when combined with clarithromycin. Second-line agents include rifabutin (300–450 mg daily), amikacin (7.5–15 mg/kg daily), and ciprofloxacin (500–750 mg bid daily). Rifabutin should not be administered to patients receiving certain antiretroviral agents (see chap. 5).

Response to therapy is generally seen within six weeks, after which the regimen should be continued indefinitely. Treatment failure is often indicative of drug resistance. If this occurs, alternate regimens containing at least two additional agents may be necessary. It is likely, though not yet established, that treatment may be discontinued in patients receiving effective ART when the CD4 lymphocyte count rises above 200/mm^3.

Patients who have completed at least 12 months of therapy and have a sustained increase in their CD4 cell count to >100 cells/mm^3 are at low risk of recurrence, and discontinuation of maintenance therapy can be considered under these circumstances, but therapy should be restarted if the CD4 cell count falls below 100 cells/mm^3 (11).

The Immune Reconstitution Syndrome and MAC Infection

A symptomatic IRIS may occur after the initiation or reinitiation of ART. For this reason, it has been suggested that ART not be initiated until at least two weeks after mycobacterial therapy has begun. Nonsteroidal anti-inflammatory agents may be effective in treating IRIS in these patients. Corticosteroids can be reserved and used in short-course regimens (4–8 weeks) in more severe cases (28).

HERPES SIMPLEX VIRUS INFECTION

Therapy

Therapeutic strategies directed at mucocutaneous herpes simplex virus (HSV) infection are dictated by the severity and chronicity of symptoms. Treatment of individual recurrences with oral valacyclovir, famciclovir, or acyclovir for 5 to 10 days is generally sufficient (11). Long-term suppressive therapy with valacyclovir should be considered for patients with severe or frequent recurrences. Severe mucocutaneous or visceral infection should be treated initially with intravenous acyclovir.

Alternative Therapy

Unfortunately, resistance to acyclovir may emerge in patients treated for several months with acyclovir and may become manifest as recurrent or expanding lesions occurring on therapy. Foscarnet (40 mg/kg intravenously three times daily) is almost always effective in such cases, although foscarnet resistance has also been described. Topical therapy with cidofovir, trifluridine, or imiquimod has reportedly been successful in some cases (11).

The Immune Reconstitution Syndrome and HSV Infection

Persistent or worsening lesions despite appropriate therapy may be indicative of the immune reconstitution inflammatory syndrome (29) in patients successfully treated with antiretroviral therapy. The optimal approach to this phenomenon has not yet been determined.

CYTOMEGALOVIRUS INFECTION

Therapy

Retinitis

The therapy of CMV retinitis has improved significantly in recent years. Previously, after induction of therapy with either ganciclovir or foscarnet, intravenous therapy with one of these agents was continued indefinitely. The observation that oral systemic therapy with valganciclovir was nearly as effective in long-term maintenance as intravenous therapy led to improvements in the quality of life for many patients.

However, two major advances beginning in the mid-1990s have had a large impact on the incidence and management of this infection. The advent of highly active antiretroviral therapy (HAART) dramatically reduced the incidence of CMV retinitis (30). In addition, the development of topical antiviral therapy of CMV retinitis, both in the form of intraocular injection of ganciclovir, foscarnet, or cidofovir and as ganciclovir ocular implants permitted high local concentrations in the eye while minimizing systemic side effects of these agents. In addition, studies have demonstrated that anti-CMV therapy can be discontinued in selected patients who have a virologic and immunologic response to HAART (31).

Ganciclovir implants have the advantages of convenience. Although they need to be replaced every six to eight months, intravenous therapy may not be necessary, and this form of therapy results in the longest delay in disease progression. Systemic therapy, in addition to ocular implants, may prevent retinitis in the contralateral eye for patients with unilateral involvement and appears to be associated with improved overall survival (32).

COLITIS

Much less information is available on the management of CMV infections other than retinitis. Colitis and esophageal infection respond in the majority of patients to oral valganciclovir, intravenous ganciclovir, or foscarnet in the induction regimens used for retinitis. The need for continued maintenance therapy is not clearly established and may vary among patients.

The Immune Reconstitution Syndrome and CMV Infection

It is not clear that ART can induce a symptomatic IRIS. For patients with nonocular involvement, it is recommended that ART be instituted at the time of diagnosis (11). Because of the possibility of an immune reconstitution inflammatory reaction causing rapid deterioration in patients with neurologic involvement, it is recommended that ART be delayed in this condition until there is clinical improvement (11).

INTESTINAL PARASITES: CRYPTOSPORIDIOSIS, MICROSPORIDIOSIS, ISOSPORIASIS

Therapy

Infection with *Isospora belli* typically responds to therapy with TMP-SMX (33) and is effectively prevented by this medication when it is used to prevent PCP. In contrast, current therapeutic agents are not usually very effective in treating cryptosporidiosis. A variety of antiparasitic drugs have been shown to be ineffective (34). These include metronidazole, diiodohydroxyquin, tetracycline, chloroquine, primaquine, and quinacrine and an number of other agents. Nitazoxanide has recently been approved for treatment of cryptosporidiosis and appears superior to placebo in HIV-negative individuals. This agent (35), as well as paromomycin, may reduce symptoms' severity in patients with HIV infection. Since sustained infection with this organism occurs almost exclusively among individuals with CD4 cell counts below $100/mm^3$, the primary approach to therapy is with effective antiretroviral regimens.

Intestinal microsporidiosis typically responds to effective ART when the CD4 cell count rises and remains above 100 cells/mm^3.

The Immune Reconstitution Syndrome and Intestinal Parasites

Symptomatic immune reconstitution inflammatory disease appears not to occur with the intestinal protozoal infections described above (11).

MYCOBACTERIUM TUBERCULOSIS INFECTION

Therapy

The response to therapy for TB is comparable to that seen in non-HIV-infected individuals (11), although several factors associated with poor response to therapy have been identified (36). These include low CD4+ cell count, MDRTB, and no use of directly observed therapy (DOT). As the incidence of multidrug resistant TB has declined in recent years, the therapy of sensitive strains of *M. tuberculosis* has received increased attention, and novel approaches to therapy have been developed. Several important principles must be incorporated into the management of TB (36).

1. Culture confirmation and susceptibility testing should be obtained in all cases of suspected TB.

2. Proven or suspected cases of pulmonary or laryngeal TB should be placed in respiratory isolation until they are no longer infectious.
3. All proven cases should be reported promptly to public health authorities.
4. HIV testing should be offered and strongly encouraged in all cases of confirmed TB.
5. DOT should be employed whenever feasible.
6. Patients with sensitive organisms should be treated for 6 to 12 months.
7. If treatment failure is suspected, two new drugs should be added to the regimen pending repeat susceptibility studies.
8. Individuals with latent TB (positive tuberculin test with no evidence of active infection) should be treated (see chap. 8).

Typically, pending susceptibility results, a four-drug initial regimen (isoniazid with pyridoxine, rifampin, ethambutol, and pyrazinamide) should be initiated. Ethambutol may be discontinued if isoniazid sensitivity to the other agents is confirmed. If cavitary disease is present and sensitivity is confirmed, isoniazid and rifampin should be continued to complete nine months of therapy. Longer courses of therapy are considered advisable in cases of central nervous system or skeletal infection (37). Corticosteroids should be initiated as early as possible in the presence of central nervous system (38) or pericardial infection.

It is recommended that patients receiving anti-TB therapy be monitored clinically on a monthly basis (in addition to DOT) for evidence of response or progression of their infection as well as for drug toxicity. For patients with pulmonary TB, monthly, or more frequent, sputum specimens should be obtained until two consecutive specimens are negative on culture (37). If cultures remain positive after four months of therapy, treatment failure is likely, and alternate regimens are designed. Drug-induced liver toxicity should be considered likely if baseline transaminases increase three fold. In designing a substitute regimen in the face of elevation of transaminases, it should be borne in mind that although all first-line drugs may produce liver toxicity, rifampin is the least of these drugs to be implicated.

The management of TB may become complicated in the setting of possible drug resistance, nonresponse, or drug toxicity. It is beyond the scope of this discussion to address all potential approaches to these issues. If possible, professionals with specific training and experience in managing tuberculosis should be consulted in the care of all patients with TB but especially those with extrapulmonary disease, suspected or proven drug resistance, or drug toxicity necessitating novel treatment strategies.

In addition, DOT should be employed whenever noncompliance is likely, and household contacts of persons with active TB, especially children under age 5 and immunosuppressed individuals should be evaluated promptly.

Resource-Limited Settings

Coinfection with TB and HIV presents extremely difficult challenges in resource-limited settings throughout the world. Effective management may become nearly impossible if appropriate laboratory facilities for culture and sensitivity testing are not available (see chap. 8).

The Immune Reconstitution Syndrome and Tuberculosis

The optimal time to initiate ART in the setting of active TB is somewhat unclear, and studies are under way to address this issue. For patients with CD4 counts below 100 cells/mm^3, it may be prudent to begin ART quickly, perhaps after two weeks of initiation of TB therapy (39). ART might be best withheld in patients with higher CD4 counts to avoid confusion regarding drug side effects. A number of studies have suggested improved survival and slowing if HIV disease progression among patients beginning ART within 30 days of TB therapy (40). Confounding these strategies is the high proportion of patients with TB who experience immune reconstitution phenomena after beginning ART, particularly within the first one to three months (41), which, although usually self limited, may produce dramatic worsening of pulmonary and extrapulmonary lesions. Nonsteroidal or corticosteroidal treatment of such reactions may be indicated.

SYPHILIS

During the last half of the 1980s, the incidence of primary and secondary syphilis, as well as congenital infection, began increasing dramatically, particularly in areas with high seroprevalence of HIV infection (42). After a decline in cases, a resurgence has been seen in recent years, particularly among homosexual and bisexual men (43).

Although the clinical and laboratory features of syphilis in HIV-infected patients are usually similar to those in uninfected patients, in some cases, the presentation of syphilis appears to be altered by concomitant HIV infection. Progression of disease, despite standard therapy (44), and both false-positive, sometimes extremely high titer, and false-negative serologic test results have been reported (45).

Diagnosis

It is appropriate that serologic testing for syphilis be performed on all patients who acquired HIV infection through sexual contact or intravenous drug use. Darkfield examination or direct fluorescent antibody staining of exudate from lesions should be performed when there is clinical suspicion of syphilis despite negative results of serologic studies.

Therapy

Early syphilis (primary, secondary, and early latent) should be treated, as in non-HIV-infected patients, with benzathine penicillin (2.4 million units intra-muscularly). Serologic testing should be performed at intervals of one, two, and three months after treatment. If titers of the Venereal Disease Research Laboratory (VDRL) or rapid plasma reagin (RPR) tests do not decrease by two fold within three months in primary syphilis or six months in secondary syphilis a lumbar puncture should be performed to exclude neurosyphilis (45).

In cases of late latent syphilis or infection of unknown duration, the CSF should be examined before therapy to exclude neurosyphilis. If there is no evidence of neurosyphilis, benzathine penicillin should be administered (2.4 million units intramuscularly weekly for three weeks). Patients with neurosyphilis, either symptomatic or asymptomatic, should receive intravenous therapy (aqueous penicillin G, 2–4 million units every four hours for 10 days).

Tetracycline (500 mg orally four times daily for 14 days) or doxycycline (100 mg two times daily for 14 days) should be used in the therapy for primary, secondary, or latent syphilis of less than one year's duration in cases of penicillin allergy. Tetracycline or doxycycline should be continued for 28 days in patients with late latent or tertiary syphilis who are unable to receive penicillin.

HEPATITIS B VIRUS

Therapy

Indications for initiation of treatment for hepatitis B for HIV/Hepatitis B virus (HBV)-coinfected patients are in a state of evolution, and a thorough discussion of the complexities of treatment strategies is beyond the scope of this text. It is not certain, for example, that combination therapy is superior to monotherapy for HBV infection among individuals not coinfected with HIV. Indications for treatment of HIV-infected patients not receiving antiretroviral therapy (ART) are identical to those for the HIV-negative patient, that is, abnormal alanine aminotransferase (ALT) and HBV DNA levels greater than 20,000 International Units (International Unit)/mL for patients who are hepatitis B e antigen (HBeAg) positive and abnormal ALT with HBV DNA levels greater than 2000 International Unit for those who are HBeAg negative. Treatment of the HIV/HBV-coinfected patient is complicated by the increased rate of progression of HBV in the setting of HIV infection, which suggests that treatment of any level of detectable viremia, particularly in the setting of significant liver histopathologic changes may be indicated (11).

A number of agents have received approval for the treatment of HBV infection. Among these are lamivudine, tenofovir, adefovir, entecavir, telvivudine, and standard interferon-α as well as pegylated interferon (pegIFN)-α. Lamivudine, although well tolerated, is associated with high rates of HBV resistance, particularly in the setting of HIV coinfection (46). For this reason and because of rapid emergence of HIV to lamivudine monotherapy, HIV/HBV-coinfected patients should never be treated with lamivudine monotherapy. The related drug, emtricitabine, should also not be used in monotherapy of coinfected patients for similar reasons. Adefovir is effective in both HBeAg-positive and HBeAg-negative patients and is associated with a slower rate of the development of HBV resistant strains in comparison with lamivudine. It can be considered for use in the HIV/HBV-coinfected patients. pegIFN-α-2a is potentially appropriate for treatment of coinfected patients as it does not have implications for choices of current or future antiretroviral regimens.

However, emtricitabine, which is often used in combination with tenofovir in the fixed drug combination agent Truvada, which forms the backbone of ART for many patients, is also active against HBV. Because of the overlap of several agents in their activity against HIV and HBV, there are some particularly convenient options for treating the dual-infected patient. Perhaps the most convenient strategy is to employ an antiretroviral regimen with tenofovir/emtricitabine as the nucleotide/nucleoside backbone. In fact, existing guidelines recommend ART for any coinfected patient meeting indications for therapy of HBV infection.

For the patient not receiving ART, treatment for HBV infection not containing interferons should be continued for 6 to 12 months after HBeAg seroconversion (see chap. 8). Interferon-based regimens are continued for 48 weeks. For patients receiving ART with activity against HBV, as discussed above, treatment for both conditions is indefinite.

The Immune Reconstitution and Hepatitis B

A flare of hepatitis can occur with immune reconstitution in the patient receiving ART (47), representing the immune reconstitution inflammatory syndrome. Such events mimic acute viral hepatitis and can be severe and even fatal and can create diagnostic confusion. Such events may also occur if antiretroviral regimens are changed such that an agent active against HBV, such as lamivudine, is withdrawn. The most appropriate approach to worsening of liver function tests after initiation of or change in antiretroviral regimen is not always clear since such events may represent worsening of viral hepatitis due to immune reconstitution or viral resistance or drug side effects. It is essential that medications effective against HBV be continued if possible. Care should involve clinicians with expertise in the management of HBV infection.

HEPATITIS C

Therapy

The goal of hepatitis C virus (HCV) therapy is to fully suppress viremia, to halt progression of liver fibrosis, and, as a result, to reduce the risk of progression to cirrhosis and risk of hepatocellular carcinoma. Combination therapy with pegIFN and ribavirin (RBV) is recommended for HIV/HCV-coinfected patients who meet indications for therapy. Most studies of therapy have employed fixed-dose RBV (800 mg/day). Recent data suggest that weight-based dosing may be more effective (48).

Nonetheless, treatment regimens carry a substantial risk of serious side effects, and the optimal timing of therapy is unclear for many patients. Of the four genotypes of HCV (1–4), treatment is most effective for types 2 and 3. With current therapeutic regimens, the response rate (sustained virologic response) is reported to be 14% to 29%, while that for types 2 and 3 is 43% to 73% (49,50). The therapy of hepatitis C is in a state of transition. Although effective treatments have been developed (49), their applicability to individuals with HIV coinfection has been challenged by some. However, an expanding body of knowledge indicates that properly timed therapy for HCV infection can be beneficial in the presence of HIV infection and that reduction in hepatic disease achieved by control of hepatitis C may have significant benefits for coinfected patients.

At present, antiviral therapy is recommended for individuals with HCV infection who have a high risk of progression to cirrhosis, are able to tolerate therapy, and have a reasonable chance of a sustained virologic response. Patients should be considered for therapy if they meet the following criteria (11): HCV genotype 2 or 3; genotype 1 with HCV RNA level <800,000 IU/mL; significant fibrosis on liver biopsy (bridging fibrosis or cirrhosis); stable HIV not requiring ART; acute HCV infection; cryoglobulinemic vasculitis or mebranoproliferative glomerulonephritis; and motivation to undergo therapy. It should be noted that these criteria are not exclusive and that other patients, particularly those receiving ART who are otherwise appropriate candidates, should be considered for therapy.

Contraindications to interferon therapy reflect side effects of these agents and include active alcohol or other substance abuse, major depression, cytopenias, hyperthyroidism, renal transplantation, and evidence of autoimmune disease. RBV may cause hemolytic anemia, bone marrow suppression, and renal failure. Because it is teratogenic, female patients must be cautioned not to become pregnant during therapy. Other situations in which risks may outweigh benefits of treatment include advanced HIV infection with uncontrolled viremia, decompensated cirrhosis, severe depression, renal insufficiency, sarcoidosis, and active, uncontrolled autoimmune disease (11).

Because of these restrictions on the use of current therapy, the need for liver biopsy, and the slow rate of progression of HCV-related liver disease in most patients, treatment decisions are challenging. In selected coinfected patients, however, control of HCV may improve quality of life and simplify the treatment of HIV infection considerably. Monitoring of the patient with HCV infection not on therapy or who has failed therapy should consist of liver biopsy every three to five years or more frequently if histology suggests significant fibrosis or bridging and imaging of the liver, perhaps annually, for indication of early development of hepatocellular carcinoma.

The Immune Reconstitution Syndrome and Hepatitis C

Analogous to HBV infection (see above), HCV infection may accelerate after the institution of ART and significant immune reconstitution. Recognizing immune reconstitution and distinguishing it from drug side effects or progression of liver disease due to HCV itself may initially be difficult. The need to discontinue therapy is rare, but the appropriate approach to immune reconstitution is currently the subject of study.

LYMPHOMA

Therapy

Chemotherapy is typically used in the treatment of non-Hodgkin's lymphoma (NHL) outside of the central nervous system, because of the advanced stage of disease at presentation in most patients. In contrast, brain irradiation is the primary form of treatment of primary cerebral lymphoma. In the early years of the AIDS epidemic, chemotherapy for extraneural lymphoma was typically conservative, consisting of low-dose regimens to minimize side effects. This approach was considered appropriate, despite the high risk of relapse, because the ultimate survival of patients after the diagnosis of lymphoma was very limited and most often related to uncontrollable opportunistic infections. As the overall prognosis of HIV infection has improved with the advent of highly active ART and the concomitant reduction in life-threatening opportunistic infections, this approach has been reevaluated and strategies designed to confer more significant long-term benefits are currently under evaluation.

KAPOSI'S SARCOMA

Therapy

Traditionally, AIDS-related Kaposi's sarcoma has been treated with local radiation, cryotherapy, surgical excision, or intralesional chemotherapy for limited disease or systemic chemotherapy or interferon-α, for widespread disease, all with mixed results. Recent data and clinical experience suggest that ART alone may lead to regression of lesions in some cases.

DISEASES OF THE TROPICS AND SUBTROPICS

A number of diseases uncommon in temperate climates are impacted by coinfection with HIV. Among these are the following.

Malaria

Malaria appears to be more frequent and more severe in the presence of HIV infection, particularly among patients with low CD4 counts (51). Standard treatment regimens appear to be as effective as in non-HIV-infected individuals.

Leishmaniasis

The parasitic infection leishmaniasis appears to be more severe among patients with HIV coinfection particularly, as in the case of malaria, among individuals with advanced immune deficiency (52). First-line treatment of visceral disease is with amphotericin, and response rates appear to be comparable to those in non-HIV-infected hosts. Immune reconstitution with worsening of systemic symptoms of leishmaniasis has been reported in association with ART (53). Long-term suppressive therapy is recommended following initial therapy. It is unclear if this therapy (e.g., amphotericin every 2–4 weeks) can be safely discontinued even after a significant rise in the CD4 cell count.

Chagas Disease

The parasitic infection Chagas disease caused by *Trypanosoma cruzi*, common in South America, may reactivate in the presence of HIV infection. It is typically treated with benznidazole or nifurtimox in the acute or chronic phase. Little is known regarding long-term suppression of Chagas disease. ART is not contraindicated in coinfected individuals, and there is no known IRIS associated with Chagas disease (11).

REFERENCES

1. Hughes W, Leoung G, Kramer F, et al. Comparison of atovaquone (566C80) with trimethoprim-sulfamethoxazole to treat *Pneumocystis carinii* pneumonia in patients with AIDS. N Engl J Med 1993; 328:1521–1527.
2. Safrin S, Finkelstein DM, Feinberg J, et al. Comparison of three regimens for treatment of mild to moderate *Pneumocystis carinii* pneumonia in patients with AIDS: a double-blind, randomized, trial of oral trimethoprim-sulfamethoxazole, dapsone-trimethoprim and clindamycin-primaquine. Ann Intern Med 1996; 124:792–802.
3. Medina I, Mills J, Leoung G, et al. Oral therapy for *Pneumocystis carinii* pneumonia in the acquired immunodeficiency syndrome: a controlled trial of trimethoprim-sulfamethoxazole versus trimethoprim-dapsone. N Engl J Med 1990; 323:776–782.

4. Wharton JM, Coleman DL, Wofsy CB, et al. Trimethoprim-sulfamethoxazole or pentamidine for *Pneumocystis carinii* pneumonia in the acquired immunodeficiency syndrome: a prospective randomized trial. Ann Intern Med 1986; 105:37–44.

5. Smego RA, Nagar S, Maloba B, et al. A meta-analysis of salvage therapy for *Pneumocystis carinii* pneumonia. Arch Intern Med 2001; 161:1529–1533.

6. Murray JF, Mills J. State of the art: pulmonary complications of human immuno-deficiency virus infection. II. Am Rev Respir Dis 1990; 141:1582.

7. Sattler FR, Cowan R, Nielsen DM, et al. Trimethoprim-sulfamethoxazole compared wwith pentamidine for treatment of *Pneumocystis carinii* in the acquired immunodefi-ciency syndrome: a prospective, noncrossover study. Ann Intern 1988; 109:280–287.

8. Toma E, Thorne A, Singer J, et al. Clindamycin with primaquine therapy for mild and moderately severe *Pneumocystis carinii* pneumonia in patients with AIDS: a mjulticenter, double-blind, randomized trial. Clin Infect Dis 1998; 27:524–530.

9. Arozullah AM, Yarnold PR, Weinstein RA, et al. A new preadmission staging system for predicting inpatient mortality from HIV-associated *Pneumocystis carinii* pneumonia in the early highly active antiretroviral therapy (HAART) era. Am J Respir Crit Care Med 2000; 161(4 pt 1):1081–1086.

10. Briel M, Buchr HC, Boscacci R, et al. Adjunctive corticosteroids for *Pneumocystis jiroveci* pneumonia pneumonia in patients with HIV infection. Cochrane Database Syst Rev 2006; 3:CD006150.

11. Kaplan JE, Benson C, Holmes KK, et al. Guidelines for prevention and treatment of opportunistic infections in HIV-infected adults and adolescents. Recommendations from CDC, the National Institutes of Health, and the HIV Medicine Association of the Infectious Diseases Society of America. MMWR Recomm Rep 2009; 58:1–198.

12. Koval C, Gigliotti FN, Demeter LM. Immune reconstitution syndrome after suc-cessful treatment of *Pneumocystis carinii* pneumonia in a man with human immu-nodeficiency virus type 1 infection. Clin Infect Dis 2002;35:491–493.

13. Katlama C, De Wit S, O'Doherty E, et al. Pyrimethamine-clindamycin vs. pyr-imethamine-sulfadiazine as acute and long-term thrapy for toxoplasmic encephalitis in patients with AIDS. Clin Infect Dis 1996; 22:268–275.

14. Saba J, Morlat P, Raffi F, et al. Pyrimethamine plus azithromycin for treatment of acute toxoplasmic encephalitis in patients with AIDS. Eur J Microbiol Infect Dis 1993; 12:853–856.

15. Katlama C, Mouthon B, Gourdon D, et al. Atovaquone as long-term suppressive therapy for toxoplasmosis encephalitis in patients with AIDS and multiple drug intolerance. Atovaquone Expanded Access Group. AIDS 1996; 10:1107–1112.

16. Torres RA, Weinberg W, Stansell J, et al. Atovaquone for salvge treatment and suppression of toxoplasmic encephalitis in patients withAIDS, Atovaquone/Tox-oplasmic Encephalitis Study Group. Clin Infect Dis 1997; 24:422–429.

17. Saag MS, Graybill RJ, Larsen RA, et al. Practice guidelines for the management of cryptococcal disease. Clin Infect Dis 2000; 30:710–718.

18. Saag M, Powderly WG, Cloud GA, et al. Comparison of amphotericin B with fluconazole in the treatment of acute AIDS-associated cryptococcal meningitis. N Engl J Med 1992; 326:83–89.

19. Zuger A, Louie E, Holzman RS, et al. Cryptococcal disease in patients with the acquired immunodeficiency syndrome: diagnostic features and outcome of treat-ment. Ann Intern Med 1986; 104:234–240.

20. Saag MS, Cloud GA, Graybill R, et al. A comparison of intracoazole versus flu-conazole as maintenance therapy for AIDS-assoicated cryptococcal meningitis. Clin Infect Dis 1999; 28:291–296.

21. Shelburne SA, Darcourt J, White AC, et al. The role of immune reconstitution inflammatory syndrome in AIDS-related *Cryptococcus neoformans* disease in the era of highly active antiretroviral therapy. Clin Infect Dis 2005; 40:1049–1052.

22. Shelburne SA, Visnegarwala F, Darcourt J, et al. Incidence and risk factors for immune reconstitution inflammatory syndrome during highly active antiretroviral therapy. AIDS 2005; 19:399–406.

23. Clifford DB, Yiannnoutsos C, Glicksman M, et al. HAART improves prognosis in HIV-associated progressive multifocal leukoencephalopathy. Neurology 1999; 52:623–625.

24. Tantisiriwat W, et al. Progressive multifocal leukoencephalopathy in patients with AIS receiving highly active antiretroviral therapy. Clin Infect Dis 1999; 28(5):1152–1154.

25. DeLuca A, Giancola ML, Ammassari A, et al. The of potent antiretroviral therapy and JC virus load in cerebrospinal fluid on clinical outcome of patients with AIDS-associated progressive multifocal leukoencephalopathy. J Infect Dis 2000; 182:1077–1083.

26. Benson CA, Williams PL, Currier JS, et al. A prospective, randomized trial examining the efficacy and safety of clarithromycin in combination with ethambutol, rifabutin or both for the treatment of disseminated *Mycobacterium avium* complex disease in persons with acquired immunodeficiency syndrome. Clin Infect Dis 2003; 37:1234–1243.

27. Chaisson RE, Benson CA, Dube MP, et al. Clarithromycin therapy for bacteremic *Mycobacterium avium* complex disease: a randomized, double-blind, dose-ranging study in patients with AIDS. Ann Intern Med 1994; 121:905–911.

28. Phillips P, Bonner S, Gataric N, et al. Nontuberculous mycobactrial immune reconstitution syndrome in HIV-infected patients: spectrum of disease and long-term followup. Clin Infect Dis 2005; 41:1483–1497.

29. Fox PA, Barton SE, Francis N, et al. Chronic erosive herpes simplex virus infection of the penis: a possible immune reconstitution disease. HIV Med 1999; 1(1)10–18.

30. Kedhar SR, Jabs DA. Cytomegalovirus retinitis in the era of highly active antiretroviral therapy. Herpes 2007; 14:66–71.

31. Jabs DA, Bolton SG, Dunn JP, et al. Discontinuing anticytomegalovirus therapy in patients with immune reconstitution after combination antiretroviral therapy. Am J Ophthalmol 1998;126:817.

32. Kempen, JH, Jabs DA, Wilson LA, et al. Mortality risk for patients with *Cytomegalovirus* retinitis and acquired immune deficiency syndrome. Clin Infect Dis 2003; 37:1365–1373.

33. Pape JW, Verdier RI, Johnson WD Jr., et al. Treatment and prophylaxis of *Isospora belli* infection patients with AIDS. N Engl J Med 1989; 320:1044.

34. Abubakar I, Aliyu SH, Arumugam C, et al. Treatment of cryptosporidiosis in immunocompromised individuals: systematic review and meta-analysis. Br J Clin Pharmacol 2007; 63:387–393.

35. Rossignol JF, Hidalgo H, Feregrino M, et al. A double-blind placebo-controlled study of nitazoxanide in the treatment of cryptosporidial diarrhea in AIDS patients in Mexico. Trans R Soc Trop Med Hyg 1998; 92:663–666.

36. Alpert PL, Munsiff SS, Gourevitch MN, et al. A prospective study of tuberculosis and human immunodeficiency virus infection: clinical manifestations and factors associated with survival. Clin Infect Dis 1997; 24:661–668.
37. Centers for Disease Control and Prevention. Treatment of tuberculosis. Morbid Mortal Weekly Rep 2003; 52(No. RR-11).
38. Thwaites GE, Gnuyen DB, Nguyen HD, et al. Dexamethasone for the treatment of tuberculous meningitis in adolescents and adults. N Engl J Med 2004; 351:1741–1751.
39. Dean GL, Edwards SG, Ives NJ, et al. Treatment of tuberculosis in HIV-infected persons in the era of highly active antiretroviral therapy. AIDS 2002; 16:75–83.
40. Dheda K, Lampe FC, Johnson MA, et al. Outcome of HIV-associated tuberculosis in the era of highly active antiretroviral therapy. J Infect dis 2004; 190:1670–1676.
41. Shelburne SA, Hamill RJ, Rodriguez-Barradas MC, et al. Immune rreconstitution inflammatory syndrome: emergence of a unique syndrome during highly active antiretroviral therapy. Medicine 2002; 81:213–217.
42. Centers for Disease Control and Prevention, syphilis and congenital syphilis: United States. Morbid Mortal Weekly Rep 1988; 37:486.
43. Williams LA, Klausner JD, Whittington WL, et al. Elimination and reintroduction of primary and secondary syphilis. Am J Public Health 1999; 89:1093–1097.
44. Berry CD, Hooton TM, Collier AC, et al. Neurologic relapse after benzathine penicillin therapy for secondary syphilis in a patient with HIV infection. N Engl J Med 1987; 316:1587–1589.
45. Centers for Disease Control and Prevention. 1998 Guidelines for Treatment of Sexually Transmitted Diseases 1998; 47(RR-1).
46. Benhamou Y, Bochet M, Thibault V, et al. Lon-term incidence of hepatitis B virus resistance to lamivudine in human immunodeficiency virus-infected patients. Hepatology 1999; 30:1302–1306.
47. Lau GK. Does treatment with interferon-based therapy improve the natural history of chronic hepatitis B virus infection? J Hepatol 2007; 46:6–8.
48. Hadziyannis SJ, Sette HJ, Morgan TR, et al. Peginterferon-alpha2a and ribavirin combination therapy in chronic hepatitis C; a randomized study of treatment duration and ribavirin dose. Ann Intern Med 2004; 140:346–355.
49. Chung RT, Andersen J, Volberding P, et al. Peginterferon alfa-2a plus ribavirin versus interferon alfa-2a plus ribavirin for chronic hepatitis C in HIV-coinfected persons. N Engl J Med 2004; 351:451–459.
50. Laguno M, Murillas J, Blanco JL, et al. Peginterferon alfa-2b plus ribavirin compared with interferon alfa-2b plus ribavirin for treatment of HIV/HCV co-infected patients. AIDS 2004; 18:F27–F36.
51. Cohen C, Karstaedt A, Frean J, et al. Increased prevalence of severe malaria in HIV-infected adults in South Africa. Clin Infect Dis 2005; 41:1631–1637.
52. Lopez-Velez R, Perez-Molina JA, Guerror A. Clinicoepidemiologic characteristics, prognostic factors, and survival analysis of patients coinfected with human immunodeficiency virus and Leishmania in an area of Madrid, Spain. Am J Trop Med Hyg 1998; 58(4):436–443.
53. Berry A, Abraham B, Dereure J, et al. Two case reports of symptomatic visceral leishmaniasis in AID patients concomitant with immune reconstitution due to antiretroviral therapy. Scand J Infect Dis 2004; 36(3):225–227.

7

Approach to substance abuse and care of the active injection drug using patient

INTRODUCTION

Injection drug use (IDU) was recognized as one of the major routes of transmission of HIV infection in the earliest days of the HIV/AIDS epidemic. In the early years of the epidemic in the United States, as many as one-third of all HIV-infected patients had acquired infection by means of IDU through needle sharing. In recent years, the number of individuals infected through IDU has declined. This decrease has been attributed both to the advent of effective antiretroviral therapy (ART) and to needle exchange programs in many areas of the country (1,2). Despite this change in the demographics and epidemiology of HIV/AIDS, however, the death rate from AIDS among injection drug users has risen (3). IDU remains an important route of transmission in other regions of the world. Eastern Europe and Central Asia saw a rapid rise in spread by this means beginning in the 1990s. The epidemic in those regions is now transforming and broadening to involve the sexual partners of injection drug users (4).

Substance use affects the diagnosis and treatment of HIV infection in ways other than direct transmission. Aside from drugs that are injected (e.g., heroin and cocaine) and pose a risk of transmission of both HIV and hepatitis C through sharing of needles, other drugs of abuse may represent an obstacle to appropriate care. Benzodiapines, marijuana, so-called club drugs such as the synthetic amphetamine MDMA ("Ecstasy"), and, of course, alcohol may all interfere with adherence to treatment and maintenance in care and contribute to a disinhibition, leading to an enhanced risk of sexual transmission of HIV. This phenomenon has been demonstrated with crack (noninjection) cocaine users (5) and alcohol abusers (6). The prevalence of substance abuse in general has been reported to be as high as 20% to 40% in general primary care settings (7), and 44% of patients entering care at the Johns Hopkins HIV clinic were found to have substance abuse disorders (8).

OBSTACLES CREATED BY SUBSTANCE USE

Active IDU poses difficult challenges for the person infected with HIV. Drug dependence and associated with neuropsychiatric disorders can interfere with adherence to therapy (9) as well as behavior modification to reduce transmission of HIV infection. Attitudes of health care workers regarding substance abusers are often negative (10). Pessimism regarding the substances user's ability to reliably take ART has been shown to influence decisions regarding the timing of therapy by HIV specialists. A survey of nearly 1000 such providers indicated that alcohol or drug use was frequently considered contraindication to initiation of antiretroviral therapy (11). Although recent data suggest that ART can be effective despite ongoing problems with addiction (12), the perception that complete abstinence from drug use must precede even attempts at treatment persists (13,14). On the other hand, of course, the requirement for strict adherence to current antiretroviral agents to maintain suppression of viral replication is no less important among injection drug users than in others, and the often disordered lifestyles of injection drug users pose great difficulties in maintaining adherence to therapy. Nonetheless, survival among injection drug users treated with ART was found to be equivalent to that of non–injection drug users in one large Canadian study (12).

Screening for Substance Abuse

In view of the high prevalence of substance abuse, including alcoholism, among HIV-infected individuals, screening on entry into care and on a regular basis, perhaps annually, has been recommended (15). If active substance use is suspected, screening should be performed immediately. The strategies for screening include the use of any of a number of established screening questionnaires that have been published (15). Such questionnaires include nonjudgmental questions regarding current or past use of recreational or prescription drugs. The provider is encouraged to ask, if appropriate, family members or associates of the patient if substance abuse is suspected. The medical history is, of course, sometimes suggestive of drug or alcohol abuse in that frequent falls, injuries, or a history of seizures, pancreatitis, hepatitis, skin, and soft tissue infections, particularly at potential injection sites, may be highly suggestive. Of course, a history of substance abuse treatment or legal problems potentially related to alcohol or other drug use identifies the patient at high risk. The patient may be unwilling to discuss prior or current drug or alcohol abuse at the initial visit, and it is important that the provider persists at subsequent visits to gain an understanding of the patient's attitudes and practices regarding substance abuse.

Comorbid Psychiatric Disorders

Patients with substance abuse disorders frequently have other psychiatric disorders. These disorders appear to be more common among HIV-infected substance abusers (16). The most common of these is major depression, which was encountered in approximately one-third of such patients in one series (17). Other psychiatric disorders including anxiety, psychosis, and dementia may also complicate substance abuse. The presence of psychiatric disorders in HIV-infected substance users creates obstacles to adherence to ART (18). The colocation of drug treatment facilities and/or mental health services with HIV services represents both a convenience for the patient and an extremely valuable resource for providers for both screening for and treating substance abuse and accompanying psychiatric disorders. Systems of care, which persist in some countries, in which patients must first be "cleared" by a mental health professional before they can be considered for treatment of HIV infection, are not justified by available data indicating that antiretroviral treatment can proceed effectively despite ongoing substance use and mental health issues (12).

Comorbid Medical Disorders

IDU places the patient at risk for other infectious complications including cellulitis at injection sites, infective endocarditis, and viral hepatitis. The treatment of these conditions, especially hepatitis C in the setting of HIV infection, introduces further complexity in the management (see chap. 6) of HIV infection and its direct complications.

Relapse of the Former Substance User

Drug abuse lends itself to relapse, and maintaining abstinence from drugs, including alcohol, may be impossible for some individuals. This reality must be recognized by the primary care provider and should reinforce the need for frequent questioning about active drug or alcohol use. Ready access to drug treatment and to mental health professionals represents an important component of modern HIV care.

TREATMENT MODALITIES FOR SUBSTANCE ABUSE

Behavioral Therapy

A number of behavioral therapeutic strategies are available to assist in the management of substance abuse. The specifics of these strategies (e.g., the health belief model, social, cognitive, and transtheoretical models) are beyond the scope of this discussion. In the setting of a comprehensive HIV program, individual and group counseling, including the involvement of peers, may be beneficial for some patients. As noted previously, a multidisciplinary team approach involving mental health professionals, social workers, nursing and medical providers, and, potentially, peers in the care of the current or former substance abuser provides the best environment of care and the greatest chance of maintenance in care and adherence to therapy.

The Role of Opiate Replacement Therapy

Abstinence from IDU has been shown to improve adherence to ART and virologic response in the Swiss HIV Cohort Study of over 8500 individuals (19). Heroin use provides an opportunity, opiate replacement therapy, for a form of treatment, which has met with controversy. While opiate replacement therapy, either with methadone or with newer agents such as buprenorphine, has been shown to enhance life expectancy (20), reduce the use of injected opiates, be cost effective (21), and, recently, represent an important component of the adherence strategy for injection drug users receiving ART in a variety of settings (22), it has not yet been accepted in some regions of the world as an appropriate strategy to treat addiction. Methadone, an opiate agonist, is administered for opiate addiction within licensed programs, which require daily visits by the patient. Interactions between methadone and a number of drugs used in HIV care including nevirapine, efavirenz, ritonavir, and rifampin, all of which can speed its metabolism and precipitate opiate withdrawal, must be taken into account.

Buprenorphine, a partial opiate agonist, may be provided by certified practitioners to a limited number of patients outside of the relatively rigid setting of a methadone maintenance program. This approach, if feasible, may carry less stigma than methadone maintenance and provide a convenient alternative. Unfortunately, the number of individuals who would benefit from opiate replacement therapy far exceed the capacity for these interventions in the United States.

The Therapeutic Approach to Nonopiate Addiction

There is no equivalent to opiate replacement therapy for individuals using cocaine, benzodiazepines, barbiturates, or other drugs of abuse. Gradual detoxification, if undertaken, should be conducted under the supervision of a professional experienced in this strategy as dangerous and even lethal reactions may occur during detoxification from benzodiazepines or barbiturates in particular. Behavioral interventions may also represent effective treatment options, although some experts use antidepressant therapy for cocaine or amphetamine addiction, and gradual transition to selective serotonin reuptake inhibitors (SSRIs) may be appropriate for some patients abusing benzodiazepines. Alcoholism may be treated through so-called 12 step programs or other behavioral modalities. Acute withdrawal syndromes are managed according to medical protocols beyond the scope of this text.

Treatment of Coexisting Mental Disorders

As indicated above, depression and other major psychiatric disorders often coexist with substance abuse and must be treated concurrently. A comprehensive discussion of the management of these disorders is beyond the scope of this text.

ANTIRETROVIRAL THERAPY IN THE SETTING OF ACTIVE SUBSTANCE USE: LESSONS LEARNED

On the basis of published literature, much of which is cited above, several conclusions can be drawn regarding the effective use of ART for the current or past substance abuser.

1. Active substance abuse is not a contraindication to ART.
2. ART is approximately as effective in the active substance user as in other HIV-infected individuals.
3. Attitudes of health care professionals toward substance abusers are often negative and pessimistic and may lead to delays in treatment of HIV infection.
4. Substance abuse is common in both the general population and the HIV-infected population.
5. Significant psychiatric comorbidities, especially major depression, often accompany substance abuse and should be addressed concurrently with HIV infection and substance abuse itself.
6. Opiate replacement therapy with methadone or buprenorphine represents an important tool in overall HIV care for individuals addicted to opiates.
7. Depriving substance users of effective therapy for HIV not only places their own health in jeopardy but also fosters transmission of infection to others, including their sexual partners and offsprings.

REFERENCES

1. Muga R, Sanvisens A, Egea JM, et al. Trends in human immunodeficiency virus infection among drug users in a detoxification unit. Clin Infect Dis 2003; 37(suppl 5):S404.

2. Maslow CB, Friedman SR, Perlis TE, et al. Changes in HIV seroprevalence and related behaviors among male injection drug users who do and do not have sex with men: New York City, 1990-1999. Am J Public Health 2002; 92:385.

3. Centers for Disease Control and Prevention. HIV Surveillance Report: Estimated rates of diagnsoses of HIV infection among adults and adolescents, by sex and race/ ethnicity, 2008—37 states with confidential name-based HIV infection reporting, 2008.

4. UNAIDS, World Health Organization. AIDS epidemic update. Joint United Nations Programme on HIV/AIDS (UNAIDS) and World Health Organization (WHO), 2009.

5. De Souza CT, Diaz T, Sutmoller F, et al. The association of socioeconomic status and use of crack/cocaine with unprotected anal sex in a cohort of men who have sex with men in Rio de Janeiro, Brazil. J Acquir Immune Defic Syndr 2002; 29:95.

6. Stein MD, Hanna L, Natarajan R, et al. Alcohol use patterns predict high-risk HIV behaviors among active injection drug users. J Subst Abuse Treat 2000; 18:359.

7. Isaacson JH, Schorling JB. Screening for alcohol problems in primary care. Med Clin North Am 1999; 83:1547–1563.

8. Lyketsos CG, Hanson A, Fishman M, et al. Screening for psychiatric morbidity in a medical outpatient clinic for HIV infection: the need for a psychiatric presence. Int J Psychiatry Med 1994; 24:103.

9. Confranceso J, Scherzer R, Tien PC, et al. Illlicit drug use and HIV treatment outcomes in a U.S. cohort. AIDS 2008; 22:357.

10. McLaughlin D, Long A. An extended literature review of health professionals' perception of illicit drugs and their clients who use them. J Psychiatr Ment Health Nurs 1996; 3:283–288.

11. Bogart LM, Kelly JA, Catz SL, et al. Impact of medical and nonmedical factors on physician decision making for HIV/AIDS antiretroviral treatment. J Acquir Immune Defic Syndr 2000; 23:396–404.

12. Wood E, Hogg RS, Lima VD, et al. Highly active antiretroviral therapy and survival in HIV-infected injection drug users. JAMA 2008; 300(5):550–554.

13. Elovich R, Drucker E. On drug treatment and social control: Russian narcology's great leap backwards. Harm Reduct J 2008; 5:23.

14. Wolfe D. Paradoxes in antiretroviral treatmentofor injecting drug users: access, adherence and structural barriers in Asia and the former Soviet Union. In J Drug Policy 2007; 18(4):246–254.

15. New York State Department of Health AIDS Institute. Substance use in patients with HIV/AIDS: HIV clinical guidelines for the primary care practitioner. New York State Department of Health AIDS Institute, 2009.

16. Chander G, Himelboch S, Moore RD. Substance abuse and psychiatric disorders in HIV-positive patients: epidemiology and impact on antiretroviral therapy. Drugs 2006; 66:769–789.

17. Ahmad B, Mufti KA, Farooq S. Psychiatric comorbidity in substance abuse. J Pak Med Assoc 2001; 51:183.

18. Avants SK, Margolin A, Warburton LA, et al. Predictors of nonadherence to HIV-related medication regimens during methadone stablization. Am J Addict 2001; 10:69–78.

19. Weber R, Huber M, Rickenbach M, et al. Uptake of and virological response to antiretroviral thrapy among HIV-infected former and current injecting drug users

and persons in an opiat substitution treatment programme: the Swiss HIV Cohort Study. HIV Med 2009; 10(7):407–416.

20. Kimber J, Copeland L, Hickman M, et al. Survival and cessation in injecting drug users:propective observational study of oubcomes and effect of opiate substitution treatment. BMJ 2010; 341:c3172.

21. Connock M, Juarez-Garcia A, Jowett S, et al. Methadone and buprenorphine for the management of opioid dependence: a systematic review and economic evaluation. Health Technol Assess 2007; 1199:1–171.

22. Armstrong G, Kermode M, Sharma C, et al. Opioid substation therapy in Manipur and Nagaland, northeast India: operational research in action. Harm Reduct J 2010; 7:29.

8

Coinfection with tuberculosis or viral hepatitis

INTRODUCTION

Coinfection with *Mycobacterium tuberculosis* [tuberculosis (TB)] and with hepatitis B and C viruses presents unique challenges in the management of the HIV-infected individuals. Globally, TB accounts for approximately 13% of deaths of individuals with AIDS (1), and interactions between rifamycins used to treat TB and some antiretroviral agents may add complexity to the treatment of both the infections. The increasing prevalence of strains resistant to conventional therapy is particularly alarming and poses great challenges, particularly in resource-limited settings where access to resistance testing is often nonexistent.

Viral hepatitis, both B and C, poses unique challenges in diagnosis and therapy. The interactions of the diseases caused by these agents and the potential bidirectional impact on natural history of HIV infection complicate treatment strategies.

For these reasons, it was felt that these infections should receive special attention.

TUBERCULOSIS AND HIV INFECTION

Infection caused by *M. tuberculosis* continues to strike enormous numbers of individuals in the developing world and, as noted above, represents a leading cause of death worldwide. The HIV/AIDS epidemic has fueled the spread of TB and has coincided with an increased proportion of highly resistant strains of *M. tuberculosis*. This convergence of two deadly infections, both of which require prolonged therapy and an exceptionally high degree of adherence to therapy, has hampered the battle against each. Approximately one-third of the HIV-infected individuals worldwide are thought to be infected with TB either in its latent or active form, and TB is regarded as the commonest curable cause of death in the world (2). Although vaccination against TB has been available for decades, its relatively poor efficacy has caused it to have little impact on the spread of disease. Thus, two global epidemics, TB and HIV/AIDS, linked by poverty and requiring complex forms of therapy and reasonably sophisticated clinical and laboratory facilities for their management, have joined forces to pose enormous challenges to systems of care in major areas of the world.

Epidemiology

TB is readily transmitted by the respiratory route. In most individuals, the infection is contained, and the organisms cease to multiply within a few weeks. A dormant phase then occurs in which viable organisms remain without causing recognizable disease, the so-called latent phase. In the normal host, active TB eventually develops in approximately 10% of cases of latent disease, typically within the first two years. Among HIV-infected individuals, however, primary disease can develop shortly after infection in as many as one-third of cases (3). In contrast to other infections associated with HIV, active TB can occur at any CD4 cell count. In the United States, cases of TB are both among HIV-infected persons and in the general population (4). Globally, the total number of cases of TB is increasing because of the increase in the world's population, but the capita rate has declined in recent years (2).

Over the past two decades, the phenomenon of multidrug-resistant TB, defined as infection with organisms resistant to both isoniazid and rifampin (MDRTB), has emerged as a global crisis. In 2007, approximately 30,000, presumed to be an underestimate, cases of MDRTB were reported to the World Health Organization (2). Three countries, Russia, China, and India, are thought to account for 57% of the world's cases of MDRTB (2). Even more concerning, in the past decade, has been the emergence of extensively resistant TB (XDRTB) in which infection with organisms resistant to all first-line agents has been reported. The complexities of treating HIV/TB coinfection are daunting under the best of circumstances, but the emergence of resistant strains of *M. tuberculosis* has greatly complicated treatment strategies, and containment measures are urgently sought, particularly in high-prevalence regions with limited laboratory capacity.

Clinical Manifestations of Active Tuberculosis in the Setting of HIV Infection

Pulmonary Tuberculosis

Among HIV-infected individuals with relatively preserved cellular immunity (CD4 cell count 350 cells/mm^3 or greater), pulmonary TB usually presents much as it does in HIV-negative persons (5) with subacute respiratory and systemic symptoms such as cough, hemoptysis, weight loss, and fever. Chest X-ray findings typically demonstrate upper lobe or apical consolidation, often with cavity formation and adjacent localized pleural thickening. Hilar lymphadenopathy may be present.

In patients with a more advanced degree of immunosuppression, the presentation may be quite atypical. Lower lobe rather than apical involvement is common; cavity formation is less frequently seen, and in some cases, there may be minimal or no abnormalities seen on chest X ray. Clinical progression in this setting may be more acute and sometimes fulminant, mimicking severe bacterial pneumonia or other respiratory opportunistic infections such as *Pneumocystis* pneumonia.

Extrapulmonary Tuberculosis

Extrapulmonary TB, which may exist without apparent pulmonary disease, appears to be more common among patients with advanced immune deficiency (4). Pleural, pericardial, central nervous system, skeletal, lymphatic, or other sites of involvement may be encountered (6).

Diagnosis

Latent Tuberculosis

Testing for latent TB is usually conducted by means of the tuberculin skin test (TST). Induration of at least 5 mm at the site after 48 to 72 hours is considered positive in the setting of HIV infection. In recent years, interferon-γ releasing assays (IGRAs), which are blood tests designed to detected interferon-γ released from cells in response to peptides specific for *M. tuberculosis*. Because of their greater specificity, IGRAs have a lower rate of false positives and are particularly valuable in patients who have received BCG vaccination and may thus have a false positive TST. Unfortunately, IGRAs also lose sensitivity at advanced degrees of immune deficiency (7), and in addition, results between IGRA testing and TST may not agree. It is recommended that all HIV-infected individuals be tested for latent TB at the time of diagnosis of HIV (see chap. 12). Patients with fewer than 200 CD4 cells/mm^3 who test negative should be retested after the CD4 count rises above 200 cell/mm^3. Annual testing should be conducted for patients remaining at high risk for exposure to TB (4). These may include prisoners, active drug users, and those living in congregate settings or in regions where TB remains highly endemic (4). Individuals testing positive should undergo chest X ray to exclude active pulmonary disease and an assessment for possible extrapulmonary disease if symptoms of physical or laboratory signs are suggestive.

Active Tuberculosis

The diagnosis of active TB can present many challenges, particularly in resource-limited settings where only microscopic examination of clinical specimens for acid-fast bacilli (AFB) may be available and no technology exists for culture confirmation or sensitivity testing. Tests for latent TB, whether TST or IGRA, are not sensitive or specific enough to establish the diagnosis of active disease. Isolation of the organism in culture for accurate identification and sensitivity testing represents the gold standard of diagnosis. Pulmonary disease is best diagnosed by the collection, examination, and culture of adequate sputum samples. The yield of this technique is improved by obtaining three morning specimens on separate days, and results are most likely to be positive in the presence of cavitary disease. In resource-rich areas, laboratories may have the availability of liquid media systems, which may produce culture results within one to three weeks, and nucleic acid amplification technology, which may be performed on clinical specimens and greatly speed the identification of *M. tuberculosis* when compared with the traditional method of solid-phase culture techniques, which typically take as long as eight weeks to provide a definitive diagnosis. However, even this technology lacks sensitivity when performed on clinical specimens that are negative by AFB staining (8).

Immune Reconstitution

TB may become manifest or may accelerate during the period of immune reconstitution, which follows successful antiretroviral therapy. This phenomenon is discussed in chapter 5.

Treatment of the Coinfected Patient

Latent Tuberculosis

Treatment of latent TB in the setting of HIV infection should be undertaken in all patients without suspicion of active TB and who have not received prior therapy for latent or active disease. Isoniazid, either daily or twice weekly for nine months (9). Treatment should also be considered for individuals with a high likelihood of exposure to TB (e.g., household contacts) regardless of the results of testing for latent infection. Patients receiving isolniazid should receive supplemental treatment with pyridoxine to reduce the risk for drug-related neuropathy. For patients unable to tolerate isoniazid or those exposed to isoniazid-resistant TB, either daily rifampin or rifabutin is recommended for four months (4) (Fig. 8.1).

Active Tuberculosis

Active TB in the setting of HIV infection is generally treated in the same fashion in which it is treated in HIV-negative hosts. Possible exceptions, which may require longer courses of therapy, include central nervous system and skeletal

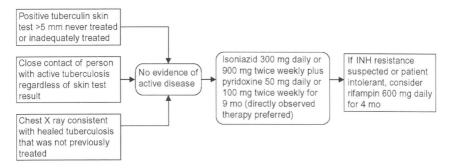

Figure 8.1 Treatment of latent tuberculosis in the setting of HIV infection.

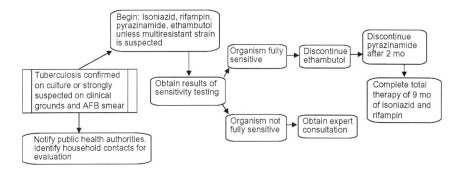

Figure 8.2 Treatment of active tuberculosis in adults with HIV infection. *Note*: See Appendix II for drug doses and side effects. Pyridoxine should be administered with isoniazid. Rifabutin 150 mg po daily should be substituted for rifampin for patients taking most protease inhibitors. Rifampin dose should be increased to 450 mg in patients taking efavirenz. *Source*: Adapted from Ref. 10.

involvement. Treatment of MDRTB and XDRTB must be individualized. Whenever possible, treatment should be administered under a system of directly observed therapy (DOT). See Figure 8.2.

Infection Control Considerations

Pulmonary TB is a highly contagious disease. For this reason, efforts must be made to isolate infected individuals during the period in which they have positive sputum AFB smears. In resource-limited settings where modern isolation techniques such as negative-pressure rooms and air-exchange and filtration systems are not available, maximum physical separation of infected from uninfected patients must be ensured.

VIRAL HEPATITIS AND HIV INFECTION

Hepatitis A, B, and C all have implications for the care of individuals infected with HIV. Hepatitis A, typically transmitted by the fecal-oral route, is particularly common among sexually active men who have sex with men (MSM). Although usually a self-limited infection not associated with chronic liver damage, hepatitis A virus (HAV) can produce fulminant disease in patients with chronic hepatitis B or C. Hepatitis B has become much less common in the United States and other countries that have implemented early childhood vaccination strategies but remains an enormous cause of morbidity and mortality in the developing would. Since routes of transmission of hepatitis B and HIV are identical, coinfection with these two viruses raises challenges throughout the developing world. Hepatitis C, transmitted most often through needle sharing by injection drug users (IDUs), progresses more rapidly in the presence of HIV infection and has become a prominent cause of morbidity and mortality in areas where effective anti-retroviral therapy has reduced the incidence of traditional AIDS-related opportunistic infections and resulted in enhanced survival. For these reasons, all HIV-infected individuals should be screened for hepatitis B and hepatitis C infection.

Hepatitis B

Epidemiology

The routes of transmission of hepatitis B virus (HBV) and HIV are identical. In addition to transmission by means of shared needles during injection drug use, it is spread by sexual contact and from mother to child far more efficiently than HIV. Despite the fact that the etiologic agent of hepatitis B was recognized long before HIV and that effective vaccination against hepatitis B is available, the global burden of this infection far exceeds that of HIV/AIDS. It is estimated that 400 million people are living with chronic hepatitis B infection worldwide (11). Further, approximately 40,000 individuals die of acute hepatitis B, and 500,000 die of cirrhosis or hepatocellular cancer resulting from this infection (11). In countries where childhood vaccination has been implemented effectively, such as the United States, the incidence of infection has fallen dramatically. Because, as is the case of hepatitis C, infection is chronic, many cases predate the vaccination era, and immigration from high-prevalence areas of the world has maintained hepatitis B as an important cause of morbidity and mortality in the United States where it is estimated that one million persons are chronically infected (a number roughly equivalent to that for HIV infection) and 2000 to 4000 deaths result annually. It is estimated that $1 billion is spent annually on hepatitis B–related hospitalizations alone (11).

Although the agent of hepatitis B was discovered long before the agent of hepatitis C and the natural history of infection is reasonably well understood, approaches to therapy are somewhat less well established than those for hepatitis C (see below). In particular, relatively little is known with certainty regarding the natural history and indications for therapy of hepatitis B in the setting of HIV infection. The reader is cautioned that what is outlined below has been established in non-HIV-infected individuals and that significant differences may exist in natural history, long-term consequences, and approaches to treatment in the setting of HIV coinfection and of combined infection HBV, hepatitis C virus (HCV), and HIV. It has been reported, however, that coinfection with HIV leads both to increased chronicity (12) and acceleration of the natural history of hepatitis B infection (13).

Natural History

The routes of transmission of HBV are listed above. Acute infection can be either symptomatic or asymptomatic, in contrast to acute hepatitis C infection, which is virtually always asymptomatic. Symptomatic infection has an incubation period of three to six months and is far more common in adults than in children infected in the perinatal period. After infection, hepatitis B surface antigen (HBsAg) is typically detectable within 4 to 12 weeks. Most adults, approximately 95%, recover spontaneously from acute infection and develop surface antibodies (anti-HBs) with clearance of antigen from the blood. In the minority who develop severe, progressive acute infection, coinfection with either hepatitis C or D virus is often present, and both represent risk factors for more severe infection with HBV. Chronic infection develops in less than 5% of adults but in almost all children infected in the perinatal period and almost half of those infected before the age of 5 (11).

Chronic Hepatitis B Infection

As is the case with HCV, chronic infection with HBV is typically insidious, featuring long asymptomatic periods. Serologic and virologic studies in this infection may be difficult to interpret and must often be repeated over time. It is recommended that HBV infection, as well as HCV and HIV infections, be managed by clinicians experienced in interpretation of diagnostic tests and knowledge about treatment indications and options. The three recognized phases of chronic HBV infection are as follows.

The immune tolerant phase. Although there is typically no evidence of active liver inflammation during this phase, viral replication within the liver continues. This phase is seen in almost all children infected in the perinatal period when it is characterized by particularly high levels of viral replication. The immune tolerant phase may last for many years during which the individual remains free of any indication of active liver disease and the liver is histologically normal. Most patients in this phase have detectable levels of hepatitis B e antigen (HBeAg), which generally correlates with high circulating levels of virus (11).

The immune active phase. As the immune response becomes stronger, most children and adults in the immune tolerant phase will progress to the immune active phase. Liver enzyme tests typically become abnormal, and histologic evidence of varying degrees of inflammation and/or fibrosis is present in the liver. HBeAg typically remains detectable in the blood. In a minority of patients, HBeAg is not detectable during any phase of infection, and these individuals follow a somewhat less predictable course.

The inactive carrier phase. Most individuals will eventually become inactive carriers. This phase is marked by the appearance of anti-HBeAg antibodies and the disappearance of HBeAg, with resolution of liver test abnormalities. Viral replication continues during this phase at lower levels, but the risk of progressive liver inflammation or fibrosis or of hepatocellular carcinoma (HCC) is much reduced. In individuals who develop anti-HBs and become HBsAg-negative, viral replication ceases or is reduced to extremely low levels, and they can be considered to have cleared the infection. Nonetheless, even these individuals continue to have active viral replication in the liver, and progressive infection can be reactivated in the presence of immune deficiency. Overall, those infected at birth or in early childhood are at much higher risk of progression of disease, even in the absence of HBeAg, than adults.

Prevention

The Approach to Hepatitis B Infection in the HIV-Infected Individual

As noted above, all HIV-infected individuals should be screened for both HBV and HCV infections. In the setting of acute hepatitis, testing for HBsAg and antibody to core antigen (anti-HBc) should be conducted. Screening for chronic infection should include these two studies as well. If either is positive, testing for HBV DNA should be performed. If evidence of chronic HBV infection is found, patients should be vaccinated against HAV if antibody tests indicate that they are susceptible since HAV infection can be far more severe in the presence of HBV or HCV infection. Patients without evidence of chronic HBV should receive HBV immunization.

Therapy

Substantial progress has been made in the therapy of hepatitis B in recent years. Although precise indications for therapy may be difficult to establish in the individual patient, the number of active agents is greater for HBV infection than for HCV infection. Treatment should be considered for patients chronically infected and with levels of HBV > 10,000 copies/mL for six months or active liver but compensated liver disease. See Table 8.1 for treatment protocols.

Table 8.1   Treatment Protocols for Hepatitis B and Hepatitis C Infections in the Presence of HIV Infection

Hepatitis B
>   Acute: No therapy recommended.
>   Chronic:
>   Antiretroviral therapy with regimens including tenofovir and either lamivudine or emtracitabine (see chap. 5). See Appendix II for other agents active against HBV if patient is unable to take tenofovir.
>   Alternative: Pegylated interferon-α-2a (see Appendix II) for 16-24 wk if HBeAg positive or 12 months or longer if HBeAg negative.

Hepatitis C
>   Acute: Treatment may be beneficial.
>   Chronic: (14)
>   Drugs:
>   Ribavirin 400 mg orally am 600 mg pm if patient is <75 kg
>   Ribavirin 600 mg orally twice daily if patient is >75 kg
>   Plus
>   Interferon-α-2a 180 μg subcutaneously weekly
>   Or
>   Interferon-α-2b 1.5 μg/kg weekly

Duration: 48 wk, but therapy should be discontinued if there is not a 1 log decrease in viral load at 4 wk and 2 log decrease at 12 wk. Retreatment should be considered for patients with recurrent viremia after completion of therapy.

HEPATITIS C

In the United States, infection with HCV occurs in approximately 30% of HIV-infected individuals (15) as is presumed to be present in as many as 90% of those whose HIV transmission factor is injection drug use. HCV prevalence rates are particularly high in African Americans and Hispanic Americans. With the reduction of deaths from traditional AIDS-associated opportunistic infections in developed countries, liver disease caused by HCV infection has become increasingly common as a cause of morbidity and mortality among those living with HIV (16).

Epidemiology

Natural History

HCV is most often transmitted through sharing of needles among IDUs. Sexual transmission also occurs but is much less efficient than transmission through needle sharing and occurs at much lower rates than those of most other sexually transmitted infections.

The natural history of hepatitis C is variable and is influenced by host and viral factors. The acute phase is usually asymptomatic, and the host response is sufficient to clear the virus from the body in a substantial proportion of immunologically normal individuals. In those who do not clear the virus and develop chronic infection, damage to the liver in the form of progressive fibrosis frequently never achieves clinical significance, and in the majority of cases, patients remain asymptomatic. In some, however, infection eventually leads to cirrhosis. These patients are at risk for the development of HCC. Progression to such clinically significant stages typically occurs over a period of 20 to 30 years in the non-HIV-infected host, and histologic damage may progress in the absence of abnormalities of liver chemistries. Between 10% and 15% of patients progress to cirrhosis within 20 years of acute infection (17). HCC occurs in 1% to 5% of patients after 20 years and 1% to 4% annually after the onset of cirrhosis. Male gender, age over 40, and alcohol use all represent added risk factors for progression of chronic HCV infection. Six genotypes of the virus have been identified. Approximately 70% of infections in the United States are caused by genotypes 1 and 4. The implications of these genotypic patterns for therapy are discussed below.

The impact of HIV infection on HCV infection has received increasing attention in recent years. HIV has several negative effects on HCV infection. Clearance of HCV is seen less often following acute infection in patients coinfected with HIV, and progression of hepatic fibrosis occurs somewhat more rapidly.

ACUTE HEPATITIS C

As noted, HCV typically causes a chronic, insidious infection, which can lead to cirrhosis and HCC. HCV infection is rarely diagnosed in its acute phase because, unlike hepatitis A and, to a lesser extent, hepatitis B, it seldom produces the typical signs and symptoms of acute viral hepatitis. In non-HIV-infected individuals, a portion, perhaps 25% to 35%, develop liver function abnormalities and/

or constitutional symptoms with acute infection. Following the acute phase, 15% to 45% of non-HIV-infected individuals clear HCV and are not at risk for progressive liver disease (18). In contrast, HCV is cleared in only approximately 11% of the time in the presence of HIV infection (18). The absence or subtlety of these findings may lead to a delay in diagnosis. Traditionally, and particularly since the advent of routine screening of donated blood for hepatitis C and the virtual elimination of transfusion-associated infection by this agent, the dominant means of transmission has been the sharing of needles among IDUs. In the context of the HIV/AIDS epidemic, it has been observed that HCV, which is more easily transmissible than HIV, is most often acquired before HIV among IDUs. Although progression of HCV is accelerated by coinfection with HIV, HCV infection and the liver damage it causes remain relatively slowly progressive in the setting of HIV infection. A distinct entity of acute, more rapidly progressive, acute HCV infection has been observed in MSM to whom HCV has been transmitted, likely through sexual activity, after the acquisition of HIV infection has recently been described (19). In these patients, presumably because immunosuppression caused by HIV infection is already present at the time of acquisition of HCV infection, histologic progression of liver disease appears to occur more rapidly. This observation may have implications for screening strategies for HCV infection in HIV-infected individuals. These efforts have traditionally focused on IDUs but may now have to be extended to sexually active MSMs.

CHRONIC HEPATITIS C

Diagnosis

The diagnosis of HCV infection is typically made by the detection of serum antibody. Activity of infection is determined by measuring serum HCV RNA level and liver function abnormalities. Liver biopsy and histologic staging establish the degree of liver damage and can be used to gauge progression of disease and timing of therapy.

Acute Hepatitis C

There are no exact diagnostic criteria for the diagnosis of acute HCV infection. Since antibody tests remain positive when infection has been cleared and measurements of viral load as well as liver function abnormalities may fluctuate widely during the course of infection, determining the timing of infection may be impossible. It has, therefore, been suggested that the diagnosis of acute infection be based on a combination of findings including documented seroconversion, significant elevation of alanine aminotransferase (ALT), and substantial fluctuations of serum HCV RNA, which are seen more commonly in acute than in chronic infection (19).

Chronic Hepatitis C

Patients testing positive for anti-HCV antibody should undergo qualitative or quantitative testing for serum HCV RNA to confirm infection and establish activity.

SCREENING STRATEGIES

Diagnosis

Although individuals infected with HIV through injection drug use have long been recognized as a group at high risk of HCV infection, screening for HCV only in this population may not be sufficient. Because of the possibility of HCV transmission through heterosexual or homosexual activity as noted above and because the implications of HCV infection are even more serious in those coinfected with HIV than in the general population, routine, baseline screening of all HIV-infected individuals for HCV infection should be conducted. Typically, this screening is performed using an ELISA antibody test. This form of testing, though highly sensitive, is not completely specific, and a positive antibody test should be confirmed with quantitative viral load testing. Some experts recommend viral load testing for HCV even in the absence of a positive antibody tests among patients with unexplained liver disease. This phenomenon may be especially likely among HIV-infected patients with advanced immune deficiency or in individuals with evidence of liver disease who may be experiencing a delayed response in measurable antibody. Periodic screening (perhaps annually) should be conducted in patients at ongoing risk of acquisition of HCV.

Although a positive quantitative (e.g., RNA PCR) test confirms infection with HCV, a negative test in the presence of antibody does not fully exclude infection since the plasma viral load may be intermittently undetectable in chronically infected individuals. For this reason, repeated quantitative testing may be necessary in some individuals who are at high risk or manifest ongoing evidence of liver disease that is otherwise unexplained. The fact that further complicates testing is that the level of detectable viremia does not correlate with the degree or activity of liver disease.

The overall value of specific screening strategies is underscored by the fact that only approximately two-thirds of HCV-infected individuals manifest laboratory evidence of liver inflammation (elevated serum ALT).

Therapy

The therapy of hepatitis C has been to focus of a great deal of research in the past decade. Unfortunately, substantial barriers to safe, convenient, and uniformly effective treatment strategies remain. The specific approach to treatment of the individual must take into account the viral genotype, the likelihood of treatment-related side effects, the willingness of the patient to fully comply with therapy and rigorous follow-up, and, at least in some instances, the histologic patterns seen on liver biopsy. The gender and racial background of the patient as well as the age at initial infection with HCV and duration of infection all appear to influence the likelihood of a sustained response. The mainstays of treatment, pegylated interferon and ribavirin, may not be tolerable to some individuals because of underlying anemia, heart disease, depression, or advanced liver disease. In these individuals, the risks of treatment may often outweigh the benefits to the point that treatment with current agents should not be considered. Despite these complexities, treatment of HCV in the setting HIV can be effective in preventing progression of disease and, presumably, the potential long-term complications of cirrhosis and HCC.

Genotypes 1 (most common in the United States) and 4 of HCV typically do not respond as well to current treatment as genotypes 2 and 3. For this reason, many experts recommend treatment of all otherwise eligible patients who are infected with genotypes 2 and 3 without a need to determine the histologic stage of disease by liver biopsy, reserving this procedure for those with genotypes 1 and 4.

The Role of Liver Biopsy

Liver biopsies are performed in patients with chronic HCV infection to determine the extent of inflammation and fibrosis and, by this means, to establish the likelihood of progression to cirrhosis and the overall prognosis. A variety of scoring systems are used to quantify the histologic abnormalities and are used to guide treatment decisions. Serial biopsies (every 2–5 years) may be necessary to establish the rapidity of progression and to aid in decisions regarding the timing of initiation of therapy. Biopsies, though invasive and not without risk, may be especially important in establishing indications for treatment in individuals infected with genotypes 1 or 4. Since these patients are less likely to respond to treatment than those infected with other genotypes, histologic assessment of severity and likelihood of short-term progression may be especially helpful in guiding treatment decisions. A discussion of significance of specific findings on liver biopsy is beyond the scope of this overview, and all treatment decisions regarding HCV should be made in consultation with clinicians experienced in the management of this infection.

TREATMENT STRATEGIES

Assessing for initiation of treatment

1. Does the patient meet medical indications for treatment without liver biopsy?
2. Does the patient require a liver biopsy?
3. What form of treatment is appropriate (drugs and duration)?
4. How should the patient be monitored for virologic suppression?
5. How should the patient be monitored for side effects?
6. How should the successfully treated patient be monitored post treatment?
7. When should retreatment be considered?
8. What form of ongoing monitoring is needed for the untreated patient?

See chapter 6 for treatment protocols.

REFERENCES

1. World Health Organization. Global tuberculosis control—surveillance, planning, financing. Geneva, Switzerland: WHO Report, 2007.
2. World Health Organization. Global tuberculosis control—epidemiology, strategy, financing. Geneva, Switzerland, WHO Report, 2009.

3. Centers for Disease Control. Treatment of tuberculosis. Morbid Mortal Weekly Rep 2003; 52(No RR-11):1–77.

4. Kaplan JE, Benson C, Holmes K, et al. Guidelines for prevention and treatment of opportunistic infections in HIV-infected adults and adolescents. Recommendations from CDC, the National Institutes of Health, and the HIV Medicine Association of the Infectious Diseases Society of America. Morbid Mortal Weekly Rep 2009; 58(RR04):1–198.

5. Perlman DC, El-Sadr WM, Nelson ET, et al. Variation of chest radiographic patterns in pulmonary tuberculosis by degree of human immunodeficiency virus-related immunosuppression. Clin Infect Dis 1997; 25:242–246.

6. Shafer RW, Kim DS, Weiss JP, et al. Extrapulmonary tuberculosis in patients with human immunodeficiency virus infection. Medicine 1991; 70:384–397.

7. Mazurek GH, Jereb J, Lobue P, et al. Guidelines for using the QuantiFERON-TB gold test for detecting *Mycobacterium tuberculosis* infection, United States. Morbid Mortal Weekly Rep 2005; 54(RR-15):49–55.

8. Nahid P, Pai M, Hopewell PC. Advances in the diagnosis and treatment of tuberculosis. Proc Am Thorac Soc 2006; 3:103–110.

9. Centers for Disease Control and Prevention. Tarteted tuberculin testing and treatment of latent tuberculosis infection. Morbid Mortal Weekly Rep 2000; 49(No. RR-6):1–54.

10. Horsburgh CR, Feldman S, Ridzon R. Practice guidelines for the treatment of tuberculosis. Clin Infect Dis 2000; 31(3):633–639.

11. Sorrell MF, Belongia EA, Costa J, et al. National Institutes of Health consensus development conference statement: management of hepatitis B. Ann Intern Med 2009; 150:104–110.

12. Hadler SC, Judson FN, O'Malley PM, et al. Outcome of hepatitis B virus infecton in homosexual men and its relation to prior human immunodeficiency virus infection. J Infect Dis 1991; 163:454–459.

13. Thio CL, Seaberg EC, Dkolasky R Jr., et al. HIV-1, hepatitis B virus and risk of liver-related mortality in the Multicenter Cohort Study (MACS). Lancet 2002; 360:1921–1926.

14. Hadziyannis SG, Sette H, Morgan TR, et al. Peginterferon-α-2a and ribavirin combination therapy in chronic hepatitis C. A randomized study of treatment duration and ribavirin dose. Ann Intern Med 2004; 140:346–355.

15. Vallet-Pichard A, Pol S. Natural history and predictors of severity of chronic hepatitis C virus (HCV) and human immunodeficiency virus (HIV) co-infection. J Hepatol 2006; 44(1 suppl):S28–S34.

16. Martin-Carbonero L, Sanchez, Somolinos M, Garcia-Samaniego J, et al. Reduction in liver-related hospital admission and deaths in HIV-infected patients since the year 2002. J Viral Hepat 2006; 13:851–857 (abstr).

17. National Institutes of Health. NIH Consensus Statement on Management of Hepatitis C:2002. NIH Consens State Sci Statements 2002; 19:1–46.

18. Piasecki BA, Lewis JD, Reddy KR. Influence of alcohol use, race, an dviral coinfections on spontaneous HCV clearance in a US veteran population. Hepatology 2004; 40:892–899 (abstr).

19. Fierer DS, Uriel AJ, Carriero DC, et al. Liver fibrosis during and outbreak of acute hepatitis C virus infection in HIV-infected men: a prospective cohort study. J Infect Dis 2008; 198:683–686.

9

Issues of aging among HIV-infected individuals

INTRODUCTION

Since its beginning, the HIV/AIDS epidemic has had its most devastating impact on the young. In recent years, and for several reasons, an increasing number of persons living with HIV/AIDS (PLWHA), whether newly diagnosed or not, have been over the age of 50, particularly in developed countries. In the United States, the proportion of PLWHA over the age of 50 increased from 17% to 24% between 2001 and 2005, a year in which 15% of new diagnoses of HIV/AIDS were among those over 50 (1). Improvements in antiretroviral therapy (ART) have brought dramatic improvements in life expectancy such that many patients diagnosed at earlier ages are now living well past 50. With the incorporation of HIV testing up to the age of 64 into routine medical care, as has been recommended by the U.S. Centers for Disease Control and Prevention (CDC) (see chap. 1), the number of infected older individuals identified may increase further.

The life expectancy of effectively treated HIV-infected patients has not yet reached that of comparable uninfected populations (2,3), however. A number of factors may be contributing to this, including delay in diagnosis of HIV infection, effects of HIV or the immune deficiency on the incidence and progression of other chronic diseases, and, perhaps, the effects of long-term ART itself. The concept of premature aging of individuals with HIV infection has been suggested, although the evidence for this hypothesis has been challenged (4).

Although the potential ramifications of the aging of the HIV/AIDS population are easy to see, little research is available to guide our approach to the treatment of the older patient. Some of the issues that may impact on the care of these patients are as follows:

Because of the age distribution of PLWHA, individuals over the age of 50 are typically underrepresented and sometimes intentionally excluded from trials of antiretroviral agents.

As a result, the expected virologic and immunologic response to therapy has
been derived from studies of younger individuals.

Complications of ART or the inflammatory state associated with HIV
infection (5) or its treatment (6,7), particularly cardiovascular and
metabolic changes, may be accelerated in the presence of established
conditions such as hypertension, diabetes mellitus, osteoporosis, and
coronary artery disease—all more common in the elderly.

In general, the social networks of individuals who are middle aged and older
have been shown to differ in significant ways from those of younger
adults (8–10), potentially creating novel obstacles to treatment adherence
and maintenance in care.

Medical disorders that are not clearly associated with HIV infection but
increase in prevalence with increasing age may complicate the overall
management strategy and come to dominate decisions regarding care.
This may be particularly evident in patients suffering from the commonest
malignancies accompanying aging.

Of course, individuals with HIV infection represent a diverse cross-section of the
population. In large categories, that is, men who have sex with men (MSM),
women who have acquired HIV infection through heterosexual contact, and
current or former injection drug users (IDU), may confront very different personal and medical issues as they age. For this reason, general guidelines to care
cannot simply be age based but must take into account life circumstances and
demographics as they do in younger adults. Nonetheless, some general observations may be helpful in tailoring systems of care to the HIV-infected older
adult.

For the purposes of this discussion, the term elderly is applied to individuals over the age of 50 because of the increase in chronic medical disorders,
which typically begins after that age, and because of the life situations
(employment, family structure, social network, etc.) that are often in transition
during that period of life.

Conditions directly associated with HIV infection (specific cancers and
metabolic disorders) are discussed elsewhere in this text. The emphasis in this
chapter is on the overall impact of aging as well as standard recommendations
for screening for common disorders not clearly caused by HIV infection directly.

THE AGING OF THE HIV/AIDS POPULATION: DEMOGRAPHICS

Between 2001 and 2007, the proportion of PLWHA over 50 rose from 19% to
25% in the United States (11). The major reason for this shift has been the aging
of previously diagnosed individuals and the prolonged life expectancy accompanying modern ART. Impressively, the cumulative number of AIDS cases
among individuals over the age of 50 had already increased fourfold between
1990 and 2001 (12). In one analysis from New York City, it was found that 64%

of PLWHA were over the age of 40 and 25% were over 50 (13). Among those over 50, 89% of individuals were non-Caucasian and 34% were women and fewer than 50% had disclosed their HIV status to friends.

General Factors

In general, older individuals are more likely to live alone and be unmarried (14). An absence of family and friends due to age and stigma as well as reluctance to disclose HIV status may also contribute to social isolation (15). Perhaps not surprisingly, one survey has indicated that older adults with HIV infection suffer more comorbid medical conditions as well as great incidence of depression (16).

Gender

The gender distribution of PLWHA over the age of 50 differs from that of younger age groups. In a recent analysis, women accounted for 22.2% of patients over the age of 60 and 12.6% of those between the ages of 30 and 49 (14). This may, in part, reflect the fact that women with HIV infection are diagnosed at an older age than men. Older women undergo HIV testing at lower rates than younger women: 16% versus 33% in one series (14).

RACIAL/ETHNIC PATTERNS

Recent U.S. data indicates that HIV infection rates are nine times higher in black women than in white women (17). Data such as these underscore the fact that African Americans as well as Hispanics are overrepresented among PLWHA in the United States. This demographic pattern must be taken into account in evaluating differences in incidence of chronic disease between populations of HIV-positive and HIV-negative individuals (4).

TRANSMISSION FACTORS AND AGE

Men Who Have Sex with Men

The dramatic advances in therapy witnessed in the past decade have resulted in MSM on treatment frequently living normal lives well past the age of 50. In the United States, incidence rates of 1% to 2% have been reported in this group, primarily reflecting the aging of individuals who acquired infection prior to the age of 50 (18). The overall prevalence of infection in this group has been reported to be 19% and 29% among older black men in the United States. The prevalence of infection among these men has remained constant in recent years (19), in large part because the high mortality, reported to be 69% (18), has offset the maturing of individuals into this age group.

Minorities

Racial disparities are dramatic among older HIV-infected individuals in the United States. In general, older MSM are more likely to be white, have health insurance, and be employed than younger MSM (20). While only 40% of older white persons with HIV infection were employed in one analysis compared with over 70% of the general white population, only 15% of the older minority group with HIV infection compared with 64% of the overall older minority population were employed (21). From these data, a picture emerges of a degree of financial inequality between white and minority individuals that would be expected to impact on access to care and overall survival.

Women

Recent data indicate that in the United States, 10% of women with HIV infection are diagnosed after the age of 50 and that this proportion had risen from 9% to 15% between 1988 and 2000 (22). In addition, one-quarter of all women in the United States infected with HIV were diagnosed after the age of 45. This undoubtedly reflects, in part, that women are more likely to be unaware of their risk of exposure to HIV due to heterosexual contact. Other data has pointed to a lower rate of HIV testing among older women, perhaps reflecting this unawareness in many cases. Sexual activity remains common in older women, but condom use is less common than in younger women, and older women have less access to HIV prevention education (22).

GENERAL HEALTH MAINTENANCE

Care of elderly patients, whether HIV infected or not, places increased focus on screening for chronic disorders such as cardiovascular disease and for cancer. Chronic disease management also plays an increasingly significant role for most individuals as they age. The impact of HIV infection on the natural history of chronic diseases such as diabetes, hyperlipidemia, and hypertension is complex and not thoroughly understood. The potential relationship between HIV infection and cancers not highly associated with HIV has been studied for a variety of common malignancies, with somewhat contradictory conclusions. Of course, effective treatment and control of HIV infection and its known complications remain central in general health maintenance for infected individuals.

QUALITY OF LIFE

As noted during the first two decades of the HIV/AIDS epidemic, the individuals most affected have been young, previously healthy adults. Conditions more associated with an older population, such as cancer and coronary artery disease, could be largely ignored by physicians caring for these individuals in favor of the more immediate complications of HIV infection and immune deficiency. As the prognosis of HIV infection improves with effective ART, other chronic disorders will become increasingly important among HIV-infected patients. Coincident with the epidemic, however, significant advances have come in the prevention and management of these other conditions, which, in some instances, may become more immediately important to the middle-aged or older adults with HIV infection.

An additional consideration is the increasing susceptibility to infection that accompanies the normal aging process (23). As the HIV/AIDS population ages, the impact of HIV infection on this so-called immunosenescence will become increasingly important.

In this chapter, strategies for routine health maintenance developed for the general population are examined, and their application to the care of HIV-infected individuals is considered. Beyond this, the impact of lifestyle changes, which come into play with advancing age, will also be addressed as they affect different subsets of the HIV/AIDS population.

The purpose of including this material in a book on the care of the HIV-infected patient is twofold. It is hoped that this inclusion will serve as an acknowledgement of the importance of routine health maintenance for these patients. In addition, since many practitioners caring for the HIV-infected do not practice general internal medicine, this overview can serve as a quick reference to current preventive strategies.

Little data exist to direct the clinician in the general approach to health maintenance in the setting of HIV infection, but several conclusions can be drawn from recent findings. Furthermore, the possibility that HIV infection itself or ART alters the natural history of cancer, atherosclerosis, dementia, or other high prevalence conditions will be discussed. In addition to screening for occult disease, the primary provider should provide routine preventive counseling regarding smoking cessation, diet, and injury avoidance.

Since medical practitioners caring for HIV-infected patients often assume responsibility for general primary care, a brief discussion of screening and counseling strategies applicable to the general population is also provided. It should be borne in mind that general health maintenance services are not accessed by all those in the general population for whom they are recommended (24) for a variety of reasons. In a recent analysis of services in the United States, it was found that low educational level, lack of health insurance, and the cost of care all represented significant barriers (24). Inadequate access to care is most dramatic among minority populations, especially blacks and Hispanics, the same groups disproportionately affected by the HIV/AIDS epidemic. As preventive services and strategies become increasingly detailed and sophisticated, the challenges confronting the primary care provider increase. It is essential that providers continue to remain informed regarding changes in recommended strategies as those mentioned in this book may change or expand in the coming years.

SCREENING STRATEGIES

Hypertension

It is recommended that blood pressure be measured in all individuals beginning at the age of 21 (25). Although the optimal screening interval has not been determined, a variety of experts have recommended every two years if the most recent blood pressure was 140/85 or less and annually if the last diastolic blood pressure was 90 mmHg or more. Blood pressure measurement is also recommended during routine visits for children and adolescents.

Although no direct association between hypertension and HIV infection has been defined, the incidence of both is disproportionately high among African American men and women. For this reason, hypertension may be encountered more often by providers serving large groups of HIV-infected patients. The evaluation and management of hypertension in the setting of HIV infection should probably parallel that seen in other patients. Although no serious interactions have been reported to occur between antiretroviral drugs and common antihypertensive agents, although the blood level of calcium channel–blocking agents may be elevated by protease inhibitors, prescribing information should be consulted for combining specific agents.

The risk of cardiovascular disease among hypertensive patients who develop hyperlipidemia secondary to ART has not been adequately defined.

CANCER

While it has long been recognized that lymphoma (including Hodgkin's disease), Kaposi's sarcoma, cervical neoplasia, and anorectal cancer are seen with increased frequency among HIV-infected individuals, some studies have suggested that a broader predilection to variety of solid tumors may also exist in these patients (26,27). The emphasis in this chapter is on screening for types of cancer and other chronic conditions not known to be directly related to HIV infection but primarily to aging and other risk factors. Screening for and evaluation of malignancies known to occur with higher incidence in the setting of HIV infection are discussed elsewhere in this book.

As expected in any medical condition as common as HIV/AIDS, a wide variety of malignancies have been described in the setting of HIV infection, which may have no clear link to HIV infection. As the HIV-infected individual ages, increasing attention must be paid to the screening for, prevention, and treatment of conditions associated with aging in the general population. Standard accepted screening strategies focus on neoplasms, which can be detected in premalignant stages, such as colon polyps and malignancies for which early detection results in a significant survival advantage with treatment. This group includes colon, prostate, and breast cancer. Individual risk based on family and personal medical history dictates specific screening strategies for the individual.

Breast Cancer

There is no conclusive data to suggest that the risk or natural history of breast cancer is different among HIV-infected women than that in the general population.

Breast cancer is the most common cancer diagnosed in women overall and the most frequent cause of cancer mortality between the ages of 15 and 54 (28). The lifetime risk of dying of breast cancer for women in the United States is estimated to be 3.6% (29). Approximately one-half of new breast cancer diagnoses occur in women under 65 years of age. Women with a first-degree female relative with breast cancer are at two- to threefold greater risk (30). Late age at first pregnancy and nulliparity are also associated with increased risk, as are high socioeconomic status and exposure to high doses of radiation.

The meaning of this observation is not clear, however, and little data are available to suggest that the natural history, clinical manifestations, or epidemiology of breast cancer are different in the setting of HIV infection.

It has long been established that the predominant risk factors for breast cancer are age, estrogen exposure, and family history. In addition, two genes, BRCA 1 and BRCA 2, increase the risk of breast cancer but are present in only a minority of women with a family history of breast cancer. Routine screening for breast cancer has received tremendous attention over the past 20 years and has been associated in many studies with earlier detection and greater overall survival. Although screening technology has become more sophisticated in recent years, the majority of women undergoing screening undergo routine mammography. The timing of screening is controversial, however. Screening beginning at the age of 40 has been recommended by The American Cancer Society (31) and a number of other organizations. The U.S. Preventive Service Task Force Screening has recommended routine screening beginning at the age of 50 (32). Screening strategies should be individualized for women deemed to be at high risk by family history or other factors.

Colorectal Cancer

Although anal cancer has been associated with HIV infection, primarily among MSM, there is no clear evidence that HIV infection increases the risk of colorectal cancer. In the general population, universal screening for colon cancer should begin at age 50 and continue until 75, in the absence of specific risk factors, such as strong family history, prior polyps, and inflammatory bowel disease, according to the U.S. Preventive Services Task Force (33). Screening may be conducted by colonoscopy (every 10 years) or computed tomographic colonography, flexible sigmoidoscopy, or double-contrast barium enema (every 5 years). Annual fecal occult blood testing, though less sensitive, should be conducted for patients unable to undergo other forms of screening.

The applicability of these guidelines in the setting of HIV infection has not been established. The incidence of colon cancer has not been shown to be higher among HIV-infected individuals than in the general population. However, the risk of anal squamous cell cancer is four- to eightfold higher among HIV-infected men, particularly those with a history of homosexual contact. Screening for this neoplasm is discussed elsewhere in this text.

Prostate Cancer

Prostate cancer is exceeded only by lung cancer as a cause of cancer-related death among American men. There is no clear link between prostate cancer and HIV infection. Controversy exists over the appropriate means of screening for prostate cancer, particularly about the role of prostate specific antigen (PSA) measurements. Originally developed as a means of following response to therapy, PSA testing has become a common means of screening for prostate cancer over the past two decades. Confounding this strategy, however, is the relative lack of specificity of PSA for cancer. Levels may be elevated in acute prostatitis and in benign prostatic hypertrophy as well as by prostate biopsy and even digital rectal examination (34,35), and sensitivity too has been problematic, typically estimated at 70% to 80% using the standard cutoff of 4.0 ng/mL. Because of the suboptimal sensitivity and specificity of PSA testing, concerns have been raised regarding both unnecessary biopsies and their attendant risks in some instances and late diagnoses in others. In recent years, several large studies have attempted to define the optimal screening strategies for prostate cancer in the general population and have come to somewhat contradictory conclusions. A large meta-analysis published in 2010 indicated that cancer diagnosis was increased but cancer mortality was not decreased in men undergoing screening (36).

No convincing association between HIV infection and prostate cancer has been demonstrated. Standard guidelines should be followed until further data regarding such issues as the incidence, natural history, and therapy of prostate cancer in the setting of HIV infection as well as the utility of screening in this population are available. A number of panels have suggested reviewing the pros and cons of screening with men as they age. The U.S. Preventive Services Task Force issued guidance in 2008, concluding that there was insufficient evidence to assess the relative risks and benefits of screening for prostate cancer in men less than 75 and recommended not screening men over 75 (37).

ATHEROSCLEROSIS AND CORONARY ARTERY DISEASE

Because of the association between hypertriglyceridemia and insulin resistance and ART, the risk of premature atherosclerosis in patients taking ART has received increasing attention in recent years. Current treatment guidelines take into account the differing degrees to which various antiretroviral drugs appear to contribute to coronary artery disease, and HIV infection itself may be as important a risk factor for the development of coronary artery disease as are hypertension and hypercholesterolemia. Reports of premature coronary artery disease associated with HIV infection appeared before the advent of modern ART. Since the early period of the HIV/AIDS epidemic, coronary endothelial abnormalities and frank atherosclerotic lesions were described in autopsy studies of young HIV-infected patients, including some children (38). Serum markers of endothelial cell dysfunction, such as von Willebrand factor and tissue plasminogen activator, may be elevated in association with HIV infection (39), and hypercoagulability may correlate with plasma HIV viral load (40). High circulating levels of triglycerides, known to accelerate atherosclerosis in non-HIV-infected individuals, were seen in association with HIV infection prior to the advent of protease inhibitors or other newer antiretroviral drugs.

Despite evidence of accelerated atherosclerosis and the presence of physiologic markers of endothelial dysfunction, the full implications of hyperlipidemia and insulin resistance associated with ART are currently not completely known. Specifically, the impact of these factors on the age of onset and natural history of coronary artery disease in the setting of HIV infection are not yet clear. An attempt was made to quantify the excess risk of coronary artery disease among patients developing hyperlipidemia in association with ART. On the basis of this analysis, an excess of 1.4 cardiovascular cases per 100,000 individuals would occur every 10 years, based on predictive criteria from the Framingham study (41).

As the full spectrum of atherosclerosis in HIV infection is elucidated, at present, it is clear that coronary risk modification addressing smoking, obesity, hypertension, and exercise should be explored with HIV-infected patients (42).

GENERAL COUNSELING STRATEGIES

Behavioral counseling for the aging HIV-infected individual must of course address issues specific to this population including adherence to ART, substance abuse treatment when indicated, and reduction in the risk of transmission of HIV. However, since the focus of this chapter is intended to be on the more general approach to the aging individual, other forms of counseling, it should be noted here that an emphasis on the same behaviors for which all patients should receive counseling is no less important for those living with HIV. In fact, in light of the associations with atherosclerosis and HIV infection outlined above, counseling regarding these behaviors in the aging HIV patient may be particularly crucial.

Smoking Cessation

The prevalence of smoking among HIV-infected MSM appears to be significantly higher than that (25%) in the general population (43). Whether this phenomenon is seen across other populations is not clear; however, a study from England found that more than 70% of HIV patients currently smoked, and few desired to stop (44).

Attempts have been made to study the impact of cigarette smoking on the natural history and clinical course of HIV infection, with conflicting results. Several studies have suggested that tobacco use accelerates the development of immune deficiency and clinical progression (45,46), while other studies have failed to confirm this (47). Specific manifestations and complications of HIV infection may be influenced by cigarette smoking. In a study comparing large groups of smokers and nonsmokers, community-acquired pneumonia, oral candidiasis, and oral hairy leukoplakia were more common in the smoking group, while progression to AIDS and the incidence of *Pneumocystis carinii* pneumonia and Kaposi's sarcoma were equal (48). Other studies have demonstrated an association between smoking and a range of oral pathology (49). The risk of heterosexual transmission of HIV infection appeared to be increased among women smokers in a study conducted in Haiti (50). Predictably, cigarette smoking is associated with accelerated deterioration of lung function among HIV-infected individuals (51).

Patients should be questioned about current and past tobacco use, efforts to quit smoking, and symptoms of nicotine withdrawal. It is recommended that all patients who smoke receive smoking cessation counseling on a regular basis. The most effective form of individual counseling is a direct statement by the provider that smoking is harmful and that all tobacco use should stop. Specific information about health risk to the individual as well as children and pregnant women living in the household should be provided and emphasized.

Data from the general population indicates that stopping smoking at any age results in a reduction of smoking-related morbidity and mortality. Stopping before the age of 50 results in a 50% reduction of the risk of dying within the following 15 years (51). The impact of smoking cessation on specific HIV-related disorders has not been evaluated.

Various means of individual and group counseling have been shown to be effective. Self-help brochures and other materials are available from a variety of sources, and smoking cessation programs are frequently available through community organizations. All such resources should be explored and made available.

All patients who smoke should be offered, as a minimum, a nicotine replacement and general advice on the value of quitting. Nicotine gum may improve cessation rates as well as appointment compliance rates (52). The nicotine transdermal patch, applied daily, may be more effective (53). Unfortunately, only a minority of patients have the motivation to stop smoking when the subject is first raised by the provider. The level of motivation may be even lower among HIV-infected individuals than it is in the general population (44).

Patients who are pessimistic about their chances of long-term survival, realistically or not, may be especially difficult to motivate. Improving motivation often requires the involvement of several types of providers. The primary care physician can provide basic, and repeated, advice that should include the firm message to discontinue smoking. Follow-up by nurses and/or social workers to encourage and reinforce cessation should also be offered if possible. Specific motivational sessions may be offered through mental health professionals and antismoking organizations. The provider should maintain a focus on smoking cessation at each encounter, discuss obstacles, and inform the patient about available nicotine substitutes.

Promoting a Healthy Diet

Nutritional considerations in HIV infection are complex and vary according to the clinical and immunologic status of the patient. A detailed dietary history should be obtained from each patient. Recommendations for the general population, such as limitation of dietary fat and cholesterol as well as consumption of fruits, vegetables, and grains, are most likely appropriate for otherwise healthy, immunologically normal HIV-infected adults.

Exercise

Regular moderate-to-intense physical activity can reduce the risk of coronary artery disease, hypertension, obesity, and diabetes. Aside from this general concept, however, specific counseling regarding exercise must be individualized. The high prevalence of disorders that impact an individual's ability to exercise (such as chronic interstitial lung disease, cardiomyopathy, malnutrition, and peripheral neuropathy) may represent obstacles to the application of standard recommendations.

REFERENCES

1. CDC. HIV/AIDS Surveillance Report 2005 vol 17. Rev ed. Atlanta US DHHS, CDC 2007:1–54.
2. Antiretroviral Therapy Cohort Collaboration. Life expectancy of individuals on combination antiretroviral therapy in high-income countries: a collaborative analysis of 14 cohort studies. Lancet 2008; 372:293–299.
3. Lohse N, Hansen AB, Pedersen G, et al. Survival of persons with and without HIV infection in Denmark, 1995-2005. Ann Intern Med 2007; 146:87–95.
4. Martin J, Volberding P. HIV and premature aging: a field still in its infancy. Ann Intern Med 2010; 153(7):477–479.
5. Lane HC. Pathogenesis of HIV infection: total CD4+ T-cell pool, immune activation, and inflammation. Top HIV Med 2010; 18(1):2–6.
6. Bicanic T, Meintjes G, Rebe K, et al. Immune reconstitution inflammatory syndrome in HIV-associated cryptococcal meningitis: a prospective study. J Acquir Immune Defic Syndr 2009; 51(2):130–134.

7. Muller M, Wandel S, Colebunders R, et al. Immune reconstitution inflammatory syndrome in patients starting antiretroviral therapy for HIV infection: a systematic review andmeta-analysis. Lancet Infect Dis 2010; 10(4):251–261.

8. Sicotte M, Alvarado BE, Leon EM, et al. Social networks and depressive symptoms among elderly women and men in Havana, Cuba. Aging Ment Health 2008; 12 (2):193–201.

9. Chan A, Malhotra C, Malhotra R, et al. Living arrangements, social Networks and depressive symptoms among older men and women in Singapore. Int J Geriatr Psychiatry 2010 Jul 30 (epub ahead of print).

10. Choi NG, Ha JH. Relationship between spouse/partner support and depressive symptoms in older adults: gender difference. Aging Ment Health 2010:1–11.

11. Martin CP, Fain MJ, Klotz SA. The older HIV-positive adult: a crtical review of the medical literature. Am J Med 2008; 121:1032–1037.

12. Mack KA, Ory MG. AIDS and older Americans at the end of the twentieth century. J Acquir Immune Defic Syndr 2003; 33(suppl 2):S68–S75.

13. Shippy R, Karpiak S. The aging HIV/AIDS population: fragile social networks. Aging Ment Health 2005; 9:246–254.

14. Emlet C, Farkas K. Correlates of service utilization among midlife and older adults with HIV/AIDS: the role of age in the equation. J Aging Health 2002; 14:315–335.

15. Chesney M, Chambers D, Taylor J, et al. Social support, distress and well-being in older men living with HIV infection. J Acquir Immune Defic Syndr 2003; 33(suppl 2):S185–S193.

16. Shippy R, Karpiak S. Perceptions of support among older adults with HIV. Res Aging 2005; 27:290–306.

17. Operskalski E, Mosley JW, Busch MP, et al. Influences of age, viral load and CD4+ count on the rate of progression of HIV-1 infectoin to AIDS. Transfusion Safety Study Group. J Acquir Immune Defic Syndr Hum Retrovirol 1997; 15:243–244.

18. Crystal S, Akincigil A, Sambamoorthi U, et al. The diverse older HIV-positive population: a national profile of economic circumstances, socal support, and quality of life. J Acquir Immune Defic Syndr 2003; 33(suppl 2):S76–S83.

19. Dolcini M, Catania J, Stall R, et al. The HIV epidemic among older men who have sex with men. J Acquir Immune Defic Syndr 2003; 33(suppl 2):S115–S121.

20. Brown D, Sankar A. HIV/AIDS and aging minority populations. Res Aging 1998; 20:865–884.

21. Joyce GF, Goldman DP, Leibowitz AA, et al. A socioeconomic profile of older adults with HIV. J Health Care Poor Underserved 2005; 16:19–28.

22. Zablotsky D, Kennedy M. Risk factors and HIV transmission to midlife and older women: knowledge, options and the initiation of safer sexual practices. J Acquir Immune Defic Syndr 2003; 33(suppl 2):S122–S130.

23. Meyer KC. The role of immunity and inflammation in lung senescence and susceptibility to infection in the elderly. Semin Respir Crit Care Med 2010; 31(5):561–574.

24. Centers for Disease Control and Prevention, State-specific prevalence of selected health behaviors, by race and ethnicity–behavioral risk factor surveillance system. Morbid Mortal Weekly Rep 2000; 49:SS-2, 1.

25. U. S. Preventive Services Task Force, Screening for Hypertension, Guide to Clinical Preventive Services. 2nd ed. Baltimore: Williams & Wilkins, 1996:39.

26. Engels EA, Pfeiffer RM, Goedert JJ, et al. Trends in cancer risk among people with AIDS in theUnited States 1980-2002. AIDS 2006; 20:1645–1654.
27. Simard EP, Pfeiffer RM, Engels EA. Cumulative incidence of cancer among individuals with acquired immunodeficiency syndrome in the United States. Cander 2010 Oct 19 (Epub ahead of print).
28. Wingo PA, Toping T, Bolden S. Cancer statistics. CA Cancer Clin 1995; 45:8.
29. Ries LAG, Miller BA, Hankey BF, et al. (eds.), SEER cancer statistics review, 1973-1991: tables and graphs, Bethesda, National Cancer Institute (NIH publication no. 94-2789), 1994.
30. Colditz GA, Willet WC, Hunter DJ, et al. Family history, age, and risk of breast cancer. JAMA 1993; 270:338.
31. Smith RA, Cokkinides V, Brawley OW. Cancer screening in the United States, 2009: a review of current American Cancer Society guidelines and issues in cancer screening. CA Cancer J Clin 2009; 59:27.
32. U.S. Preventive Services Task Force. Screening for breast cancer: U.S. Preventive Services Task Force recommendation statement. Ann Intern Med 2009; 151:716.
33. U.S. Preventive Services Task Force. Screening for colorectal cancer: U.S. Preventive Services Task Force recommendation statement. Ann Intern Med 2008; 149:627.
34. Yuan JJ, Coplen DE, Petros JA, et al. Effects of rectal examination, prostatic massage, ultrasonography and needle biopsy on serum prostate specific antigen lefles. J Urol 1992; 147:910.
35. Nadler RB, Humphrey PA, Smith DS, et al. Effect of inflammation and benign prostatic hyperplasia on elevated serum prostate specific antigen levels. J Urol 1995; 154:407.
36. Dulbegovic M, Beyth RJ, Neuberger MM, et al. Screening for prostate cancer: systematic review and meta-analysis of randomized controlled trials. BMJ 2010; 341:c4543.
37. U.S. Preventive Services Task Force. Screening for prostate: U.S. Preventive Services Task Force recommendation statement. Ann Intern Med 2008; 149:185.
38. Joshi VV, Pawel B, Connor E, et al. Arteriopathy in children with AIDS. Pediatr Pathol 1987; 7:261–275.
39. Blann A, Constans J, Dignat-George F, et al., The platelet and endothelium in HIV infection. Br J Haematol 1998; 100:613–614.
40. Karochine M, Ankri A, Calvez V, et al. Plasma hypercoagnulability is correlated to plasma HIV load. Thromb Haemost 1998; 80:208–209.
41. Grunfeld C, Doerrler W, Pang M, et al. Abnormalities of apolipoprotein E in the Acquired immunodeficiency syndrome. J Clin Endocrinol Metab 1997; 82:373.
42. Carr A, Samaras K, Thorisdottir A, et al. Diagnosis, prediction and natural course of lipodystrophy, hyperlipidemia and diabetes mellitus: a cohort study. Lancet 1999; 353:2093–2099.
43. Arday DR, Erdin BR, Giovino DA, et al. Smoking, HIV infection and gay men in the United States. Tobacco Control 1993; 2:156.
44. Niaura R, Shadel WG, Morrow K, et al. Smoking among HIV-positive persons. Ann Behav Med 1999; 21(suppl):S116.
45. Royce RA, Windelstein W, Bacchetti P. Cigarette smoking and incidence of AIDS. Int Cont AIDS 1990; 6:143.

46. Nieman RB, Fleming J, Coker RJ, et al. The effect of cigarette smoking on the develo-pment of AIDS in HIV-1-seropositive individuals. AIDS 1993; 7:705.
47. Craib KJ, et al. The effect of cigarette smoking on lymphocyte subsets and progression to AIDS in a cohort of homosexual men. Clin Invest Med 1992; 15:301.
48. Conley LJ, Bush TJ, Buchbinder SP, et al. The association between cigarette smoking and selected HIV-related medical conditions. AIDS 1996; 10:1121.
49. Palmer GD, Robinson PG, Challacombe SJ, et al. Aetiological factors for oral manifestations of HIV. Oral Dis 1996; 2:193–197.
50. Mitchell DM, Fleming J, Pinching AJ, et al. Pulmonary function in human immunodeficiency virus infection. A prospective 18-month study of serial lung function in 474 patients. Am Rev Respir Dis 1992; 146:745–751.
51. Department of Health and Human Services, The health benefits of smoking cessation: a report of the Surgeon General, Rockville, MD, 1990 (Pub. No. DHS (CDC-90-8416).
52. Lam W, Sze PC, Sacks HS, et al. Meta-analysis of randomized controlled trials of nicotine chewing gum. Lancet 1987; 2:27–30.
53. Fiore MC, Smith SS, Jorenby DE, et al. The effectiveness of the nicotine patch for smoking cessation: a meta-analysis. JAMA 1994; 271:1940.

10

Issues confronted by women

INTRODUCTION

HIV infection in women raises specific issues that have long been recognized as critical in the societal response to the HIV/AIDS epidemic. In the developing world, approximately half of all HIV infections are seen among women. In the United States, women account for approximately 25% of reported cases (1). Because heterosexual contact is the most frequent route of transmission of HIV infection to women in the United States (1) and in the developing world, infection may go unsuspected and unrecognized more often among women since they are less likely than men who have sex with men or injection drug users to recognize that they are at risk. The possibility of transmission of HIV from mother to unborn child adds another dimension to the epidemic in women, and this route of transmission accounts for the vast majority of pediatric HIV/AIDS cases. Child care and other family responsibilities shouldered disproportionately by women often stand in the way of their medical care. In this chapter, the impacts of these various factors on women are discussed.

EPIDEMIOLOGY OF HIV INFECTION IN WOMEN

Recent Epidemiological Trends in the United States

It is estimated that between 120,000 and 160,000 adult and adolescent women are currently living with HIV infection in the United States. However, the number of individuals, including women, with HIV infection in the United States is not known with certainty. In evaluating epidemiological data regarding HIV infection, a distinction must be drawn between individuals testing positive for the virus since only 37 states gather name-specific data reflecting this and those meeting the case definition for AIDS, a relatively precise national figure published by the Centers for Disease Control and Prevention. Approximately 200,000 women had been diagnosed with AIDS in the United States between the beginning of the epidemic through 2008 (1). Among the 37 states with confidential name-based HIV infection reporting, approximately 9000 new cases of

HIV infection were reported among women annually between 2005 and 2008 (1). After a sharp rise in the incidence and prevalence of HIV infection among women during the 1980s and 1990s, recent years have seen a stabilization of the rate of HIV infection and slight decrease in the rate of AIDS diagnosis (1).

In 2008, women accounted for approximately 26% of newly reported AIDS cases and approximately 25% of newly reported HIV infections (1). The route of transmission of HIV infection to women has shifted dramatically in the past decade. During the period 1991 to 1998, injection drug use accounted for 48% of HIV infections among women. However, by 1998, only 28% of reported women were infected by this route (2), and in 2008, this proportion fell to an estimated 15% (1) among newly reported women. Another important trend has been the increasing shift of the burden of HIV infection into minority populations, both male and female. In 1998, for example, AIDS accounted for 13% of deaths among black women compared with 2% among Caucasian women (2). As of 1999, 57% of women living with AIDS were African American, 20% were Hispanic, and 23% were Caucasian. The epidemic has also increasingly affected women living in poverty or conditions of social upheaval. More than 80% of women with AIDS lived in households with annual income less than $10,000 (2), 86% were unmarried, and 23% lived alone. Half had at least one child below the age of 15. The majority are unemployed and lack health insurance. The geographical distribution of female AIDS cases has trended somewhat away from traditional high prevalence areas of the north-east: in 1998, more new cases were reported from the south than from any other area of the country. Among newly diagnosed cases of AIDS in 2008, 46% lived in the south, 22% in the north-east, 19% in the west, and 11% in the midwest (1).

Racial and Ethnic Patterns of HIV Infection in the U.S. Female Population

African American and Hispanic women are disproportionately impacted by the HIV/AIDS epidemic in the United States (1). In 2008, the most recent year for which data has been published, Black African American women accounted for nearly 60% of women with HIV infection and Hispanic/Latino women comprised approximately 15%.

Global Epidemiological Trends

The total number of individuals living with HIV infection in the world has risen steadily over the past 20 years. This reflects dramatic successes and discouraging failures. The success of antiretroviral therapy in prolonging life has had a substantial impact despite the fact that the majority of individuals who would benefit from therapy cannot currently access it. It is estimated that over 11 million years of life have been added worldwide (7.2 million in Western Europe and North America) since 1996 because of effective therapy (3). Unfortunately, the continued transmission of HIV in all regions and the resultant large number of newly infected individuals each year also contribute to this rise, although the estimated number of new cases has trended downward in recent years. Approximately 2.2 million adults and 370,000 children under 15 were newly infected in 2009 (4). There is of course great geographical variation in the distribution of cases of HIV/AIDS. Approximately two-thirds of persons living with HIV/AIDS live in sub-Saharan Africa. In this region, seven countries (Botswana, Lesotho, Malawi, South Africa, Swaziland, Zambia, and Zimbabwe) (3) have a seroprevalence greater than 10%. In Botswana, Lesotho, and Swaziland, this figure exceeds 20%. Latin America, Eastern Europe, and East Asia have witnessed significant increases in the number of infected individuals between 2001 and 2008 (3).

Of the estimated 33 million individuals living with HIV in the world, approximately 16 million (48%) are women. The impact is seen most dramatically in sub-Saharan Africa, where it is estimated that 60% of all cases are currently among women (3). Contributing to this heavy burden is sexual violence (5) and the widely held belief in some countries of the region that women do not have the right to refuse sexual intercourse with husbands or boyfriends (6).

TRANSMISSION OF HIV INFECTION TO WOMEN

Sexual transmission of HIV infection from men to women accounts for the vast majority of reported AIDS cases among women worldwide and an increasing number of AIDS cases and new HIV infections in the United States. HIV can be isolated in semen, both in cell-free fluid and in mononuclear cells (7). Overall, the likelihood of transmission from male to female appears to be in the range of 0.05% to 0.15% per sexual contact and is significantly greater than the likelihood of female-to-male transmission.

Risk Factors for Sexual Transmission

Several risk factors for increased HIV replication in vaginal secretions have been identified. Bacterial vaginosis caused by *Gardnerella vaginalis* is associated with increased transmission of HIV (8) and increased vaginal HIV production (9). It has also been noted that HIV levels in cervical and vaginal fluids rise shortly before and during menses, independent of plasma levels (10).

A number of other risk factors that are thought or known to increase the likelihood of transmission of HIV infection from men to women have been identified. Among these are the following:

Active sexually transmitted disease
Lack of circumcision in the male partner
The use of spermicides
Cervical ectopy
Bleeding (including menstrual bleeding) during intercourse
Receptive anal intercourse

Advanced HIV infection in the male partner
Specific HIV clades

Reducing Heterosexual Transmission to Women

Proper use of male condoms is highly, although not completely, effective in preventing transmission of HIV during heterosexual intercourse. For example, no instances of transmission were identified between discordant couples using condoms consistently after 15,000 episodes of intercourse in a large European study (11). The rate of transmission in couples not using condoms or using them intermittently was 13%.

It has been observed since the early days of the HIV/AIDS epidemic that heterosexual transmission between some discordant couples never occurred even when condoms were not used. More insight into this phenomenon has been gained in recent years. Strong cytotoxic T-cell response was found in the majority of uninfected partners with frequent exposure to HIV in one small study (12). Specific viral virulence factors and coreceptor (e.g., CCR5) status of the uninfected partner may also play a role in protection against heterosexual transmission.

Finally, antiretroviral therapy has been shown to reduce HIV shedding in semen (13). It is assumed, probably correctly, that this ultimately reduces male-to-female transmission. However, the proportion of men actually rendered noninfectious by therapy is unknown, and any HIV-infected man must, on the basis of the present state of knowledge, be assumed to be capable of transmitting HIV even if he is receiving effective antiviral therapy with complete suppression of plasma viremia. Of course, viral resistance to antiretroviral drugs may result in high concentrations of virus in semen, even in some men receiving therapy.

MOTHER-TO-CHILD TRANSMISSION

HIV infection may be transmitted from mother to child during pregnancy, at the time of delivery or during the postnatal period through breast-feeding. Such vertical transmission has accounted for the majority of cases of AIDS in children. Specific risk factors for transmission have been identified in recent years, and strategies of prevention have been refined. The most important predictor of transmission to the fetus is maternal plasma viral load.

Prospective studies have generally indicated that in the absence of anti-retroviral therapy, approximately one-sixth to one-third of children born to HIV-infected women will be infected (14). In contrast, a combined approach of maternal antiretroviral therapy in the antepartum period and during labor and delivery, combined with elective Caesarian section (ECS) in selected women, avoidance of breast-feeding, and treatment of the infant with six weeks of zidovudine (AZT) prophylaxis, has been demonstrated to reduce the risk of transmission to less than 2% (15).

Risk Factors for Mother-to-Child Transmission

Maternal Viral Load

Maternal viral load has been shown to correlate with the likelihood of transmission (16,17), although no lower limit of viral load has been established below which transmission cannot occur. High concentration of virus in maternal cervicovaginal secretions and, as a result, a relatively large viral load innoculated into the oropharynx of the infant may be even more important determinants of transmission (18,19). In a U.S. study of nearly 500 women who received AZT during pregnancy, it was found that 107 women had undetectable viral loads (<500 copies/mL) at the time of delivery (17). Similar results were seen in a comparable study from Zimbabwe (20) and another U.S. study in which high maternal plasma viral load at any time during pregnancy was correlated with the risk of transmission (16). As might be expected from these findings, levels of HIV RNA in vaginal secretions correlate closely with plasma levels and fall with antiretroviral therapy (21). Maternal host factors may also facilitate or hinder transmission. In a study of 75 women, suppression of HIV by CD8 cells was shown to reduce the risk of transmission (22).

Other factors that appear to increase the risk of transmission include cigarette smoking and premature rupture of the membranes (23).

PREVENTION OF MATERNAL-TO-CHILD TRANSMISSION

Overview of the Role of Antiretroviral Therapy

In early 1994, an interim analysis of a double-blind prospective (AIDS Clinical Trials Group protocol 076) indicated that AZT given to pregnant women reduced the likelihood of mother-to-child transmission of HIV infection (24). The treatment group in this study began AZT therapy (100 mg orally five times daily) between 14 and 34 weeks gestation and continued therapy intravenously (2 mg/kg loading dose followed by 1 mg/hr) through labor and delivery. Infants born to these mothers received AZT syrup (2 mg/kg every six hours) for the first six weeks of life. The transmission rate in the treatment group was 8.3%, compared with 25.5% in the placebo group, a difference that was highly statistically significant.

In 1994, it was demonstrated that AZT given to the mother through the perinatal period reduces mother-to-child transmission by approximately 75% (25). Subsequent studies have confirmed this and established the efficacy of other antiretroviral regimens in this regard. Since this initial report, the administration of antiretroviral therapy in this manner has become a standard practice in the United States. The dramatic effectiveness of such preventive therapy has led to enhanced programs of prenatal testing of women and postnatal testing of their infants for HIV infection in many areas. Despite these findings, approximately 1000 are born with HIV infection each day worldwide primarily because of the lack of both prenatal HIV testing and antiretroviral therapy for pregnant HIV-infected women.

As newer antiretroviral agents have become available since 1994, including all of the protease inhibitors and nonnucleoside reverse transcriptase inhibitors and as highly active antiretroviral therapy (HAART) has become more widespread, a number of issues have arisen regarding the optimal strategy for prevention of perinatal transmission. Since single-drug therapy with AZT or any other antiretroviral agent is not currently recommended in any other setting, the safety, efficacy, and long-term consequences of therapy with other agents have come under scrutiny. In addition, since resistant virus may be transmitted despite appropriately administered antiretroviral therapy treatment regimens for women who are suspected or proven to have developed AZT-resistant, viral strains have been developed. Finally, more cost-effective approaches have been sought, which can be applied to large numbers of women living in developing countries. See chapter 5 for specific recommendations regarding antiretroviral therapy to prevent mother-to-child transmission.

The widespread use of antiretroviral therapy in resource-rich countries to prevent vertical transmission has occurred rapidly. As a result, dramatic reductions in perinatal transmission and, thus, of pediatric AIDS in the United States occurred by the late 1990s (26). Recent data indicate that 50% of HIV-infected pregnant women take antiretroviral therapy and that the overall rate of transmission is less than 3%. Such observations raise the prospect that vertical transmission could be completely eliminated in the United States (27) and other developed countries.

For current guidelines regarding antiretroviral therapy to prevent maternal-to-child transmission, see chapter 5.

Method of Delivery

Caesarian section has long been proposed as a means of reducing or eliminating the risk of transmission of HIV during delivery (28). In the United States, ECS is recommended if the maternal viral load remains above 1000 copies/mL near term (29). Because of the low risk of HIV intrapartum transmission when the viral load of the mother is less than 3000 copies/mL, the appropriateness of this method of delivery has been challenged when the maternal plasma viral load is low or undetectable (30). In resource-limited settings, where ECS may not be safe or available, it has been suggested that vaginal delivery may be safer and more cost-effective among women receiving antiretroviral therapy while achieving similar success rates in prevention of maternal-to-child transmission (31).

Breast-Feeding

HIV can be transmitted from mother to child during breast-feeding. In a study from Africa, 7% of infants born to HIV-infected mothers who had not received antiretroviral therapy to prevent vertical transmission acquired HIV infection through breast-feeding (32). Transmission of HIV was likeliest during the first five months, but was documented throughout the 24 months of follow-up. Especially alarming is a study from Kenya indicating that 44% of cases of perinatal transmission result from breast-feeding (33). Other data suggest, however, that rates of HIV infection may be roughly equal in breast-fed and bottle-fed infants (34). These conflicting data have made reaching a consensus about the advisability of breast-feeding difficult to achieve. Some feel that breast-feeding is advisable in developing countries where infant nutritional status may otherwise be in jeopardy, while others feel that women should be strongly counseled against breast-feeding, as they are in the United States. In 2010, The World Health Organization revised its recommendations regarding breast-feeding by HIV-infected women in recognition of the obstacles presented by bottle-feeding in resource-deprived areas. Under the current guidance, all HIV-infected pregnant women should receive antiretroviral therapy during pregnancy to prevent transmission to the child. Supported by on data indicating that breast-feeding is safe and protective of the infant if the mother is receiving anti-retroviral therapy (35,36), and as an acknowledgement of the overall health benefits of breast-feeding, the 2010 guidelines include the recommendation that infants born to HIV-infected women who are receiving antiretroviral therapy be breast-fed for the first 12 months of life (37).

Diagnosis of HIV Infection in the Neonatal Period

Confirmation of HIV infection in the neonate requires direct evidence of circulating viral antigen. This is because passive transfer of maternal HIV antibody results in detectable antibody in the infant for the first 15 months of life even in the absence of HIV infection. Adding to the diagnostic confusion is the phenomenon of late seroconversion, which results in some infected infants initially having antibody-negative test results. In one reported case in a child who tested HIV negative after 6 months, detectable antibody developed at 22 months of age. Such problems of diagnostic ambiguity have been largely overcome by the use of the polymerase chain reaction technique for measuring viral RNA or proviral DNA. Such studies performed in the first 48 hours of life can detect over 30% of infected infants. Sensitivity of these tests improves rapidly over the first two weeks such that virus can be detected in over 90% of infected children by 14 days. Infants initially testing negative should be retested at three to six months. HIV infection can be almost completely excluded in infants testing repeatedly negative at this point; however, antibody tests should be repeated periodically until negative.

Because of the possibility of preventing transmission to the fetus, calls for routine prenatal screening of women have intensified, and this practice has become more commonplace. In developing countries, particularly in Africa, however, transmission during pregnancy remains common, and an increasing number of children are born HIV infected. The HIV-infected woman caring for an infected child represents one of the most poignant images of the AIDS epidemic, particularly in the setting of extreme poverty where it usually occurs. As her own health may be failing, she must face the emotional trauma and logistic and financial burden of her child's sickness and death. Even in the United States, it is clear that the needs of an infected and ill child often prevent the mother from seeking adequate care for herself.

CLINICAL MANIFESTATIONS OF HIV INFECTION IN WOMEN

Primary Infection

The signs and symptoms of primary HIV infection have been elucidated primarily in studies using male cohorts (see chap. 2). In a recent series describing female sex workers in Kenya, several symptoms were found to statistically associated with HIV seroconversion; these included fever, arthralgia, myalgia, diarrhea, vomiting, and noninguinal lymph node enlargement.

Opportunistic Infections and Malignancies

The patterns and relatively frequencies of AIDS-defining conditions are similar in men and in women with three exceptions.

- Cervical neoplasia (38) complicating human papillomavirus infection (HPV) is an AIDS-defining condition among women.
- Vaginal candidiasis is common as an early manifestation of HIV infection.
- Kaposi's sarcoma is more common among men.

Cervical Neoplasia

Cervical neoplasia, both cervical cancer and cervical intraepithelial neoplasia (CIN), are associated with HPV infection. HPV infection is more common in the presence of HIV infection, especially with significant immunodeficiency (38) or high HIV viral load (39) as are some HPV-related cervical neoplasms (40,41). In a study of over 2000 HIV-infected women, it was found that 40% had abnormal Pap smears, including atypical squamous cells of unknown significance (ASCUS) as well as squamous intraepithelial lesions (SIL) and CIN, compared with 17% among HIV-negative controls. Thirty percent of infected women had SIL compared with 7% of controls (42).

Vaginal Candidiasis

In one large early series from North America (43), vaginal candidiasis was the most common initial manifestation of HIV infection in women.

Disease Progression and Survival

Data regarding the relative rates of disease progression and overall prognosis of men and women have often been ambiguous. While disease progression appears to be comparable, women tend to present later in the course of HIV infection. For example, death was the first reported clinical event in 27.5% of women and 12.2 % of men without prior clinical HIV progression (44).

Some reports suggest that women may have lower levels of viral RNA (often in the range of 35–50% lower) in the plasma than men at similar stages of disease (45,46). Clinically, this may indicate a higher risk of disease progression among women with a given viral load than among their male counterparts. The clinical significance of these observations is not clear, and other series have failed to demonstrate a significant gender difference, particularly for women who acquired infection by the heterosexual route (47).

Response to Therapy

Women have been underrepresented in clinical trials of new antiretroviral agents. For this reason, data from these trials must generally be extrapolated to women with some uncertainty. A number of studies have indicated that the effectiveness of combination antiretroviral therapy in lowering the plasma viral load in women is approximately equal to that in men. Nevertheless, pharmacokinetics of these agents may differ in men and women. For example, hormonal changes associated with the menstrual cycle may lead to variability in absorption and clearance (48).

PRIMARY CARE OF HIV-INFECTED WOMEN

Disease Staging

Clinical and immunological staging of HIV infection in women, as it does in men, permits rational decisions regarding antiretroviral therapy and prophylaxis of opportunistic infection. Although some studies have suggested that women tend to have lower levels of viral load than men at similar CD4 cell counts (see above), the clinical significance of this observation is unknown, and staging (see chap. 5) should be performed as it is in men.

Antiretroviral Therapy

Men have far outnumbered women in clinical trials of antiretroviral drugs. Because of this, concern has been raised that the pharmacokinetic properties and toxicity profile of these agents are largely unstudied. Gender differences in absorption and metabolism as well as body weight and fat distribution may have clinical significance. In addition, the hormonal changes associated with the menstrual cycle and with pregnancy may also impact on the safety and efficacy of these agents in women.

Prevention of Opportunistic Infection

The patterns and incidence of AIDS-related opportunistic infections appear to be similar between the genders. Indications for preventive therapy directed at *Pneumocytis carinii* pneumonia, *Mycobacterium avium* complex, and tuberculosis are the same for men and women.

General Health Maintenance

As survival improves with current combination antiretroviral therapy, issues of general health maintenance are expected to become more important in the care of HIV-infected individuals. Both cardiovascular disease and cancer will most likely become more common in the coming years. Screening for hypertension and hypercholesterolemia should be carried out as it is for male patients (see chap. 9).

Screening for Cervical Neoplasia

As discussed above, because of the high incidence of CIN among HIV-infected women (49) and concern about progression to cervical carcinoma (50), screening for cervical neoplasia is strongly recommended for HIV-infected women (49). Of note, both CIN and cervical cancer have been linked to infection with HPV, which is exceptionally prevalent and persistent in HIV-infected women. In one series, the prevalence of HPV infection was 58% and 26% in HIV-positive and HIV-negative women, respectively (51). Furthermore, HPV infection is independently associated with high HIV plasma viral load and low CD4+ cell counts.

For these reasons, it is recommended that HIV-infected women undergo a gynecological examination with Pap smear at baseline six months and annually thereafter if the results are normal (49). It is advisable that women with a history of abnormal Pap smear be monitored every six months. If inflammation with reactive squamous cell changes is detected, the Pap smear should be repeated in three months. Women in whom ASCUS are found can be monitored annually. Patients with SIL should be considered for colposcopy and biopsy, particularly if the lesion is high grade. Women with invasive carcinoma should undergo colposcopy with biopsy or conization. Therapeutic options (radiation or surgery) should be considered.

It should be remembered that the sensitivity of Pap smears for SIL is in the range of 80% to 85%. For this reason, certain high-risk patients may require routine colposcopy.

Screening for Breast Cancer

The incidence of breast cancer is not known to be influenced by HIV infection. As the mean age of HIV-infected women increases because of improvements in therapy and longer survival, an increasing number will become candidates for routine screening mammography (see chap. 9).

OBSTACLES TO CARE FACED BY HIV-INFECTED WOMEN

Access

It has been demonstrated that HIV-infected women tend to enter care later than their male counterparts and are less likely to receive medical care, including effective antiretroviral therapy (52).

Treatment Adherence

Women often face more obstacles to care and to adherence with antiretroviral therapy than men do. Family responsibilities may lead to poor compliance with appointments, less tolerance of medication side effects, and a tendency to sacrifice one's own health for the health of a child or other loved ones.

Potential Gender Bias in the Understanding of HIV Infection

Most of the current understanding of the clinical manifestations and immunologic features of HIV infection has come from studies of men, particularly homosexual and bisexual men. In addition, almost all data regarding the effectiveness of antiretroviral therapy, as well as therapy of opportunistic infections and malignancies, have been accumulated through large clinical trials that have enrolled few women. This is true despite obvious differences in male and female heterosexual transmission and several important contrasts in the clinical features of HIV infection between men and women.

Possible sources of gender bias include the following:

There is a higher incidence of AIDS in men in developed countries where most research has been conducted.

There is a low level of recruitment of women into clinical trials of new therapies.

Intravenous drug use among HIV-infected women in the early years of the epidemic was predominant. Women in this heterogeneous group have often been perceived as poor candidates for clinical trials and have lacked the unified advocacy groups that represented male homosexuals in the planning of and recruitment for these trials.

Access to health care for HIV-infected women is generally less than that of men (53,54).

Biological differences between genders may impact negatively on the response to antiretroviral therapy among women (55,56), although the evidence of consistent differences between men and women in this regard is generally lacking.

REFERENCES

1. Centers for Disease Control and Prevention. Estimated rates of diagnoses of HIV infection among adults and adolescents by sex and race/thnicity, 2008—37 states with confidential name-based HIV infection reporting. HIV Surveillance Report, 2008. Available at: http://www.cdc.gov/hiv/topics/surveillance/resources/reports. Published June 2010.

2. Centers for Disease Control and Prevention, HIV/AIDS Surveillance Report 2000, 11(2):5.

3. UNAIDS/World Health Organization. 09 AIDS epidemic update. Joint United Nations Programme on HIV/IDS(UNAIDS and World Health Organization (WHO), 2009.

4. WHO Global Report. Global summary of the AIDS epidemic/2009. Available at: http://www.who.int/hiv/data/2009_gobal_summary.png.

5. Khobotlo M, Tshehlo R, Nkonyana J, et al. Lesotho: HIV prevention response and modes of transmission analysis. Maseru, Lesotho National AIDS Commission, 2009.

6. Andersson N, Ho-Foster A, Mitchell S, et al. Risk factors for domestic physical violence: national cross-sectional household surveys in eight southern African countries. BMC Womens Health 2007; 7:11.

7. Gupta P, Mellors J, Kingsley L, et al. High viral load in semen of human immunodeficiency virus typ1-infected men at all stages of disease and its reduction by therapy with protease and nonnuclesoide reverse transcriptase inhibitors. J Virol 1997; 71:6271–6275.

8. Taha TE, Hoover DR, Dallabetta GA, et al. Bacterial vaginosis an ddisturbances of vaginal flora: association with increased acquisition of HIV. AIDS 1998; 12:1699–1706.

9. Hashemi FB, Ghassemi M, Roebuck KA, et al. Activation of human immunodeficiency virus type 1 expression by *Gardnerella vaginalis*. J Infect Dis 1999; 179:924–930.

10. Reichelderfer PS, Coombs RW, Wright DJ, et al. Effect of menstrual cycle on HIV-1 levels in the peripheral blood and genital tract. AIDS 2000; 14:2101–2107.

11. Devincenzi I for the European Study Group on Heterosexual Transmission of HIV. A longitudinal study of HIV transmission by heterosexual partners. N Engl J Med 1994; 331:341.

12. Bienzle D, MacDonald KS, Smaill FM, et al. Factors contributing to the lack of human immunodeficiency virus type 1 (HIV-1) transmission in HIV-1-discordant partners. J Infect Dis 2000; 182:123.

13. Barrosi PF, Schechter M, Gupta P, et al. Effect of antiretroviral therapy on HIV shedding in semen. Ann Intern Med 2000; 133:280–284.

14. Andiman WA, Simpson BJ, Olson B, et al. Rate of transmission of human immunodeficiency virus type 1 infection from mother to child and short term outcome of neonatal infection: results of a prospective cohort study. Am J Dis Child 1990; 144:758–766.

15. Anderson BL, Cu-Uvin S. Pregnancy and optimal care of HIV-infected patients. Clin Infect Dis 2009; 48(4):449–455.

16. Garcia PM, Kalish LA, Pitt J, et al. Maternal levels of plasma human immunodeficiency virus typ 1 RNA and the risk of perinatal transmission. N Engl J Med 1999; 41:394–402.

17. Mofenson LM, Lambert JS, Stiehm ER, et al. Risk factors for perinatal transmission of human immunodeficiency virus type 1 in women treated with zidovudine. N Engl J Med 1999; 341:385–393.
18. Mwanyumba F, Gaillard P, Verhofstede, et al. The influence of HIV-1 shedding in the genital tract and moth-to-chld HIV infection. 13th International Conference on AIDS, Durban, 2000.
19. Chuachoowong R, et al. Determinants of HIV RNA in newborn nasal/oral secretions and association with risk for perinatal HIV transmission. 13th International Conference on AIDS, Durban, 2000.
20. Katzenstein DA, Mbizvo M, Zijenah L, et al. Serum level of maternal human immunodeficiency virus (HIV) RNA, infant mortality and vertical transmission of HIV in Zimbabwe. J Infect Dis 1999; 1790:1382–1387.
21. Hart CE, Lennox JL, Pratt-Palmore M, et al. Correlation of human immunodeficiency virus type 1 RNA levels in blood and the female genital tract. J Infect Dis 1999; 179(4):871–882.
22. Plaeger S, Bermudez S, Mikyas Y, et al. Decreased CD8 cell mediated-viral suppression and other immunologic characteristics of women who transmit human immunodeficiency virus to their infants. J Infect Dis 1999; 179:1388–1394.
23. Burns DN, Landesman S, Muenz LR, et al. Cigarette smoking, prmature rupture of membranes, and vertical transmission of HIV-1 among women with low CD4+ levels. J Acquir Immune Defic Syndr 1994; 7:718–726.
24. Connor EM, Sperling RS, Gelber R, et al. Reduction of maternal-infant transmission of human immunodeficiency virus type 1 with zidovudine. N Engl J Med 1994; 331:1173–1180.
25. Centers for Disease Control and Prevention. Recommendations of the U.S. Public Health Service Task Force on the use of zidovudine to reduce perinatal transmission of human immunodeficiency virus. Morbid Mortal Weekly Rep 1994; 43(RR-11):1.
26. Lindegren ML, Byers RH Jr, Thomas P, et al. Trends in perinatal transmission of HIV/AIDS in the United States. JAMA 1999; 182:531–538.
27. Mofenson LM. Can perinatal HIV infection be eliminated in the United States? JAMA 1999; 282:577.
28. The European Mode Of Delivery Collaboration. Elective caesarean-section versus vaginal delivery in prevention of vertical HIV-1transmission: a randomized clinical trial. Lancet 1999; 353:1035.
29. AIDSinfo. Home page. Available at: http://AIDSInfo.nih.gov.
30. Stronger JS, Rouse DJ, Goldenberg RL. Prophylactic caesarean delivery for the prevention of perinatal human immunodeficiency virus infection: the case for restraint. JAMA 1999; 281:1946.
31. Murkherjee K. Cost-effectiveness of childbirth strategies for prevention of mother-to-child transmission of HIV among mothers receiving nevirapine in India. Indian J Community Med 2010; 35(1):29–33.
32. Miotti PG, Taha TE, Kumwenda NI, et al. HIV transmission through breastfeeding: a study in Malawi. JAMA 1999; 282:744–749.
33. Nduati R, John G, Mbori-Ngacha D, et al. Effect of breast feeding and formula feeding on transmission of HIV-1: a randomized clinical trial. JAMA 2000; 283:1167–1174.

34. Coutsoudis A. Method of feeding and transmission of HIV-1 from mothers to children by 15 months of age: prospective cohort study from Durban. 13th International Conference on AIDS, Durban, 2000.

35. Shapiro RL, Hughes MD, Ogwu A, et al. Antiretroviral regimens in pregnancy and breast-feeding in Botswana. N Engl J Med 2010; 362(24):2282–2294.

36. Kesho Bora Study Group. Eighteen-month follow-up of HIV-1-infected mothers and their children enrolled in the Kesho Bora study observational cohorts. J Acquir Immmune Defic Syndr 2010; 54(5):533–541.

37. World Health Organization. Guidelines on Infant Feeding 2010. Available at: http://www.who.int/child_adolescent_health/documents/9789241599535/en.

38. Delmas M, Larsen C, van Benthem B, et al. Cervical squamous intraepithelial lesions in HIV-infected women: prevalence, incidence and regression. AIDS 2000; 14:1775–1784.

39. Luque AE, Demeter LM, Reichman RC. Assoication of human papillomavirus infection and disease with magnitude of human immunodeficiency virus type (HIV-1) RNA plasma level among women with HIV-1 infectino. J Infect Dis 1999; 179:1405.

40. Wright TC, Ellerbrock TV, Chiasson MA, et al. Cervical intraepithelial neoplasia in women infected with human immunodeficiency virus: prevalence, risk factors and validity of Papanicolaou smears. Obstet Gynecol 1994; 84:591–597.

41. Klein RS, Ho GY, Vermund SH, et al. Ris factors for squamous intraepithelial lesions on Pap smear in women at risk for HIV infection. J Infect Dis 1994; 170:1404–1449.

42. Barkan SE, Melnick SL, Preston-Martin S, et al. The women's interagency HIV study: WIHS collaborative study group. Epidemiology 1998; 9(2):117–125.

43. Carpenter CCJ, Mayer KH, Stein MD, et al. HIV infection in North American women: experience with 200 cases and a review of the literature. Medicine (Baltimore) 1991; 70:307–325.

44. Melnick SL, Sherer R, Louis TA, et al. Survival and disease progression according to gender of patients with HIV infection. JAMA 1994; 272:1915–1921.

45. Katzenstein DA, Hammer SM, Hughes MD, et al. The relation of virologic and immunologic markers to clinical outcomes after nucleoside therapy in HIV-infected adults with 200 to 500 CD4+ cells/mm3. AIDS Clinical Trials Group Study 175, Virology Study Team. N Engl J Med 1996; 335:1091–1098.

46. Evans JS, Nims T, Cooley J, et al. Serum levels of virus burden in early-stage human immunodeficiency virus type 1 disease in women. J Infect Dis 1997; 175:795–800.

47. Junghans C, Ledergerber B, Chan P, et al. Sex differences in HIV-1 viral load and progression to AIDS. Lancet 1999; 353:589.

48. Fletcher CV, Acosta EP, Strykowski JM. Gender differences in human pharmacokinetics and pharmacodynamics. J Adolesc Health 1994; 15:619.

49. Aberg JA, Kaplan JE, Libman H, et al. Primary care guidelines for the management of persons infected with human immunodeficiency virus: 2009 update by the HIV Medicine Association of the Infectious Diseases Society of America. Clin Infect Dis 2009; 49:651–681.

50. Mandelblatt JS, Fahs M, Garibaldi K, et al. Association between HIV infection and cervical neoplasia: implications for clinical care of women at risk for both conditions. AIDS 1992; 6:173–178.

51. Palefsky J, Minkoff H, Kalish LA, et al. Cervicovaginal human papillomavirus infection in human immunodeficiency virus-1 (HIV)-positive and high risk HIV negative women. J Natl Cancer Inst 1999; 91(3):226–236.
52. Shapiro MF, Morton SC, McCaffrey DF, et al. Variations in the care of HIV-infected adults in the United States: results from the HIV Cost and Services Utilization Study. JAMA 1999; 281:2305–2315.
53. Hellinger FJ. The use of health services by women with HIV infection. Health Serv Res 1993; 28(5):543–561.
54. Stein MD, Piette J, Mor V, et al. Differences in access to zidovudine (AZT) among symptomatic HIV-infected persons. J Gen Intern Med 1991; 6(1):35–40.
55. Mave V, Gahunia M, Frontini M, et al. Gender differences in HIV drug resistance mutations and virological outcome. J Womens Health 2010; [Epub ahead of print].
56. Squires KE, Johnson M, Yang R, et al. Comparative gender analysis of the efficacy and safety of atazanavir/ritonavir and lopinavir/ritonavir at 96 weeks in the CASTLE study. J Antimicrob Chemother 2010; [Epub ahead of print].

11

Systems of care: the model HIV program

INTRODUCTION

From the earliest days of the HIV/AIDS epidemic, it was clear that individuals infected with HIV frequently presented not only with complex medical disorders but also with an array of psychological and social problems, which required a comprehensive and thoughtful approach to care. As the epidemic has continued and the life expectancy of individuals with HIV infection has steadily improved, additional "nonmedical" obstacles to care as well as the wealth of secondary problems associated with the virus, its treatment and newly defined requirements for treatment adherence, and avoidance of complex drug interactions have continued to emerge. In areas with sophisticated systems of care, these needs have further emphasized the need for interdisciplinary cooperation among a variety of health care providers. In the developing countries, confronting poor access to antiretroviral therapy (ART) and other elements of care, this interdisciplinary approach is no less essential, although it may be particularly difficult to achieve.

As ART has become increasingly sophisticated and effective, HIV infection and its direct complications have become less of an immediate cause of morbidity and mortality among patients achieving viral suppression and immune reconstitution. This dramatic shift in the landscape of care has led to an increased emphasis on aligning the long-term health maintenance goals of HIV-infected individuals with those established for everyone. As is discussed in chapter 9, the aging of the HIV population has brought new challenges and necessitated modifications of the overall approach to care. A variety of groups have provided recent updates regarding the components of comprehensive primary care, which include both strategies to enhance the impact of ART and those to reduce the risk and impact of those chronic diseases to which the entire population is at risk.

The HIV/AIDS epidemic has posed an enormous challenge to the development of adequate systems of care. First, it has been most devastating among young adults in their most productive years and in the time of life when family responsibilities are typically at their greatest. Second, the increasingly complex medical needs of HIV-infected individuals, some of which have been amplified by the aging of the successfully treated patients and others by the side effects of ART itself necessitate more comprehensive medical care. Third, the broad medical needs created by HIV infection require equally broad expertise among physicians and other health care personnel, including nurses, social workers, psychologists, counselors, and clinical pharmacists in addition to peer counselors and administrative staff. This breadth of expertise is lacking in all but the most sophisticated and well-financed systems.

This chapter will address the requirements of a comprehensive system of care from the time of entry of the HIV-infected individual placing the emphasis on the ambulatory setting. The approach to initial diagnosis of HIV infection and strategies to expand testing are discussed in chapter 1.

Others chapters in this book address quality assurance and specific obstacles confronting resource-limited settings. In this discussion, the focus will be on the key elements needed to deliver quality care including how they may be adapted to settings in which staffing, training, and equipment shortages represent sometimes insurmountable problems.

THE ELEMENTS OF CARE

Since HIV infection has far-reaching implications for the physical and emotional well-being of the individual, the elements of care, though involving various disciplines, must be carefully integrated if a stable and healthy living situation is goal. This discussion will assume that the individual has entered into care medically stable though not necessarily asymptomatic.

Medical Assessment and Appropriate Plan for Medical Follow-up

As discussed in earlier chapters, this must include not only establishing and recording essential information regarding HIV infection specifically (viral load, CD4 lymphocyte count, etc.) but also the status of disorder directly or indirectly related to HIV infection. These include other infections, including other sexually transmitted diseases, viral hepatitis, and tuberculosis as well as renal insufficiency. Strategies for evaluation and screening for these conditions are discussed elsewhere in this text.

In addition, age- and risk-appropriate screening for chronic diseases including hypertension, diabetes, dyslipidemia, as well as malignancies, particularly breast, cervical, prostate, and colon cancer, should be initiated.

Mental Health Assessment

A variety of mental health issues may confront an individual with HIV infection. Major depression as well as anxiety disorders are particularly common, and a relatively high rate of suicide has been documented among certain risk groups. Bipolar disorders as well as schizophrenia and personality disorders are encountered as in the general population. Of course, the immediate trauma and disruption of receiving a diagnosis of HIV infection, particularly if it comes during a significant illness, often has an enormous impact on the emotional well-being even among individuals without a defined psychiatric disorder.

For these reasons, mental health assessments, particularly depression scales, are important in the initial and repeated evaluation of each patient. The integration of mental health professionals into a comprehensive system of care is essential, although the primary care provider must remain knowledgeable about the psychosocial stresses and needs of their patients.

Social Services Need Assessment

Stable housing has been demonstrated to be critical for HIV-infected individuals to receive effective care. Homelessness in particular may pose nearly insurmountable problems to the individual attempting to adhere to appointment schedules, obtain and take medication appropriately, and maintain good nutrition.

Family Needs

HIV infection does not eliminate the family responsibilities of affected patients. Women in particular may often place the needs of their children ahead of their own care. As understandable as this is, such altruistic and purely practical neglect of scheduled appointments, medication adherence, and even proper nutrition may quickly lead to clinical deterioration. For these reasons, the family situation of each individual must be thoroughly explored. In resource-rich areas where systems of care have become increasingly sophisticated and with the remarkable advances in therapy seen over the past decade, it is likely that fewer infected individuals are struggling to balance their own medical needs with responsibilities. However, most of world's population, particularly those living with HIV infection, do not yet have the advantages of such systems, and family concerns may far outweigh the needs of the individual.

Where resources permit, the provision of daycare, respite care, parenting classes, and child life care may help relieve some of the stress associated with family responsibilities.

Transportation to Services

Transportation to services, clearly an enormous problem in many resource-deprived areas, may raise problems in developed countries, particularly in rural regions. Attention must be paid to the transportation needs of each individual even in urban settings where bus or subway fare as well as clinical condition may pose sometimes hidden barriers to care.

Employment

A diagnosis of HIV infection may have an immediate effect on an individual's employment. In areas where early diagnosis and effective treatment have become commonplace, this impact has been greatly reduced. The reduction in stigma, which has been accomplished in many developed countries, has resulted in less concern regarding the safety of employing persons with HIV and, in many areas, legal protection against termination. However, when diagnosis is delayed until the individual becomes significantly symptomatic or requires very frequent clinic or office visits for any reason, employment may be quickly impacted. This fact is compounded by the relatively high rate of unemployment among certain high-risk populations, particularly active injection drug users.

For some, job training may be appropriate. Our program, located in New York City, has offered computer training and English-as-a-second-language courses to facilitate entry or reentry into the job market.

The loss of employment and income has obvious and far-reaching effects. In addition to its place as one of life's most stressful events under any circumstances, it brings immediate financial problems as well as stigma and sometimes rejection by friends and family. The impact on health insurance, if the employer provided it, and the need to qualify for public assistance compound the situation further and may add to feelings of hopelessness. As in the case of family obligations and housing and transportation needs, the effects of joblessness may be completely unapparent to caregivers and manifest simply as failure to keep appointments or fill prescriptions, or emotional or psychiatric issues. The key role of social services in examining these issues on an individual basis and periodically reassessing all of these factors is obvious. The comprehensive HIV/AIDS program cannot reach its potential and fully care for all of its patients if these issues are not systematically and effectively addressed.

Partner Notification

Notification of sexual partners who may have become infected may be an extremely difficult process for some. It is the responsibility of care givers and of the program as a whole to facilitate effective and documented partner notification. Of course, because of the long latent period of HIV infection, during which transmission may occur, it may be impossible even for well-intentioned patients to identify and notify all potentially exposed partners. All efforts (as local laws permit and mandate) must be made to notify current and prior spouses, however, as well as other current or former partners who can be identified. Because of the delicate and traumatic nature of this important task, individuals may ask for assistance in notifying a partner, or, as a last resort, public health authorities, depending on local practices, may provide anonymous notification. Partner notification, accompanied by the provision of easy access to HIV counseling and testing, is a vital strategy in reducing the number of infected individuals who are unaware of their HIV status. This group, predominantly female in the United States, are not only potential candidates for the full range of HIV-related services described in this chapter but also represent a reservoir of infection with the potential for further transmission.

Advance Directives

Advance directives, including health care proxies where available, plans to care for children in the event of the death of a parent, wills, and other instruments are vitally important for any adult, particularly those with responsibility for others. For the individual with advanced HIV infection, these issues may suddenly become immediate concerns. There is every reason to openly discuss advance directives early in the care of all patients and to systemically record and periodically reevaluate the status of their wishes.

Prevention and Harm Reduction

It has been demonstrated that an individual's knowledge that they are HIV infected typically reduces sexual transmission by that individual (Oguabugu presentation). Nonetheless, high-risk behaviors, both that foster transmission to others and that are harmful to the individual, may continue. In a system of care for HIV-infected patients, prevention of transmission and reduction of harm to self are directly linked with each other.

PROGRAM STRUCTURE

The emphasis of the chapter is on ambulatory services. Traditional obstacles to be overcome in the ambulatory care of HIV-infected individuals include access to care, convenient referral among disciplines and medical specialties, and efficient record-keeping among others.

Staffing

Since the bulk of HIV care takes place in the outpatient setting, staffing of a system of care should ideally include a diversity of professionals and, perhaps, nonprofessional peer support staff designed to provide the breadth of care and meet the challenges of the ambulatory patient.

Physicians and Other Staff Providing Direct Clinical Care

At the center of an adequate system of care lies the physician, nurse practitioner, or physician's assistant capable of conducting a through clinical assessment and designing screening, treatment, preventive, and follow-up medical plans for patients at all stages of HIV/AIDS. In the past decade, the concept of the HIV Specialist (1) has emerged and is supported by a number of professional societies. In well-resourced areas, the majority of care of HIV-infected individuals is provided by such professionals. As life expectancy increases and changes in retroviral therapy become a less frequent necessity, generalists, including primary care internists, family practitioners and hospitalists may take on an increasing share of the care, but at this time the pace of change in HIV care strategies is such that a clinician with a specific emphasis on HIV and its ramifications is probably optimal where feasible. This clinician is typically has specific training in all aspects of HIV care and is required to maintain sufficient credentials through patient volume and continuing medical education (CME) to demonstrated a state-of-the- art knowledge of the basics of HIV care. The ability to remain current regarding treatment guidelines as well as the experience and training to recognize the symptoms of HIV itself, complicating infections as well as side effects of ART and other medication is critical to the effective long-term management of patients in care. Ideally, the clinician should have a manageable number of patients on a standing panel who are followed longitudinally as well as the time and facilities to evaluate patients newly entering care and to fill in for colleagues in the temporary management of their patients when necessary.

Nurses

The role of the nurse knowledgeable in HIV care is indispensible in comprehensive systems of care. In the role of administering medications, providing instructions to patients regarding medication use and lifestyle issues and representing a bridge to the clinician provider, the HIV nurse has assumed a role as essential as that in all fields of medicine. Far beyond these traditional functions, however, the nurse in a comprehensive and well-integrated HIV program provides specific guidance to the patient on the logistical issues, which can often seem insurmountable to the patient entering or maintaining himself/herself in care perhaps, especially in resource-limited settings (2,3). Specialty and subspecialty referrals, telephone triage, follow-up of patients' care needs and comprehension of their often complex care requirements can be readily facilitated by a nurse trained in the issues that these patients confront. It is not unusual for the nurse in such a program to become the primary contact person for the patient between visits to the clinician and the link between the patient and their HIV specialist provider. In the final chapter of this book, some of our group's specific findings and experiences in collaborating with HIV/AIDS programs in Russia (4,5) and in Ethiopia are outlined. In both of these diverse cultural and medical environments, it was quickly recognized that the role of the nurse could and should be raised above the carrying out of traditional tasks. An intake clinic for initial assessment, including laboratory studies, education, and orientation of patients newly entering outpatient care, is largely based on the nurses in our and other programs to enhance efficiency of the first provider visit and to help the patient understand the structure of services. In our program in a large hospital-based HIV/AIDS clinic in New York City, this intake clinic, staffed both by nurses and social workers, has served an invaluable purpose in helping patients to overcome the initial impact of the HIV diagnosis, its potential stigma, and to understand the seemingly complex array of services, some needed, some not, available through insurance and entitlement programs. As in the case of all HIV care providers, the nurse must maintain a manageable workload to function effectively.

Social Workers and Social Service Staff

The skills of social workers and related staff bridge the mental health and logistical needs of the patient in countless ways. From assisting the recently diagnosed patient in coping with the emotional impact and family ramifications of his/her diagnosis to performing early screening for depression and other mental illness, to helping the patient navigate the complex world of entitlements and other services that they have entered, the HIV-trained social service staff hold a special place in the comprehensive model of an HIV/AIDS program for ambulatory and hospitalized patients. Mental health interventions beyond initial screening individual and group therapy may also fall under the purview of this component of staff. Interactions between the base program and community agencies devoted to providing services to HIV-infected individuals, including housing, nutrition, and additional mental health and logistical support, are also typically the province of these professionals. As was the case in collaborations between by the Elmhurst Hospital Center AIDS Program and programs in Russia and in Ethiopia, social workers, in short supply in both locations, were found to be underutilized and confined to traditional roles. In resource-limited settings, the value of all professionals willing to accept training in HIV care and assignment to centers providing services to these patients is greatly magnified, and the utilization of social service staff can be indispensible even in areas where central clinical care is underresourced (4,5).

Clinical Pharmacy Staff

Several factors have emerged over the course of the HIV/AIDS epidemic to elevate the role of clinical pharmacists in the overall structure of a comprehensive HIV/AIDS program:

- The proliferation of antiretroviral agents with their attendant side effects and drug interactions
- The aging of the HIV/AIDS population with the inevitable need for additional medications to treat such disorders as coronary artery disease, diabetes and cancer, further complicating ART management
- The recognition that medication errors are a frequent cause of adverse outcomes in both the inpatient and outpatient settings

Clinical pharmacists who become particularly knowledgeable in the management of HIV infection can form an indispensible component of an effective treatment adherence program and can counsel and advise patients on the proper timing of dosing of their medications as well as practical strategies in avoiding or managing side effects. Ma and colleagues demonstrated a significant impact of clinical pharmacists in reducing pill burden (6). A system of care in which pharmacy staff review all newly prescribed medications for potential drug interactions and assist in counseling patients at every change in ART is a valuable asset to the patients and the clinical staff. As in the case of nurses and social service staff, the pharmacist can serve as an accessible and knowledgeable resource for the patient after and between provider visits. Once again, efficient services with pharmacy staff with manageable case loads are essential to maintain patient satisfaction with pharmacy services as described here (7).

Peer Group Intervention

Although little data are available to assess the effectiveness of involving peers (HIV-infected individuals) in various aspects of comprehensive HIV/AIDS programs, the value of selected individuals in the overall care strategy may be great. Many programs in both resource-rich and resource-limited settings (8,9) involve peers in strategies to educate and encourage patients and to assist in maintenance in care and medication adherence.

Care Management

Case management and care management have been recognized in recent years as potentially important strategies in coordinating services, both inpatient and outpatient, for patients with chronic disease. Data regarding the impact of these modalities on HIV care so far is sparse. It is hoped that individual care coordinators working in collaboration with the rest of the team of a comprehensive HIV/AIDS team can effectively facilitate linkage into the various aspects of care that many patients require (10,11).

Patient Advisory Groups

The value of small, representative groups of patients attending and HIV/AIDS program can be significant. Views of individual patients regarding efficiencies, attitudes of staff, cleanliness of the clinic, and other issues that may not be apparent to the clinical staff may be extremely valuable in maintaining overall patient satisfaction and, thereby, encouraging maintenance in care and confidence in providers. The input of such patient groups may also be sought in the selection or design of clinical trials or other forms of research into practices at the facility.

Access to Care

Entry into Care

Regardless of the urgency to institute antiretroviral or other types of therapy, referral into the system of care should come as quickly as possible after the initial diagnosis of HIV infection. Systems of outreach to patients not attending their initial or subsequent appointments are essential to an effective comprehensive program. In the most resource-deprived areas of the world, such outreach represents one of the most difficult barriers to effective treatment. Lack of convenient and affordable transportation to services represents a completely insurmountable barrier in some regions and creates an environment where progression of disease and drug resistance as well as spread of infection are unavoidable.

Specialty Referral

Specialty care has represented an extremely important component of comprehensive HIV care since the beginning of the epidemic. As noted above, in recent years, national organizations have offered HIV specialist designation based on CME in specific care of HIV infection and its complications as well as practical experience in treating a minimum number of patients. This reflects the unique and increasingly complex body of knowledge required to navigate issues in ART as well as screening and management of the host of medical issues involved. Specific specialties, such as gynecology, neurology, ophthalmology, gastroenterology, psychiatry, and dermatology, have long played a vital role in the screening and management of patients for complications of disease and therapy. As the HIV/AIDS population has aged and ART has become increasingly effective, chronic diseases and other conditions associated with aging have become an ever-growing aspect of comprehensive care. Thus, additional specialties such as geriatrics, cardiology, nephrology, oncology, and hepatology have taken on important roles in the ongoing management of many patients, including those who have long achieved complete viral suppression and immune reconstitution.

Record Keeping

Accurate and thorough maintenance of medical records is of course essential to comprehensive care of any individual. HIV treatment requires particularly thorough documentation of CD4 cell counts, viral load, and resistance assays as well as ART treatment histories. As many individuals currently in care have progressed through various treatment regimens and viral mutants resistant to previously used agents may impact on the effectiveness of future therapeutic strategies, an understanding of treatment history is extremely important to effective care.

New guidelines and recommendations regarding screening for chronic conditions and malignancies have recently been promulgated (12). Since these guidelines typically recommend screening for, as an example, latent tuberculosis or cervical neoplasia, on specific timetables, records of prior screening studies must be maintained accurately.

Again, the aging of the HIV population in care and the complex metabolic consequences of HIV infection and ART now necessitate close attention to traditional risk factors for vascular disease in particular (e.g., hypertension and dyslipidemia). Screening for other conditions, some of which are impacted by HIV infection, such as osteoporosis, and some that are apparently not impacted, such as breast neoplasia, also require that schedules of screening tests be adhered to and documented.

Of course, unique challenges in accurate maintenance of records are presented by individuals under evaluation and/or treatment for viral hepatitis or tuberculosis.

SUMMARY

The model HIV program in well-resourced areas may take various forms. In resource-rich areas where major free-standing, private, or hospital-based programs provide ready access to services, certain components should be consistently provided. These include the following:

1. Access to rapid testing
2. Access to CD4 count, viral load, and genotypic resistance testing
3. Immediate referral into care for the HIV-infected individual
4. Care by a provider and team trained and skilled in the management of HIV infection at all stages, ART, and complications of disease and treatment
5. Convenient access to appropriate specialty and subspecialty referral
6. Ready referral for psychiatric evaluation when appropriate and psychosocial support
7. A means of referral or provision of substance abuse treatment
8. Full access to antiretroviral agents
9. A developed adherence program
10. A program of nutritional assessment and management
11. Provision for transport to services and, when necessary, home care and other forms of outreach
12. Meticulous record keeping and portability of records
13. A program for maintenance in care
14. Strategies for informing contacts and potential contacts

THE CONCEPT OF THE MEDICAL HOME

In recent years, the concept of a "medical home" for all patients has been promulgated as a means to avoid fragmentary care among multiple specialties, to enhance communication among caregivers, and to assure that basic preventive services as well as evidence-based prevention and care of all patients are provided in an organized and efficient fashion. In many areas of the developed world, since the early years of the HIV/AIDS epidemic, interdisciplinary teams of HIV physician specialists and specially trained nurses, social workers, and a variety of other personnel as well as dedicated subspecialists have developed systems aligned with this model.

Developed by the American Academy of Family Physicians (www.aafp. org) and other organizations, the components of a medical home span the elements of a system of care from registration procedures that feature easy access and availability of appointments, centralized and comprehensive problem lists and laboratory result tracking, thorough and accurate medication information for each patient, as well as continuous performance evaluation, quality improvement, and evidence-based decision support regarding treatment and prevention strategies. Out-of-office or home monitoring of patients' progress as well as home services should be provided where needed. Perhaps, most importantly, the strategy includes specific goals set for each individual patient with collaborative monitoring of attainment of those goals.

Embedded in this model is creation of core measures of performance and a clear understanding between the health care provider and the patient as to the goals of care.

Many structured approaches to care of individuals with HIV infection have been proposed and continuously refined. As an example, the New York State Department of Health sets criteria for HIV facilities to be recognized as designated AIDS centers (DACs) using much of the philosophy underlying the medical home concept.

RESOURCE-LIMITED AREAS

Unfortunately, most of the world's population do not have access to the system of comprehensive care referred to here. In fact, in the countries most impacted by the HIV/AIDS epidemic, staff, facility, and equipment shortages make the concept of comprehensive care and the medical home impossible to achieve as described above. Many of these countries remain plagued by inadequate and/or inconsistent supplies of antiretroviral agents, a lack of sufficient staff in all categories, inadequate systems of record keeping and quality assurance, insufficient transportation and outreach, an absence of care coordination, and a desperate shortage of trained specialists and subspecialists. Nonetheless, heroic efforts in many communities and regions most impacted have led to the development of programs that include some of the elements mentioned above. As antiretroviral drug supplies have gradually become more available, systems to allow for scaling up of service delivery have evolved in parallel. Where physician shortages exist, the role of nurses has, in some cases, been enhanced. Additional staff, including social service professionals and staff focused on treatment adherence and care coordination, have been employed in a variety of settings. Peer involvement, although somewhat unproven but relatively inexpensive, has emerged as a model of care coordination, education, and linkage to services in some resource-deprived areas. Issues confronting resource-deprived areas are myriad, and potential strategies to provide adequate care in absence of full laboratory, pharmaceutical support and appropriate staffing are addressed in chapters 12 and 13. Nonetheless, despite the remarkable advances made in the treatment of HIV/AIDS in resource-rich countries, it remains a grim fact that most of the world's HIV-infected individuals in need of antiretroviral treatment by all criteria remain untreated and destined to progress.

REFERENCES

1. Kasten MJ. Human immunodeficiency virus: the initial physician-patient encounter. Mayo Clin Proc 2002; 77(9):957–962.
2. Chen WT, Shiu CS, Simoni J, et al. Optimizing HIV care by expanding the nursing role: patient and provider perspectives. J Adv Nurs 2010; 66(2):260–268.
3. Mapanga KG, Mapanga MB. A modern African perspective on the role of the clinical nurse specialist. Clin Nurse Spec 2008; 22(5):226–230.
4. Komarov N, Gerasimov V, Mikhaylov S, et al. Improving HIV-related care and support through a partnership between a New York city AIDS and an AIDS center in the Russian Federation. AIDS 2006-SVI International AIDS Conference: Abstract no. CDB1272.
5. Komarov N, Gerasimov V, Mikhaylov S, et al. Utilizing a healthcare twinning partnership between a New York City municipal hospital AIS program and a regional health administration to develop social services for PLWHA in Orenburg, Russia. AIDS 2006—SVI International AIDS Conference Abstract no CDB1297.
6. Ma A, Chen DM, Chau FM, et al. Improving adherence and clinical outcomes through an HIV pharmacist's interventions. AIDS Care 2010; 22(10):1189–1194.
7. Karunamoothi K, Rajalakshmi M, Babu SM, et al. HIV/AIDS patients's satisfactory and their expectations with pharmacy service at specialist antiretroviral therapy (ART) units. Eur Rev Med Pharmacol Sci 2009; 13(5):331–339.
8. Medley A, Kennedy C, O'Reilly K, et al. Effectiveness of peer education interventions for HIV prevention in developing countries: a systematic review and meta-analysis. AIDS Educ Prev 2009; 21(3):181–206.
9. Norr KF, Norr JL, McElmhurry BJ, et al. Impact of peer group educaton in HIV prevention among women in Botswana. Health Care Women Int 2004; 25(3):210–226.
10. London AS, LeBlanc AJ, Aneshensel CS. The integration of informal care, case management and community-based services for persons with HIV/AIDS. AIDS Care 1998; 10(4):481–503.
11. Vargas RB, Cunningham WE. Evolving trends in medical care-coordination for patients with HIV and AIDS. Curr HIV/AIDS Rep 2006; 3(4):149–153.
12. Aberg JA, Kaplan JE, Libman H, et al. Primary care guidelines for the management of persons infected with human immunodeficiency virus: 2009 update by the HIV Medicine Association of the Infectious Diseases Society of American. Clin Infect Dis 2009; 49:651–681.

12

Quality management in the care of HIV-infected individuals

INTRODUCTION

In the United States and other developed countries, the cost of care for individual HIV-infected patients has fallen since shortly after the advent of modern antiretroviral therapy (ART) largely because of decreased rates of hospitalization and reduced hospital stays (1). The focus of care has moved increasingly into the outpatient setting. Almost simultaneously, managed care systems have proliferated in the United States, placing increased emphasis on standardization of treatment for chronic disease. Quality management as a discipline in health care has also come to the fore in recent years. The focus in this chapter will be on issues in quality management of the HIV-infected patient. Strategies to approach the diagnosis of HIV are included in chapter 1. Specific issues relevant to the elderly patients and to women are addressed in chapters 9 and 10, respectively. The final portion of this chapter is devoted to the unique issues confronted in resource-limited settings in establishing and measuring meaningful quality indicators.

During the past decade, there has been an increasing emphasis on the quality of health care delivered in the United States and other developed countries. The Institute of Medicine report Crossing the Quality Chasm (2) released in 2001 underscored the potential impact of establishing measurable standards and outcome of care in hospitals. Other data pointed to inconsistent adherence to professional standards in disease management (3).

Efforts to measure and standardize the quality of care provided to individuals infected with HIV had begun during the 1990s. Data indicating that practitioners and hospitals experienced in the management of HIV infection and its complications achieved better clinical outcomes had been noted early in the epidemic (4). In part because of the rapidly changing approach to the management of HIV/AIDS during that period, national standards embodying broad aspects of care were not fully promulgated until recent years (5,6).

Over the course of the HIV/AIDS epidemic, health care facilities in many countries have focused increasingly on quantitative measures of the quality of care delivered for all patients. As the full spectrum of issues confronting the individual with HIV/AIDS has become clear, specific quality measures appropriate for their care have come into sharper focus. Indicators of quality of care can be divided in several categories. These include the following:

1. Therapeutics: Provision of appropriate ART as well as measures to prevent opportunistic infections when applicable
2. Surveillance: Screening for HIV-associated disorders and other chronic conditions seen with increased frequency in the setting of HIV infection
3. General medical screening and chronic disease management
4. Mental health assessment and therapy when indicated
5. Nutritional counseling
6. Treatment adherence counseling
7. Social support
8. Patient satisfaction

In this chapter, strategies to define and assess quality of care will be reviewed and explored. Quality improvement strategies may take a variety of forms, but measurement of specific indicators and evaluation of measures instituted to improve care are central to these efforts. Much of the material covered here is most easily applied to developed countries possessing resources to dedicate multidisciplinary staff to the care of individuals infected with HIV. However, most of the most heavily affected regions of the world cannot devote vast resources to a single disease. In light of this fact, efforts to measure and achieve the highest attainable quality of care in resource-deprived areas will also be addressed. The reader is referred to chapter 14 for discussions of measures adopted in underserved areas to provide prevention and treatment of HIV/AIDS. Quality measures must, of necessity, go beyond these critical goals, however, and must also address the additional elements listed above. Among the many turning points faced in the three-decade global battle against the HIV epidemic, the currently emerging emphasis on provision of comprehensive care of the highest quality possible regardless of setting is clearly the most challenging and the most crucial of those that lay ahead.

QUALITY MANAGEMENT

The impact of quality monitoring has not been extensively evaluated. Nonetheless, the complexity of the care of individuals with HIV/AIDS necessitates the development and monitoring of quality indicators within all systems of care provided to these patients. The specific quality indicators most associated with favorable outcome can be debated, but the need for monitoring is indisputable.

It is clear that the availability and quality of care offered to HIV/AIDS patients is variable, even in sophisticated health care systems. For example, access to new antiretroviral agents and other treatment advances has been shown to vary from region to region (7).

High-quality medical care of HIV-infected patients requires several basic components.

1. Ready access into a comprehensive program of primary care from the time an individual is initially diagnosed with HIV infection
2. Easy availability and appropriate use of markers of disease stage, that is, viral load and T-cell subset analysis
3. Access to new antiretroviral therapies
4. Access to entitlement information when appropriate and facilitation of the application process for entitlement services, including drug assistance plans
5. A system that permits a prompt, comprehensive medical assessment including thorough history, physical examination, and mental health assessment as well as screening diagnostic studies (complete blood count, renal function tests, electrolytes, liver function tests, hepatitis A, B, and C as well as serologic tests for syphilis and toxoplasmosis, chest X ray, and tuberculin skin test)
6. Efficient referral to the care of a provider qualified and experienced in the care of individuals with HIV infection
7. Ready availability of specialty subspecialty consultation in the following areas: ophthalmology, dentistry, neurology, dermatology, gastroenterology, gynecology, psychiatry, and general surgery

Selecting Quality Indicators

In establishing a program of quality assessment, it is important to set defined, measurable goals (8). Some examples are as follows.

Volume Indicators

Volume indicators such as number of visits, newly enrolled patients, missed appointment rates, and demographic data may provide insight into the effectiveness of a program in reaching the community it attempts to serve and of its success in retaining patients once enrolled. Such data is typically the simplest to obtain but gives only indirect information about medical outcomes.

Process Indicators

These indicators measure services offered such as numbers of influenza vaccines, Pap smears, or patient education sessions. Although they provide insight into structural problems and staffing needs, they do not fully reflect outcomes.

Outcomes Indicators

In general, the most difficult data to extract, outcomes indicators provide the best measure of overall program effectiveness. Indicators such as hospitalization rates, opportunistic infection prevention, rates of viral suppression, provider competence, patient satisfaction, and treatment adherence, if measured accurately, provide a basis for redirecting, expanding, or modifying services. Because it is vitally important that adherence with ART be kept at a very high level to avoid the emergence of drug resistance, appointment compliance and treatment adherence represent paramount quality outcomes indicators.

Hospitalization rates. Combination ART has had the effect of dramatically reducing the need for hospitalization of patients with HIV/AIDS. In a large care system in Massachusetts, the hospital admission rate fell by 70% between 1995 and 1996 (9). Rates of and indications for hospitalization should be monitored concurrently. Such information can be used to evaluate the effectiveness of prevention of opportunistic infections and adherence to ART. Hospital length of stay data can provide insight into efficiency of inpatient care systems. Patient satisfaction with inpatient care should be monitored systematically.

Provider experience. Provider experience is related to outcome in the care of HIV-infected patients. In a New York state study, patients followed in clinics caring for at least 100 patients had a 50% decrease in relative hazard of death (10).

If possible, patients should be under the direct care of providers with specific training and/or significant experience in treating HIV infection and its complications (e.g., 20 patient years). Such qualifications have been developed to define the so-called HIV specialist by managed care organizations and governmental bodies (11).

Because of the rapidly changing nature of HIV care, providers should be committed to continuous educational activities. Inexperienced providers should be supervised by HIV specialists for a period of at least several months. If any of these criteria cannot be met, indirect supervision should be arranged whereby an HIV specialist reviews care indicators at regular intervals and is readily available for consultation.

Prevention of opportunistic infections. The rates of most opportunistic infections have declined substantially among patients receiving effective ART. Some of these infections, such as *Pneumocystis carinii* pneumonia (PCP) and toxoplasmosis, are almost entirely preventable in patients at risk by appropriate use of prophylaxis. For these reasons, adherence to guidelines for such prophylaxis represents a critical quality indicator for any program or provider caring for HIV-infected patients.

Consensus Measures of Quality: United States

In 2007 in the United States, a work group of HIV clinical experts was convened by the National Committee for Quality Assurance with the purpose of achieving consensus on measures of quality of HIV care (Box 12.1) (12). Prior efforts by the New York State Department of Health AIDS Institute, the Veterans Administration, and others formed a significant basis for the selection of specific measures. The processes through which care was delivered as well as outcomes and accountability for the quality of care were taken into account, and performance measures were proposed (12). The measures selected were endorsed by the American Medical Association, the Infectious Diseases Society of America, the HIV Medicine Association (HIVMA), and other bodies. Practice guidelines have been developed by HIVMA, incorporating these performance measures (see chap. 2) (13) as pilot testing of the specific performance measures takes place.

Box 12.1 Recommended Quality Measures

1. Retention in care[a]
2. CD4 cell count[b]
3. Gonorrhea/chlamydia screening[c]
4. Syphilis screening[d]
5. Injection drug use screening[d]
6. High-risk sexual behavior screening[d]
7. Tuberculosis screening[c]
8. Hepatitis B screening[c]
9. Hepatitis C screening[c]
10. Influenza immunization[d]
11. Pneumococcal immunization[c]
12. Hepatitis B vaccination first dose (if appropriate)
13. Hepatitis B vaccination series completed (if appropriate)
14. *Pneumocystis carinii* pneumonia prophylaxis (if CD4 count $<200/mm^3$
15. Appropriately prescribed antiretroviral therapy
16. Achieving maximal viral control if receiving antiretroviral therapy
17. Treatment plan documented if maximal viral control not achieved

---

[a] seen at least twice annually at least 60 days apart

[b] at least twice annually

[c] at least once

[d] annually

Source: Adapted from Ref. 6.

Measuring Quality in Resource-Limited Settings

The cost of providing high-quality services to HIV-infected individuals in resource-limited settings represents an enormous obstacle in the global effort against HIV/AIDS. In this section, a series of questions are posed regarding specific elements of care, and relevant data is presented illustrating strategies that have been proposed or implemented to overcome obstacles in achieving these elements. In some instances, the reader is referred to other sections of this book for a more complete discussion of the issues.

How Is Antiretroviral Therapy Initiated?

If drug supplies are limited or unpredictable. Inadequate and unpredictable supplies of antiretroviral drugs remain an enormous global dilemma, and only a small minority of individuals requiring therapy are receiving it (see chap. 14) despite the fact that the cost of many drugs has been reduced dramatically in recent years and a number of resource-limited countries manufacture or purchase generic versions of some of them. The negative impact of the inevitable rationing of resources when drug supplies are inadequate can be partially mitigated by providing therapy to those most in need (CD4 cell count below 200 cells/mm^3) to enhance survival until worldwide supply issues can be resolved.

If viral load and resistance testing are not available. Decisions regarding the initiation of ART can be made in the absence of viral load and resistance testing technology. Although more definitive data regarding the optimal point at which to initiate therapy awaits the results of ongoing clinical trials (see chap. 5), the CD4 cell count currently guides this decision in almost all cases. Many resource-deprived regions do possess the technology to measure CD4 counts. Recent guidelines based on clinical outcomes data have suggested that therapy be initiated at relatively high CD4 cell counts. Walensky and colleagues (14) projected improved survival and reduction in opportunistic infections when ART was initiated at counts of 350 cells/mm^3 when compared with later initiation.

Viral load monitoring by means of the technology in use in developed countries is expensive. The high cost, in addition to the equipment and training required to perform these assays, is prohibitive for many areas in the developing world. One cost reduction measure that has been proposed is the use of pooled testing of large numbers of blood specimens divided into matrices or cohorts. Tilghman and colleagues (15) reported substantial cost savings over individual viral load testing using this strategy.

Less expensive techniques for measuring viral load, such as ultrasensitive p24 and the reverse transcriptase assay, are available but are also difficult to use in resource-limited settings. Newer methods, which take advantage of recent developments in nanotechnology, are in development (16).

If adherence to therapy and retention in care cannot be assured. A high level of adherence to antiretroviral treatment is necessary to delay virologic failure. Although modern first-line regimens are simpler and likely associated with greater patient adherence than earlier regimens (see chap. 5), 95% adherence remains the difficult target for most patients. Data demonstrating substantially lower levels of treatment adherence is abundant in many populations. In resource-limited settings, antiretroviral drugs are typically in very particularly limited and often sporadic supply, and monitoring of therapeutic response is particularly difficult because of limited availability of CD4 cell and viral load testing. Many potential barriers to 95% compliance with therapy exist in these environments. Working in India, Venkatesh and colleagues (17) found increased odds of poor adherence among: individuals with CD4 cell counts greater than 500 cells/mm^3, those who had been on therapy for more than two years, and individuals with poor perception of their own health. Although such characteristics are likely associated with poor adherence in many regions, data such as this suggests that there are specific medical and psychosocial situations that are predictive of early virologic failure. In other resource-limited settings, characteristics of individuals struggling with treatment adherence may be identifiable, allowing for focused adherence counseling.

Weekly SMS messaging through the use of mobile phones was found to result in higher rates of treatment adherence and viral suppression by Lester and colleagues (18) working in Kenya.

How Can the Effect of Therapy Be Monitored?

If CD4 lymphocyte counts are not available. If CD4 counts cannot be measured, the total lymphocyte count on a routine complete blood count may aid in identifying patients with low CD4 counts who require preventive therapy for opportunistic infections. It has been suggested that the CD4+ lymphocyte count can be estimated within broad limits if only the total lymphocyte count is obtainable. In a study in India, Srirangaraj and colleagues (19) demonstrated 88% sensitivity and 35% specificity of a total lymphocyte of <1200 cells/mm^3 for a CD4 count of <200 cells/mm^3. Sensitivity rose to 95% and specificity to 100% among patients with active tuberculosis.

Low-cost technology for determining CD4 cell counts (20), when compared with World Health Organization staging algorithms, was projected to result in a 90% increase in cost-effectiveness, comparable to that seen with routine CD4 count measurement methodology.

If viral load monitoring is not available. The lack of availability of viral load assays is commonplace in resource-limited settings throughout the world.

Clinical evaluation and CD4 lymphocyte counts represent the only means of evaluating response to therapy in many countries.

Although first-line therapy in treatment-naïve therapy can be initiated in the absence of baseline viral load measurements when necessary, changing to second-line regimens is particularly challenging. Clinical and immunologic evaluation may overestimate virologic failure and result in premature changes in ART and limitation of future therapeutic options. In a government-sponsored program in India in which viral load monitoring was employed to confirm treatment failure, 25% of patients with clinical and immunologic decline were found to have adequate virologic suppression (21).

If viral resistance monitoring is not available. Viral resistance testing, used to guide initial and subsequent choices of therapy in the United States and other countries in which the technology is widely available, is not currently being performed in most of the countries most impacted by HIV/AIDS. One key obstacle to the more widespread availability of resistance testing is the difficulty in obtaining plasma specimens required for genotypic assays from individuals living in remote areas. The use of dried blood spot for such resistance testing has been found to correlate well with assays using plasma (22) and represents a means of obtaining and transporting appropriate specimens to reference laboratories. This technique, however, requires rapid transport of specimens under proper conditions of heat and humidity (23).

REFERENCES

1. Shaw-Taylor Y, Andrulis DP. AIDS in the developed world: implications for the provision and financing of care. AIDS 1997; 11:1305.
2. Committee on Quality of Health Care in America, Institute of Medicine. Crossing the quality chasm: a new health system for the 21st century. Washing, DC: National Academy Press, 2001.
3. McGlynn EA, Asch SM, Adams J, et al. The quality of health care delivered to adults in the United States. N Engl J Med 2003; 348:2635–2645.
4. Bennet CL, Garfinkle JB, Greenfield S, et al. The relation between hospital experience and in-hospital mortality for patients with AIDS-related PCP. JAMA 1989; 261:2975–2979.
5. Bozette SA. Quality of care for patients infected with HIV. Clin Infect Dis 2010; 516 (6):739–740.
6. Horberg MA, Aberg JA, Cheever LW, et al. Development of national and multi-agency HIV care quality measures. Clin Infect Dis 2010; 51(6):732–738.
7. Birkhead G, Agins BD, Jemiolo DJ, et al. Access to combination antiretroviral therapy (CART) among different populations: implementation of new guidelines for treatment of HIV infection. Int Conf AIDS 1998; 12(abstr 22333):329.
8. Valenti WM. Managing HIV/AIDS: HIV, managed care, and outcomes. Drug Benefit Trends 2000; 12:25.

9. Gallagher D, Helliger JA, Master RJ, et al. The CMA experience: applying combination antiretroviral therapy in a U.S. inner city, advanced AIDS population. Will viral rebound translate to increased costs. Int Conf AIDS 1998; 12:603.

10. Laine C, Markson LE, McKee LJ, et al. The relationahip of clinic experience with advanced HIV and survival of women with AIDS. AIDS 1998; 12:417.

11. Simmon J. Maximizing AIDS expertise. Healthplan 1997; 38:11.

12. Horberg MA, Aberg JA, Cheever LW, et al. Development and multiagency HIV quality care measures. Clin Infect Dis 2010; 51(6):732–738.

13. Aberg JA, Kaplan JE, Libman H, et al. Primary guidelines for the management of persons infected with human immunodeficiency virus: 2009 update by the HIV Medicine Association of the Infectious Diseases Society of America. Clin Infect Dis 2009; 49(5):651–681.

14. Walensky RP, Wolf LL, Wood R, et al. When to start antiretroviral therapy in resource-limited settings. Ann Intern Med 2009; 151(3):157–166.

15. Tilghman MW, Guerena DD, Licea A, et al. Pooled nucleic acid testing to detect antiretroviral treatment failure in Mexico. J Acquir Immune Defic Syndr 2010; [Epub ahead of print].

16. Wang S, Xu F, Demirci U. Advances in developing HIV-1 viral load assays for resource-limited settings. Biotechnol Adv 2010; 28(6):770–781.

17. Venkatesh KK, Srikrishnan AK, Mayer KH, et al. Predictors of nonadherence to highly active antiretroviral therapy among HIV-infected South Indians in clinical care: implications for developing adherence interventions in resource-limited settings. AIDS Patient Care STDS 2010; 24(12):795–803.

18. Lester RT, Ritvo P, Mills EJ, et al. Effects of a mobile phone short message service on antiretroviral treatment adherence in Kenya (WelTel Kenya1): a randomized trial. Lancet 2010; 376(9755):1838–1845.

19. Srirangaraj S, Venkatesha D. Total lymphocyte count as a tool for timing opportunistic infection prophylaxis in resource-limited settings: a study from India. J Infect Dev Ctries 2010; 4(10):645–649.

20. Athan E, O'Brien DP, Legood R. Cost-effectivness of routine and low-cost CD4 T-cell count compared with WHO clinical staging of HIV to guide initiation of antiretroviral therapy in resource-limited settings. AIDS 2010; 24(12):1887–1895.

21. Rewari BB, Bachani D, Rajasekaran S, et al. Evaluating patients for second-line antiretroviral therapy in India: the role of targeted viral load testing. J Acquir Immune Defic Syndr 2010; [Epub ahead of print].

22. Bertagnolio S, Parkin NT, Jordan M, et al. Dried blood spots for HIV-1 drug resistance and viral load testing: a review of current knowledge and WHO efforts for global HIV drug resistance surveillance. AIDS Rev 2010; 12(4):195–208.

23. Garcia-Lerma JG, McNulty A, Jennings C, et al. Rapid decline in the efficiency of HIV drug resistance genotyping from dried blood spots (DPS) stored at 37 degrees C and high humidity. J Antimicrob Chemother 2009; 64(1):33–36.

13

The global effort against HIV/AIDS: issues in resource-deprived areas

INTRODUCTION

Although the HIV/AIDS epidemic first came to the attention of the public and the medical community in the United States and, shortly afterward, in other developed countries, the most hard-hit regions of the world have been the impoverished countries. Sub-Saharan Africa was quickly recognized as the focal point and likely origin of the epidemic and still accounts for approximately two-thirds of estimated cases (1). Some countries of the Caribbean basin were almost equally affected at first. In the decades since, poor- and middle-income countries of Southeast Asia, the horn of Africa, and, most recently, India, China, Russia, and other countries of the former Soviet Union both in eastern Europe and in central Asia have seen the rapid emergence of HIV/AIDS as a public health calamity.

Although the preexisting health care systems in these regions differed greatly in their ability to contend with a new widespread epidemic and political considerations influencing the response to HIV/AIDS varied widely, some common themes have emerged. Specifically, the need to rapidly incorporate prevention of transmission of HIV infection and to implement the increasingly sophisticated and complex strategies of antiretroviral therapy (ART) has posed ongoing challenges. Funding from various international sources has resulted in improved access to care for significant numbers of infected individuals but has, in some instances, imposed structures of delivering this care for which existing health care systems were ill suited. The cost of first-line ART has been drastically reduced, and the production of generic versions of antiretroviral (ARV) agents has permitted some countries to broaden treatment efforts. Nonetheless, the cost of these drugs remains far beyond the reach of the vast majority of individuals who need them.

In this chapter, summary information, including examples of successes and failures from various regions of the world, will be presented in conjunction with the author's personal experience in working with systems of care in Ethiopia and in the Russian Federation. By this means, an attempt will be made to highlight the most critical of the challenges facing the dedicated individuals, including health care professionals, consumers, and their advocates who are engaged in the global fight against HIV/AIDS.

INTERNATIONAL EFFORTS TO COMBAT HIV/AIDS

The advent of effective ART in the mid-1990s led to an acceleration of international efforts to provide treatment to large numbers of infected individuals. Over the past ten years, in particular, these efforts, described in some detail below, have resulted in vast amounts of money distributed in multilateral (countries contributing to central funding sources, which would determine how resources would be distributed) as well as bilateral (individual nations donating funds to specific nations) programs. Despite the remarkable advances in ART development, however, the global epidemic continues to spread and prevalence figures are rising in some of the most heavily populated regions of the world. This fact has led some to the conclusion that efforts to reduce transmission must take precedence over funding to expand treatment of those already infected. The rising death toll of AIDS, however, makes systems to provide care to those infected an essential component of the global strategy. Because of the limited success seen so far, the amount of international funding that has been devoted to the fight against HIV/AIDS has been considered inadequate by some (2) but also to represent an overemphasis on one disease by others (3).

The international effort to treat and prevent HIV infection has become impressive in scale, but specific goals have not been fully met, and the majority of individuals requiring treatment still do not have access to appropriate care. In the poorest and most heavily impacted countries of sub-Saharan Africa, even programs to prevent mother-to-child transmission (PMTCT), a goal that has been largely achieved in the most developed countries, have not succeeded in providing this essential form of care to the majority of HIV-infected pregnant women. Tensions between strategies geared toward prevention and those focused on treatment have led to delays in the development of fully integrated programs incorporating both strategies. The so-far discouraging results of efforts to develop an effective vaccine have complicated efforts further, leaving difficult behavioral and cultural interventions as the only available strategies to reduce transmission.

The HIV/AIDS epidemic has unique features, which distinguish it from other diseases that afflict large numbers of individuals. This uniqueness of the medical and social consequences of HIV infection has been held out as justification for increased funding (4). Among these are the stigma associated with the behaviors associated with infection, the ease with which entire families may be stricken, the absence of a cure or vaccine, and the complexity of therapy. For these and other reasons, it has been difficult in most countries to incorporate HIV care into general medical care. Finally, the establishment and measurement of specific outcomes of efforts aimed at prevention and treatment have been elusive. As a result, the global fight against this disease consists not of a single campaign comparable to that which resulted in the eradication of smallpox but of a mosaic of strategies more or less adapted to a variety of health care systems. In many regions, the seroprevalence of HIV in the general population has not even been accurately determined. This is due not only to the difficulty of obtaining accurate information from the most remote areas of many countries but also to the methodology used to measure seroprevalence. Much of the statistical data collected globally reflects rates of infection among pregnant women or among blood donors. Both of these sources of information present biases and difficulties in making projections to the general population. Pregnant women represent young, sexually active individuals of a single gender, while blood donors in many countries represent either the extremely indigent who donate blood for money or family donors of patients undergoing surgical procedures who may require blood transfusions. Neither of these groups directly reflects the remainder of the population. As voluntary counseling and testing has gradually become more routine for the general population in some countries, prevalence figures have come into sharper focus.

As can be seen from the examples that follow, the ideal approach to the fight against HIV/AIDS has not yet been identified.

Regions have varied greatly in their capacity to address these challenges, and in this chapter, examples of successes and failures in existing approaches will be briefly outlined.

It is hoped as well, however, that lessons learned in all regions of the world fighting HIV/AIDS can be adapted to local circumstances and capacities effectively. Barring an effective and practical vaccine, a prospect that remains elusive, such complex strategies represent the only hope of finally turning the global tide of the HIV/AIDS epidemic.

INTERNATIONAL PROGRAMS TO COMBAT HIV/AIDS

The U.S. President's Emergency Plan for AIDS Relief

The U.S. president's emergency plan for AIDS relief (PEPFAR) is an example of bidirectional funding for HIV/AIDS in which the United States identified a group of countries in most need of assistance and provides direct funding for prevention and care efforts. The program was launched in 2003 with an initial commitment of $15 billion over a five-year period and reauthorized by the U.S. Congress in 2008 with an increase in funding to $48 billion over the subsequent five years (H.R. 5501 the Tom Lantos and Henry J. Hyde United States Global Leadership Reauthorization Act of 2008), and President Barack Obama reiterated the administration's commitment to sustaining PEPFAR in 2009 while signaling a potential shift in strategy with less emphasis on treatment and more on prevention. At the time of its initiation, approximately 1% of HIV-infected individuals in Africa who required ART were receiving it (5), while effective treatment had become widely available and had achieved remarkable success in reducing mortality from AIDS in developed countries.

PEPFAR funding has been directed almost exclusively to 16 countries of sub-Saharan Africa. It has focused on scale-up for distribution of ART in resource-deprived areas as well as on a restrictive form of prevention efforts. Critics of the program have raised doubts as to the effectiveness of scale-up for treatment within systems of care with too few providers and lacking the capability of providing adequate laboratory monitoring of HIV viral load and CD4+ lymphocyte counts. The prevention efforts endorsed by PEPFAR have also drawn criticism because they have traditionally emphasized abstinence over efforts aimed at commercial sex workers and needle exchange strategies.

By early 2008, approximately 1.7 million individuals had received ART as a result of PEPFAR funding (6), and this total had topped two million by 2010. President Obama's plan includes strategies to provide treatment to 12 million and to reduce mother-to-child-transmission by 50% by 2014. Although the bidirectional structure of the program created concerns regarding duplication and interference with multidirectional efforts such as The Global Fund and Joint United Nations Program on AIDS (UNAIDS), PEPFAR has funded multidisciplinary efforts at the governmental levels of the countries receiving funding in an effort to complement multidirectional strategies aimed at the development of country-specific systems of care. PEPFAR funding has also been expanded to train a wider variety of health care professionals and to target funding toward TB and malaria.

As with all international efforts aimed at stemming the spread of the epidemic and getting treatment to those desperately in need of it, the PEPFAR program faces a daunting task of simultaneously expanding access to medications, a task accomplished largely through expanded use of generic ARV drugs (7), while fostering the creation of an infrastructure to maintain patients in appropriate care and reduce transmission.

The following countries and regions have received various amounts of funding through PEPFAR to date: Angola, Botswana, Cambodia, Caribbean region, Central America region, China, Ivory Coast, Democratic Republic of the Congo, Dominican Republic, Ethiopia, Ghana, Guyana, Haiti, India, Indonesia, Kenya, Lesotho, Malawi, Mozambique, Namibia, Nigeria, Russia, Rwanda, South Africa, Sudan, Swaziland, Tanzania, Thailand, Uganda, Ukraine, Vietnam, Zambia, and Zimbabwe.

After 2005, a transition from brand name to generic formulations of ARV agents broadened distribution of both first- and second-line ARVs to many of the countries receiving PEPFAR support (7).

The Global Fund to Fight AIDS, TB and Malaria

The Global Fund to Fight AIDS, TB and Malaria (The Global Fund) was created in 2002 as a multilateral entity combining public and private funding and efforts to combat these diseases in the developing world. Unlike PEPFAR, the Global Fund is multinational, receiving support from many developed countries and providing support to programs in 144 countries (8). The Fund currently provides $19.3 billion to 572 programs including approximately one-quarter of HIV/AIDS funding globally. The funded programs support the provision of antiretroviral drugs as well as the development of infrastructure to improve systems of care.

The Global Fund arose in parallel with UNAIDS, World Health Organization (WHO), and PEPFAR efforts at combating HIV/AIDS. Initial discussions regarding the most appropriate agency to house the Fund focused on the U.S. government, UNICEF, WHO, and the World Bank. Eventually, the Fund became an independent corporation with administrative support from WHO, receiving funding commitments from both public and private sources. The Fund subsequently severed administrative ties with the WHO in 2009. The United States provides some funding through this mechanism but distributes the majority of its funding of efforts to combat HIV/AIDS through the bidirectional PEPFAR program to selected countries. France, Germany, and Japan are also large contributors. Support from the Global Fund is distributed in the form of grants, rather than loans, tailored to local needs and health care systems. Since the Fund is primarily a source of revenue rather than an organization oriented toward implementation of the projects that it funds, it is heavily dependent on governmental and non-governmental experts to effectively administer the funded programs. For this reason, monitoring and evaluation of programs represent a challenge for the organization.

UNAIDS

After years of various international strategies to develop a multilateral approach to HIV/AIDS in the developing world, the UNAIDS was conceptualized in 1992. UNAIDS was intended to streamline efforts of a number of UN agencies, which had been working on various strategies to combat HIV/AIDS since the 1980s. With the WHO left as the leader in developing global health policy, UNAIDS was eventually launched in 1996 following extensive consensus building among various organizations. Initially, four UN agencies agreed to combine efforts in this new entity. Later in 1996, the World Bank, which had funded a number of programs of its own in developing countries, also joined. UNAIDS remains intact and has succeeded in maintaining the place of HIV/AIDS high on the agenda of the UN (9).

The World Bank

The World Bank was among the first international entities to direct funding toward HIV/ADIS. Founded in 1944, the World Bank had a long history of providing loans to developing countries, including support for funding of health infrastructure, before the advent of the HIV/AIDS epidemic. Historically, in addition to funds, the Bank has provided analysis of infrastructure for individual countries and guidance for achieving its primary goal: the reduction of poverty. Currently, several dozen developed countries contribute funds to the Bank for distribution in this manner. Funding targeted to HIV/AIDS began in the late 1980s with screening of donated blood in Niger. Funding initiatives broadened during the 1990s to include thousands of community-based projects within governmental programs and incorporated HIV/AIDS care into broader development needs. Between $6 billion and $9 billion were committed to HIV/AIDS projects between 1990 and 2007 (4). The World Bank has been criticized for its decision-making process regarding distribution of HIV/AIDS funds (4), and, as is the case with other international efforts to combat the epidemic, the balance between funding of treatment, prevention, and development has been contentious at times.

Private Foundations and Industry Support

In recent years, a substantial amount of funding directed at HIV/AIDS care and research has come through philanthropic support from private foundations, most based in the United States, and from industry. Prominent among the private foundations have been the Bill and Melinda Gates Foundation and the Rockefeller, Ford and Clinton Foundations as well as the Elizabeth Glaser Pediatric AIDS Foundation. Industry support has come from the Merck, Pfizer and Bristol-Meyers Squibb Foundations among others.

Global Nongovernmental Organizations

Global nongovernmental organizations (NGOs) such as Doctors Without Borders, Oxfam, and Save the Children have both raised funds through contributions for HIV/AIDS programs they sponsor as well as provided specialized expertise to government and private organizations.

THE GLOBAL IMPACT OF AIDS IN THE 21ST CENTURY

All regions of the world have been impacted by HIV/AIDS. What follows is a summary of this impact by region including illustrative examples of conditions in specific countries. The richest and most developed nations, those of Western Europe as well as the United States, Japan, and Australia have generally marshaled their financial resources to provide effective treatment for those with HIV. Although even these countries have encountered problems to varying degrees in providing care to all segments of society and despite the fact that individual responses have varied depending largely on the form of public and private funding of health care in each nation, the emphasis in this discussion will be on the areas of the world where the epidemic continues to expand quickly and/or where poor- or midlevel-income countries have developed strategies unique to their political and health care systems.

Since the author's international work has been largely conducted in Russia and Ethiopia, these countries will be discussed in somewhat greater detail, heavily influenced by personal observations.

Africa

The countries of Sub-Saharan Africa have witnessed a degree of devastation resulting from the HIV/AIDS epidemic that was impossible to imagine prior to the 1980s when the epidemic's full impact became apparent. Country after country has seen hard-fought victories over other communicable diseases and a steady improvement in life expectancy completely reversed and overwhelmed by HIV/AIDS. Nonetheless, some countries, even some with the highest seroprevalence of HIV infection, have made substantial strides toward prevention and treatment, while others have had far less success. Botswana and Senegal represent examples of successful strategic planning and genuine progress. Nigeria is an example of a country in which progress has been considerably slower in coming. What follows are some general outlines of individual country responses. The essential elements of the specific strategies, without an attempt to cover all aspects of care, are described in an effort to draw distinctions among a variety of measures and their relative effectiveness. It is recognized that the countries of sub-Saharan Africa differ vastly in social structure, although most are among the poorest countries in the world, and that efforts appropriate to one society may not be feasible or as efficient in another.

Botswana

Since early in the HIV/AIDS epidemic, Botswana has been recognized as having one of the highest rates of infection in the world. The prevalence among pregnant women in 2003 was 37% (10). The country has made the development of strategies for prevention and treatment a priority, particularly since 2002. As is the case in the rest of sub-Saharan Africa, heterosexual spread has been the primary mode of transmission, and educational efforts directed at encouraging abstinence and condom use appear to have been largely ineffective (10), although male condoms are widely available. Botswana, on the basis of its mineral resources, is less impoverished than many of its neighbors. This, coupled with substantial international financial support and a strong federal commitment, has enabled the country to make ART available to a larger proportion of the population than countries with less coordination between governmental and international efforts. Botswana continues to struggle against an almost incomprehensible prevalence of infection, and projected death rates from AIDS over the coming years still point to a social crisis of drastic proportions. Nonetheless, the country represents an example of an effective top-down effort to spread treatment efforts effectively.

Senegal

The program of treatment and prevention of HIV infection in Senegal, one of the poorest countries on Earth, has been held out as one of the most effective in the developing world. In comparison to many of its neighbors, Senegal has had a low measured prevalence of HIV infection, estimated at approximately 1% (11) in the early years of the 21st century. Its population is overwhelmingly Muslim, and many religion-based NGOs have traditionally been involved in local development efforts, including those related to HIV/AIDS. Early in the epidemic and particularly after the advent of effective ART in the late 1990s, the country has focused on the widespread availability of medications as well as laboratory facilities for the monitoring of care with CD4 lymphocyte counts and viral load measurements. Efforts were not exclusively organized in a top-down fashion so that local health centers were enabled to offer testing and treatment in recent years, free of charge. The combination of cooperation between governmental and nongovernmental efforts and the early recognition of the need to decentralize care has enabled Senegal to maintain a low seroprevalence of HIV infection. Although the fact that the country traditionally has a low rate of sexually transmitted infection (STI) and the impact of strong involvement by religious institutions cannot be overlooked, the country has, nonetheless, so far, contained its HIV epidemic at a relatively low level despite its extreme poverty.

Nigeria

Nigeria witnessed a steady increase in HIV seroprevalence throughout the 1990s with levels reaching 10% in some areas of the country (12). As was the case in Botswana, an early emphasis was placed on education regarding HIV and its prevention. The federal government began its response early in the epidemic but was largely dependent on international sources for financing and technical assistance. Efforts were organized primarily at the federal level. During the early years of the 21st century, measures to obtain generic antiretroviral drugs and to scale up distribution of treatment were intensified. Through 2006, however, the reach of these efforts was relatively modest (12), and there had been little involvement by NGOs to assist in decentralizing care. Nigeria continues to struggle with its strategy to combat HIV/AIDS. The subtle differences between this country and Botswana where the prevalence of infection is considerably higher but the impact of governmental efforts appears to be more dramatic are difficult to understand. With its vast population (over 120 million) and despite its substantial income from oil resources, Nigeria continues to struggle in its efforts to apply international and national funding to its health care system to accelerate its response to the AIDS epidemic.

Ethiopia

Ethiopia is one of the poorest countries in the world with a per capita gross domestic product of only US$800. Approximately 85% of its roughly 70 million inhabitants live in rural areas. Infant mortality is over 100 per 1000 live births, and the life expectancy at birth is approximately 50 years. It is a remarkably diverse country with a population approximately 60% Christian and 35% Muslim. Geographically, it has features of tropical countries and lies only 7° latitude above the equator but, because much of its land is above 1500 m in altitude, its climate lends itself to diseases of subtropical and temperate climates as well. It has a rich and diverse history and, unlike most of the countries of Africa, avoided European colonization. Ethiopia's health care system suffers from a severe lack of hospital beds and of physicians. Please see the description below (Box 13.1) of our partnership between a U.S. hospital and an Ethiopian hospital for further details.

Box 13.1 Reflections on Our Ethiopian Partnership

Since 2007, Elmhurst Hospital Center has been partnered with Debre Berhan Hospital (DBH) in Ethiopia under a contract with the American International Health Alliance (AIHA) supported by the U.S. Centers for Disease Control and Prevention. The partnership has been on a twinning model structured in a fashion comparable to the Russian project described in Box 13.2. Each year, following the development of a jointly-agreed-upon work plan, exchanges of teams of health care personnel have made one-week visits several times to the others' hospital. After initial needs assessment visits, specific interventions and goals were developed for implementation at the Ethiopian site. The partnership has focused on scale-up of antiretroviral therapy and organization of delivery of care for individuals with HIV/AIDS. In addition, other areas of need have been identified with steps taken to address them. Among these have been hospital infection control, development of quality assurance processes, incorporation of nurses more directly into care, and the identification of key indicators of organizational effectiveness in a variety of areas.

For the sake of brevity, some aspects of the interactions between the two institutions will be omitted from this description. It should be noted, however, that general capacity building for the hospital and staff rapidly emerged as an essential component of strategies focused on HIV/AIDS care.

Initial Impressions of Debre Berhan Hospital

A group of physicians, nurses, and social workers made the initial site assessment visit to DBH in 2007. DBH is in the city of Debre Berhan, a community of approximately 100,000 approximately 60 miles north of the Addis Ababa. It is a general hospital providing medical, surgical, gynecologic, obstetrical, pediatric, and emergency care and provides inpatient and extensive outpatient services dedicated to the care of individuals with HIV/ AIDS. The complement of physicians is quite small, with approximately 8 representing a number of specialties. Nurses are more plentiful, and some staffing is provided by public health officers who serve as physician extenders.

Lessons Learned

1. Despite severe shortages in equipment, supplies, and staff, professionals working at DBH had created a system of integration of extensive HIV testing and linkage to care.
2. General infrastructural issues such as the relatively unreliable electrical system, the lack of laboratory diagnostic equipment, and limited Internet access represented barriers to be overcome despite extremely limited funds.
3. Collaboration to develop a hospital-wide infection control program modeled on the Elmhurst Hospital program met with no resistance on the part of hospital leadership.
4. Similarly, a desire to develop and also to come into compliance with standardized quality indicators was evident and led to rapid identification of specific goals to enhance services.
5. The data demands imposed by governmental authorities and required for eligibility for other international funding were and remain substantial and pose a daunting task for hospital leadership.
6. Significant barriers to retention of HIV/AIDS patients in care result from the large geographical area served by DBH and the lack of effective means of transportation and communication for some of the patients.
7. Creation of specific services related to HIV/AIDS, particularly oph-thalmologic and gynecologic services, proved extremely worthwhile and could be accomplished by trainings of appropriate staff and purchase of dedicated equipment.

Other Countries of Sub-Saharan Africa

It is beyond the scope of this discussion to review the efforts and results of the fight against HIV/AIDS in all of the countries of this hardest-hit region. Uganda has seen a substantial reduction in HIV prevalence rates and has been one of a relatively small number of countries that have imported generic antiretroviral drugs, particularly from India. South Africa, a mid-level country in terms of gross domestic product, saw a rapid rise in HIV seroprevalence from less than 1% in 1992 to more than 25% in 2002 (13), with AIDS accounting for 40% of all deaths among individuals between 15 and 49 years of age by the early 21st century. The disparity of wealth within South Africa is substantial, and this has been pointed to as one of the reasons why the HIV/AIDS epidemic, largely afflicting the poorest sectors, accelerated so dramatically. The country continues to struggle with the application of national and international resources to address this crisis.

South America

The countries of South America have all been heavily impacted by HIV/AIDS. As in most of the rest of the world, the epidemic was recognized in the early to mid-1980s throughout the continent. Several countries of the region mounted a more effective fight against the epidemic than was seen in the poorest regions of the world.

Brazil

With a relatively moderate estimated adult seroprevalence of HIV infection of 0.7% and an aggressive and centralized approach to prevention and treatment, Brazil is often held out as an example of a developing country where strategies were brought to bear early to treat infected individuals and combat the spread of disease (14). However, while ART became available relatively early in the large metropolitan areas of the country, the size of Brazil and economic diversity of its large population continue to frustrate efforts at providing adequate care for all of those who are infected. In fact, overall life expectancy lags behind several other countries in South America with lower per capita gross domestic product (GDP). Private health insurance, which often means superior standards of care, is affordable by approximately one-quarter of the population. Nonetheless, universal access to ART became available in the mid-1990s, and, as in the developed countries, AIDS mortality has declined steadily since that time (15). The adoption of national standards and care and the availability of a wide variety of antiretroviral agents, some manufactured locally in generic form, have contributed substantially to this trend. Newly diagnosed HIV cases have been seen increasingly among the lower socioeconomic groups. Efforts at prevention of transmission through mass media educational campaigns as well as harm reduction programs such as needle exchange have been robust.

Argentina

In comparison to its neighbor Brazil, Argentina responded relatively slowly to the emergence of the HIV/AIDS epidemic in the 1980s. This, coupled with political instability, has hampered efforts to fully implement international standards of care despite a governmental commitment to address treatment and prevention. Modern ART, however, was introduced promptly in the mid-1990s as it has resulted in a steady decline in the number of newly reported cases (16). Access to care in this large country remains a substantial obstacle, particularly for those living in rural areas.

The Caribbean

Countries in the Caribbean basin have been among the most impacted by the HIV/AIDS epidemic. Shortly after AIDS was recognized, Haitians living in the United States and in Haiti appeared to be disproportionately affected. Briefly, speculation that routes of transmission unique to Haitian culture existed. As the full picture of HIV infection in the Caribbean nations came into focus, however, it became obvious that infections among Haitians resulted from the same means of transmission and seen in other countries.

Haiti

Haiti is among the world's most impoverished countries. As indicated above, the HIV/AIDS epidemic was recognized early among Haitians, and the country continues to have the highest prevalence of HIV infection, estimated to be approximately 3%, outside of Africa. The epidemic was recognized early in Haiti, in part because of cases of HIV/AIDS seen among Haitian immigrants in the United States in the early 1980s. Steps to reduce transfusion of tainted blood were taken quickly, and public education campaigns and widespread availability and effectiveness of condoms (17) helped to reduce transmission. International governmental support and the efforts of nongovernmental organizations, including universities in the United States, also began early in the epidemic and were aided by research on patterns of disease (18). Training of health care workers was also enhanced greatly by these efforts. The impact of the catastrophic earthquake that struck Port-au-Prince in 2009 on the systems of care for HIV/AIDS has yet to be fully determined.

Cuba

The health care system in Cuba is frequently given as an example of the effective deployment of limited resources. In addressing the HIV/AIDS epidemic, which has been modest in scale in comparison to other Caribbean nations, the system of universal free care and an effective national system for surveillance of disease most likely helped to limit the scope and impact of AIDS. A work group functioning under the authority of the national ministry of health led to the development of diagnostic tests (19) and the reduction in the use of imported blood products and in the development or purchase of needed medical diagnostic equipment. Wholesale testing of Cubans who had travelled outside the country with subsequent contact tracing was also employed early in the epidemic. Production of a variety of generic antiretroviral compounds enabled early widespread access to treatment and reduced the rate of maternal-to-child transmission effectively. In summary, the response of Cuba was swift and decisive. Governmental and societal structure likely permitted measures that are more difficult to sustain in other nations, however.

Southeast Asia

Thailand

Thailand is considered a lower middle-income country, considerably above the poorest countries of sub-Saharan Africa in measures of GDP with a high rate of literacy, a life expectancy of 69.3 years (20), and a relatively strong health infrastructure. HIV seroprevalence has fluctuated but has generally been declining in recent years, and strategies to prevent maternal-to-child transmission have been widely implemented. Strong governmental support of condom use, especially by sex workers, has been credited as a major reason for declining rates of transmission. Thailand is often held out as an example of the effectiveness of a combination of strong government leadership in prevention measures and adequate health care facilities to provide treatment to those who are infected. Funding of these efforts has come largely from internal sources with substantially less dependence on multinational or binational sources or support. As in most of the developing world, the cost of antiretroviral drugs has represented a major impediment to further progress, but this has been partly offset by generic drug manufacture.

Cambodia

The HIV epidemic was first recognized in Cambodia in 1991 during a period of governmental instability and in which the health care system was in a state of virtual collapse. The epidemic rapidly accelerated over the ensuing decade, with seroprevalence reaching approximately 3% by 1997. Prevalence measures indicate a significant decline since that time. As is the case in Thailand, this decline has been largely attributed to the widespread uptake of condom use and periodic health assessments by sex workers (21). As in most of the world, however, the epidemic spread from sex workers and their clients to female and male partners of clients and children has achieved the familiar generalized pattern. Efforts aimed at female sex workers and their clients, however, have not been matched by strategies to decease transmission among men who have sex with men, a heavily stigmatized segment of the population, and prevention of mother-to-child-transmission has not been as successful as hoped. Cambodia received substantial international support for its efforts at containing the epidemic. Unlike its neighbor, Thailand, Cambodia has not developed a system for the manufacture of generic antiretroviral drugs and is dependent on international sources of funding to provide even partial access to care for infected individuals. The differences in the response to HIV/AIDS between these two neighboring countries appear to reflect the relative strengths of the health care infrastructures at the beginning of the epidemic and the great capacity to address prevention and, to some degree, treatment needs in Thailand.

South Asia

India

HIV was first reported in India in the mid-1980s and was particularly focused on female sex workers and their clients, including truck drivers. This pattern, as seen in other countries, fostered the spread to other populations, including pregnant and nonpregnant women, children, injection drug users (IDUs), and their sexual partners. This sequence has resulted in the relatively rapid infection of a large number of people because of the nation's vast population. In recent years, it is estimated that over five million individuals are currently infected (22). The outpatient health care in India is provided by the private sector. Because of the large and diverse population and the profound poverty of many, effective and standardized treatment of HIV/AIDS has represented an unusually difficult challenge. On the positive side, India has developed a robust manufacturing program of a variety of antiretroviral drugs for internal use and for export. This has, in recent years, dramatically reduced the cost of treatment. Nonetheless, the potential for a continued rapid escalation of the epidemic in the world's second most populous country remains, and the capacity of the public health infrastructure to effectively prevent this will continue to be strained.

China

The HIV/AIDS epidemic in China, first detected in the mid-1980s, has followed a familiar pattern. The majority of early cases were among IDUs. Rapid spread to female sex workers and their clients, bisexual men and female partners of infected men, and, ultimately, children. As has been the case in India, the vast population and size of the country has rendered prevention and treatment efforts extremely difficult. Until the early years of the present century, a shortage of HIV-trained providers as well as the laboratory and clinical facilities needed to provide care slowed the response. Beginning in 2003, the country launched a five-year program to address HIV/AIDS more broadly. The program, entitled China Comprehensive AIDS Response Programme (China CARES), provides services to approximately 83 million people in 127 sites. Within these sites, a number of impressive accomplishes have been reported, including eliminating transmission by blood transfusion and improvements in prevention of mother-to-child transmission, overall counseling, testing, and awareness levels (23). Nationwide accurate prevalence figures are difficult to access and likely vary greatly across the geographical regions and social strata. Local production of several antiretroviral agents as well as successful governmental negotiations to lower the price of other imported agents have enhanced drug availability. As is the case in India, however, the situation in China raises great concern for global control.

Eastern Europe/Former Soviet Union

Although spared from the full brunt of the HIV/AIDS epidemic until the mid-1990s, the Russian Federation and other countries of the former Soviet Union have witnessed a rapid increase in the number of infected individuals and have moved quickly to redesign existing health care systems to address the medical and social consequences.

Ukraine

Of the countries of the former Soviet Union, Ukraine has been among the hardest hit by the HIV/AIDS epidemic. Although HIV infections were documented during the 1980s, an abrupt increase in infections, primarily among IDUs, was seen in the mid-1990s, a pattern seen also in Russia (see below). As in all societies in which HIV is introduced, infection was subsequently seen among female sex workers, homosexual and bisexual men, female partners of infected men, and children by virtue of vertical transmission. As has been the case of many of the countries of Eastern Europe and the former Soviet republics of Central Asia, the HIV epidemic arrived in Ukraine with such explosive force that the systems of care in place as well as attitudes toward IDUs have added to the difficulty in scaling up for treatment and expansion of prevention efforts (24). The country has enlisted assistance from multinational sources, and an active network of NGOs have contributed to these efforts as well, but the challenge of addressing the epidemic, which reached large numbers of people in a short period of time, has been daunting.

Russia

The HIV/AIDS epidemic began to accelerate quickly in Russia after the fall of the Soviet Union. In the mid-1990s, it was concentrated in the western population centers of Moscow and St. Petersburg. Over the ensuing decade, the epidemic spread into Central Russia, fueled in large part by the traffic in heroin into this region from countries to the south. The Russian federal response to the spreading crisis was to develop AIDS centers in each of its 89 local oblast governmental units. Since the national epidemic was initially concentrated among IDUs, a group traditionally heavily stigmatized and criminalized in Russia, access to care was hampered by several elements: reluctance of patients at risk of HIV infection to present for testing and care and reluctance on the part of health care providers to reach out to this group because of the entrenched stigma and lack of experience with this relatively new and complex disease.

Greatly compounding the difficulties in the national response to the epidemic in Russia have been the outlawing of opiate substitution therapy, such as methadone and buprenorphine, well established as an effective strategy at maintaining IDUs in care and reducing transmission by this route in other countries (25). In addition, the top-down system encountered in many countries around the world in which specialized AIDS centers were created and set apart from related facilities such as tuberculosis centers, STI clinics, and drug treatment institutions has fostered a fragmentation of care as well as difficulties in identifying those infected with HIV.

See below (Box 13.2) for a description of our partnership, including lessons learned, with an HIV/AIDS center in Russia.

Box 13.2 Reflections on Our Russian Partnership

What follows is a brief, and somewhat incomplete, description of a five-year partnership between HIV/AIDS staff of a U.S. hospital and their counterparts in an HIV/AIDS center in the Russian Federation. For the sake of brevity, only the HIV/AIDS and related services are described as well as the efforts to share information and strategies to assist in the scale-up of ART in a specific region of Russia.

Beginning in 2004, the HIV/AIDS Program at Elmhurst Hospital Center, a municipal hospital in New York City academically affiliated with the Mount Sinai School of Medicine, entered into a twinning partnership with the AIDS Center in the city of Orenburg in Russia. The partnership was sponsored by a contract with the AIHA and funded by the U.S. Agency for International Development. Over the ensuing five years, through a series of exchange visits between the two sites, staff of both HIV/AIDS programs observed procedures and staffing patterns that had been developed to serve the needs of the communities they serve.

The program at Elmhurst Hospital Center had begun in 1985 and had expanded through a series of federal, state, and city funding to a system involving a dedicated staff of HIV-trained physicians, nurses, social workers, counselors, support staff, patient volunteers, and subspecialists in gynecology, mental health, and endocrinology. The program comprised an outpatient clinic in a wing of the hospital and took full responsibility for the outpatient needs of all HIV-infected individuals identified among patients seen in the hospital or referred for counseling and testing from community sources. The clinic at Elmhurst Hospital was and is run in conjunction with a large tuberculosis outpatient clinic and program as well as a clinic dedicated to treatment of viral hepatitis.

The AIDS Center in Orenburg had been established by the Russian government along with centers throughout the nation to serve the rapidly growing population of HIV-infected individuals. It is a free-standing clinic occupying an entire building providing outpatient services to HIV-infected individuals referred from physicians in the region, local medical facilities, and community sources. It was staffed with physicians, nurses, and support staff and contained a laboratory for CD4 count monitoring and other blood tests. In the city of Orenburg, a municipality of approximately 500,000, there was also a municipal and regional tuberculosis hospital providing inpatient and outpatient services to patients with active or latent TB as well as a narcology hospital and a facility for the treatment of sexually transmitted infections with outreach capability.

Initial Impressions of the Orenburg HIV/AIDS Center

A group of physicians, nurses, and a social worker made an initial visit to Orenburg, a city in the foothills of the Ural Mountains near the border between Europe and Asia in December, 2004. The HIV/AIDS center had enrolled several hundred patients, although relatively few had yet begun ART. The staff of the clinic consisted primarily of physicians and nurses. The majority of patients had been injection drug users (IDUs) or their sexual partners. The dedicated staff of experienced clinicians had established a process by which patients would be considered eligible for therapy on the basis of CD4 count and clinical stage as well as an assessment of individuals' commitment and ability to adhere to therapy. Supplies of antiretroviral drugs were initially quite limited and unpredictable. Since the visit had followed a visit by Orenburg staff to the Elmhurst Hospital Center and its HIV/AIDS program, initial efforts were designed to identify practices in place at Elmhurst which might be adaptable to the relatively new center in Orenburg. Chief among the efforts which were encouraged on the basis of this comparison were the expansion of the role of nurses at Orenburg to include more direct patient assessment, education and ongoing contact. In addition, it was felt that addition of at least one social worker, a mental health professional and a TB specialist to work onsite at the Orenburg program would facilitate maintenance of patients in care and the management of co-infected (HIV and TB) patients in collaboration with the municipal and regional TB hospitals. It was also decided to establish a cohort of 50-100 patients followed in Orenburg whose care over time could be reviewed by providers at both sites in the hope of identifying opportunities for further interventions. Of note, the Orenburg site did not have access to viral load or resistance testing so that clinical decisions were made on the basis of CD4 lymphocyte counts and clinical stages.

During subsequent exchanges, efforts were made to develop new means of communication between the related but independent HIV, TB, and narcology facilities in Orenburg so that referral and follow-up mechanisms could be enhanced. Educational materials and many oral presentations regarding all aspects of HIV care were made during exchanges to both Orenburg and Elmhurst over the ensuing years. Shortly after the initiation of the partnership, officials at the Orenburg Medical Academy became involved in developing an educational program for the staff of the HIV/AIDS center as well as for infectionists working in the region to provide updated guidelines and strategies for treatment of HIV infection. Close, professional relationships formed between U.S. and Russian counterparts, particularly physicians and nurses and a variety of educational and organizational efforts, under the guidance of the AIHA bore fruit.

Initially, relatively intense stigmatization of IDUs, particularly those still actively engaged in drug use, was evident among the staff at the AIDS center in Orenburg. Efforts were made to address these long-standing attitudes by providing examples from the Elmhurst programs as well as international data regarding the effective treatment and maintenance in care of this hard-to-reach population, and attitudes changed somewhat. An effective program of prevention of mother-to-child transmission (PMTCT) was developed in Orenburg and the surrounding region.

Lessons Learned

1. Initial misunderstanding and, to some extent, mistrust were largely overcome through the development of close professional ties and an acknowledgement by the U.S. partners that their Russian counterparts were combating both an epidemic that was expanding at a rapid rate and a disease that was relatively new to even the most experienced health care professionals.
2. Specific structural differences were relatively easily overcome. This was especially true of the incorporation of nurses more directly into care and the placement of limited social service staff and a TB specialist at the HIV/AIDS center.
3. The overall goal of the program: educational scale-up for the use of antiretroviral therapy was largely achieved through educational efforts, both didactic and case based, with the assistance of the local Medical Academy. Despite this, supplies of antiretroviral agents continued to be a difficult obstacle to fully overcome.
4. Communication between site visits was difficult and largely ineffective because of limited Internet capabilities for videoconferencing.
5. Collaborative follow-up of the cohort of patients described above was a difficult process and did not lead directly to any specific interventions.
6. Collaboration between the AIDS center, the TB centers, and the narcology hospital required consensus among the key leadership at each facility. The need for this degree of collaboration, although acknowledged as potentially important for the collaborative treatment of patients, was underestimated and continued to be a work in progress at the end of the five-year project.
7. Time-limited collaborations consisting of the twinning model can be extremely valuable in planting ideas for subsequent discussion and possible implementation.
8. Monitoring and evaluation of the accomplishments of the partnership are a difficult task, which should be designed and agreed upon at the beginning of such arrangements.

SUMMARY: MAJOR OBSTACLES CONFRONTED IN RESOURCE-DEPRIVED AREAS

Of course, not all regions that lack the resources of the wealthiest in combating HIV/AIDS suffer from obstacles of equal magnitude. Nonetheless, several themes are commonly encountered as countries in regions without fully developed systems to confront the challenges presented by the epidemic. Among the most prevalent of these themes are the following.

Ineffective Measures to Control Spread of HIV Infection

Efforts to control the spread of HIV infection have encountered difficult obstacles in all of the affected regions of the world. In many areas where transmission among IDUs is common, strategies to combat addiction have been difficult to implement. For opiate users, the lack of substitution therapy in some countries with agents such as methadone or buprenorphine has left many of these individuals with no effective alternative to heroin. This dilemma persists despite evidence that such therapy can diminish the spread of HIV infection and help to keep individuals in care. Efforts to reduce heterosexual transmission, the most frequent route of infection, have met logistical, cultural, and religious barriers in many countries. Strategies to prevent maternal-to-child transmission require availability of appropriate antiretroviral agents and workers dedicated to developing effective systems of treatment.

Stigma Among the Public and the Health Care Profession Regarding Infected Individuals

The presence of HIV infection in a community often leads to a complex array of barriers between infected individuals and appropriate care. In the earliest stages of the epidemic in the United States, both fear of contagion on the part of the public and some in the health care professions as well as bias toward high-risk groups resulted in discrimination in housing, hiring, and health care. With time and the fact that novel modes of transmission of HIV have not been identified, such fears have lessened, but some level of discrimination confronts many of those who are infected. In the developing world, these same obstacles have been encountered. In the poorest countries, the basic health care needs associated with HIV infection have been impossible to address adequately. Stigmatization of infected individuals has further compounded this desperate situation.

Inadequate Supplies of Antiretroviral Agents

Lack of adequate supplies of antiretroviral agents continues to plague many countries. Although the cost of first-line therapy has been dramatically reduced, many countries do not have access to a continuous supply of appropriate combinations of drugs, and newer agents for first-line treatment and salvage therapy may be completely unavailable. Some countries have developed substantial capacity to produce generic versions of commonly used antiretrovirals, but the numbers of patients requiring treatment have overwhelmed these sources in many regions, and of course, newer agents remain inaccessible in much of the world.

Inadequate Access to Antiretroviral Therapy for Large Segments of the Affected Population

Access to appropriate therapy poses barriers in addition to adequacy of the drug supply. Transportation to services, adequate storage of drugs and monitoring for and managing of side effects, and the availability of hospitalization and specialty services amount to a virtually insurmountable problem in many areas of the world.

Ineffective Systems for Prevention of Maternal-to-Child Transmission

Prevention of maternal-to-child transmission (PMTCT) of HIV infection has been one of the most resounding successes in the fight against HIV/AIDS. Strategies to identify pregnant women who are infected with HIV and to provide ART before and during delivery to the mother and to the infant after birth coupled with Caesarian section in cases where ART for the mother has not achieved sufficient viral suppression at term as well as discouragement of breast-feeding have resulted in nearly complete elimination in this key route of trans-mission and almost complete elimination of pediatric AIDS in developed countries. Unfortunately, maternal-to-child transmission continues in regions lacking the medications and systems of care to intervene successfully. In most of the countries with the highest seroprevalence among pregnant women, this form of therapy has not made sufficient inroads.

Insufficient Laboratory Resources to Stage HIV Infection and to Diagnose Opportunistic Infections and Malignancies

Thirty years into the HIV/AIDS epidemic, most of the poorest countries of the world do not have sufficient laboratory facilities to measure virologic response to ART directly. Although technology to measure CD4+ lymphocyte counts has become relatively widespread, the lack of information regarding viral suppres-sion and viral resistance creates barriers to effective management of individual patients and results, inevitably, in the more rapid emergence of drug resistance as partially effective regimens are prescribed blindly. Furthermore, the means to make specific diagnoses of common AIDS-related infections such as *Pneumo-cystis carinii* pneumonia and tuberculosis results in delays in effective therapy for these and other lethal coinfections. In the case of tuberculosis, in particular, the lack of availability of rapid culture techniques and drug susceptibility testing both of which plague much of the developing world has fueled the emergence of multidrug-resistant TB (MDRTB) and extensively resistant TB (XDRTB) in many regions.

Insufficient Numbers of Health Care Professionals Trained and Experienced in the Management of HIV/AIDS and its Complications

The care of individuals with HIV/AIDS requires specific training in the proper use of ART, including monitoring for effectiveness and for toxicity, as well as the ability to recognize, diagnose, and treat complicating infections and malignancies. Although resources for such training have been made widely available through the Internet and other sources in recent years, there is a global lack of health care professionals with the desire and experience required to manage HIV/AIDS. Many developing countries lack sufficient numbers of physicians and nurses generally. Other health care professionals who provide a key link to the patient in comprehensive systems of care, for example, social workers, mental health experts, pharmacists, and others, are either lacking or have not been incorporated into such systems for HIV/AIDS in much of the world. Clearly, the inability to provide adequate staff not only to prescribe and dispense ART but also to assist patients in reducing the risk of transmission, maintaining themselves and, in many instances, their children in care and supporting the overall needs of the individual and family, creates an environment that cannot be fully addressed by the simple provision of medications.

Inadequate Means of Case Finding and Rapid Testing for HIV Infection

The vast and diverse populations infected by HIV present difficulties for any system of care. Identification of infected individuals and their linkage to adequate and consistent care mean confronting a host of barriers in the most affected countries. In the severely impoverished regions of Africa and other areas, simply providing physical access to HIV care centers is impeded by lack of transportation. Systems of communication relied upon in developing countries to remain in contact with patients between visits are typically lacking. Amplifying such obstacles to access remains the stigma associated with HIV infection. This social stigma represents a barrier to case finding in many regions and, perhaps, most clearly where injection drug use and homosexual behavior are criminalized and volunteering for testing brings with it the threat of incarceration.

Inadequate Systems for and Referral of Patients to Substance Abuse Treatment

In regions where injection drug use remains a prominent route of transmission of HIV through the use of shared needles and syringes, substance abuse treatment is a vital component of reducing spread of infection and maintaining infected

individuals in treatment. Opiate substitution therapy with methadone or buprenorphine has been demonstrated to be an effective component of care for these
individuals. In some areas of the world, most notably Russia where injection
drug use led to an explosion of the HIV epidemic in the mid-1990s, such therapy
is unavailable. Other means of addressing injection drug use purely through harm
reduction efforts and detoxification are rendered less effective in the absence of
such substitution therapy.

Insufficient Mental Health Facilities and Limited Access to Mental Health Expertise

Depression and a host of other psychiatric disorders are common among individuals infected with HIV. Adequate and humane assessment of mental illness
is simply not available in many of the countries most affected by HIV. The
psychosocial support provided through mental health professionals as well as
social workers and care managers in many comprehensive systems of care in
developed countries has not yet arrived in much of the developing world. The
absence of such systems of support and of medications to treat psychiatric
disorders represents an impossible barrier to effective HIV care for many
individuals.

Obstacles in Housing

Failure to meet the basic survival needs of individuals infected with HIV may
render ART irrelevant. In many countries, including some of the most
developed, discrimination in housing against persons with HIV/AIDS has
resulted in a high incidence of homelessness. The failure to provide adequate
living conditions represents an obstacle in all other aspects of care including
the basics of simply taking medications and keeping appointments.

Inadequate Infection Control Procedures, Particularly Regarding Methods to Prevent Transmission of Tuberculosis Within Clinics and Hospitals

In the United States, it was recognized in the early 1990s that transmission of
tuberculosis among HIV-infected individuals, often with lethal consequences,
was occurring with hospitals. As a result, high-level isolation techniques,
including negative-pressure rooms employing filtered, circulated air and the use
of highly efficient personal protective equipment by hospital staff, have been
widely implemented. Most countries burdened by high prevalence of HIV
infection are also highly endemic for tuberculosis. Sophisticated isolation procedures like those employed in the United States and other developed countries
for proven or suspected cases of tuberculosis are simply too expensive for many
of these countries. As a result, transmission of tuberculosis within health care
facilities continues to represent a high-level risk against a backdrop of sustained

high rates of transmission in the community. Patients coinfected with HIV and TB require coordinated systems of care including rapid diagnosis and susceptibility testing. HIV infection is perhaps the most effective facilitator of transmission of tuberculosis known, and yet the areas where both infections are most prevalent continue to struggle to develop and sustain systems of care for either.

Poverty and the Inability of Infected Individuals to Afford all of the Elements of Comprehensive Care

As is demonstrated by most of the above barriers to care, individual and national poverty represent a common theme as obstacles in combating HIV/AIDS on a global level. Vast amounts of money from a variety of international sources have been devoted to providing treatment and prevention services and strategies to the countries most in need. Of course, most of these countries suffer from an inability to provide adequate health and social services to their people, and individual median incomes fall far below the minimum required for individuals to support the health care needs of themselves and their families. Famine, malnutrition, and a host of diseases confront the poorest nations in the world. The fight against HIV/AIDS must continue in environments where the daily struggle for survival remains for many at the forefront.

Some of these obstacles have been effectively overcome in regions with substantial numbers of infected individuals. All represent ongoing challenges, however. Progress in some domains may indeed lead to greater obstacles in others. Improvement in access to ART, when not accompanied by enhanced ability to monitor the effectiveness of therapy through viral load and resistance testing, for example, may rapidly exhaust available therapeutic alternatives and result in large numbers of patients requiring antiretroviral agents that are not currently available. Limited or no access to laboratory facilities to provide rapid diagnosis of tuberculosis, to accurately establish resistance patterns, and to provide directly observed therapy may severely undermine efforts to improve the survival of persons with HIV/AIDS as tuberculosis remains the commonest cause of death among those infected with HIV in the countries and regions experiencing the highest prevalence of HIV infection.

The solutions to this broad array of problems must also include enhanced emphasis on HIV care in the training of the coming generation of health care workers. Although the obstacles presented by the effective treatment of the complex disorder with all of its medical and social ramifications are genuinely daunting, there is no doubt that a great number of lives have been saved and many more prolonged by the efforts devoted to the care of individuals with HIV/AIDS in many of the most affected countries.

Beginning in 2004 and continuing to the time of this writing, the staff of the HIV/AIDS program at Elmhurst Hospital Center in New York City have been engaged in twinning partnerships with AIDS programs in Russia and in Ethiopia under the auspices of the American International Heath Alliance with funding from the U.S. Agency for International Development and the United States Centers for Disease Control and Prevention. What follows are brief descriptions of these twinning partnerships including lessons learned, some positive, some less so. It is hoped that these examples might prove helpful to readers who wish to become engaged in the international fight against HIV/AIDS by participating directly in other countries.

REFERENCES

1. Joint United Nations Programme on HIV/AIDS (UNAIDS) 2009. 2008 UNAIDS annual report: towards universal access.
2. Henry J, Kaiser Family Foundation. Finaincing the response to HIV/AIDS in low and middle income countries: funding for HIV/AIDS from the G7 and the European Commission. Washington, D.C.: Henry J Kaiser Family Foundation, July 2005.
3. England R. The writing is on the wall for UNAIDS. Br Med J 2008; 336:1072.
4. Lisk F. Global Institutions and the HIV/AIDS Epidemic. Responding to an international crisis. New York: Routledge, 2009.
5. El-Sadr WM. The President's Emergency Plan for AIDS Relief—is the emergency over. N Engl J Med 2008; 359:553–555.
6. The United States President's Emergency Plan for AIDS Relief. Home page. Available at: http://www.Pepfar.gov.
7. Holmes CB, Coggin W, Jamieson D, et al. Use of generic antiretroviral agents and cost savings in PEPFAR treatment programs. JAMA 2010; 304(3):313–320.
8. The Global Fund. About the Global Fund. Available at: http://www.theglobalfund.org/en/about.
9. Political Declaration on HIV/AIDS, United Nations General Assembly resolution 60/26, 22 June 2006.
10. Masupu K, Seiphone K, Roels T, et al., eds. Botwana 2003: HIV surveillance reports. Gabarone: National AIDS Corrdinating Agency, 2003.
11. WHO/UNAIDS. Report on the Global AIDS epidemic. Geneva: WHO, 2004.
12. Ogundiran A, Fatunmbi B, Costantinos BT. Nigeria. In: Beck EJ, Mays N, Whiteside AW, et al., eds. The HIV Pandemic. Local and Global Implications. Oxford: Oxford Medical Publications, Oxford University Press, 2008.
13. McCoy D, Wood R, Dudley L, et al. South Africa. In: Beck EJ, Mays N, Whiteside AW, et al., eds. The HIV Pandemic. Local and Global Implications. Oxford: Oxford Medical Publications, Oxford University Press, 2008.
14. D'Adesky A. Moving Mountains. The Race to Treat Global AIDS. London, New York: Verso, 2004.
15. Petersen ML, Travassos C, Bastos FI, et al. Brazil. In: Beck EJ, Mays N, Whiteside AW, et al. eds. The HIV Pandemic. Local and Global Implications. Oxford: Oxford Medical Publications, Oxford University Press, 2008.
16. Hamilton G, Falistococco C, Cahn P, et al. Argentina. In: Beck EJ, Mays N, Whiteside AW, et al., eds. The HIV Pandemic. Local and Global Implications. Oxford: Oxford Medical Publications, Oxford University Press, 2008.
17. Peck R, Fitzgerald DW, Liautaud B, et al. The feasibility, demand and effect of itegrarting primary care services with HIV voluntary counseling and testing:

evaluation of a 15-year experience in Haiti, 1985-2000. J Acquir Immune Defic Syndr 2003; 33(4):470–475.

18. Deschamps MM, Pape JW, Hafner A, et al. Heterosexual transmission of HIV in Haiti. Ann Intern Med 1996; 125(4):324–330.

19. Cuban Ministry of Public Health. National strategic plan for the prevention of HIV/AIDS/STI. Havana: Ministry of Public Health, 2002.

20. United Nations Development Programme (UNDP). International Human Development Indicators, 2010. Available at: http://hdrstats.undp.org/en/countries/profiles/THA.html.

21. National Center for HIV/AIDS Dermatology and STDs. Behavioral Surveillance Survey 2003. Phnom Penh: USAID, 2004.

22. WHO/UNAIDS. Country update: India. Epidemiological fact sheets on HIV/AIDS and sexually transmitted infection. Geneva: WHO/UNAIDS, 2004.

23. Han M, Chen Q, Hao Y, et al. Design and implementation of a Chena comprehensive AIDS response programme (China CARES), 2003-2008. In J Epidemiol 2010; 39 (suppl 2):ii47–ii55.

24. Wolfe D, Carrieri MP, Shepard D. Treatment and care for injecting drug users with HIV infection: a review of barriers and ways forward. Lancet 2010; 376 (9738):35–66.

25. Metzger DS, Woody GE, O'Brien CP. Drug treatment as HIV prevention: a research update. J Acquir Immune Defic Syndr 2010; 55(suppl 1):S32–S36.

Appendix I

Antiretroviral drugs

DRUG COMPENDIUM

What follows is a compendium of antiretroviral agents used in the treatment of HIV-infected patients. Dosing guidelines given are for adults with normal renal function. Many drugs listed require dose adjustments for renal insufficiency and some for hepatic insufficiency. The manufacturer's package insert should be reviewed for dose adjustment recommendations. Updated treatment guidelines and the package insert information should be consulted before prescribing these agents.

Antiretroviral Agents

Antiretroviral agents are used in combination regimens dictated by the clinical situation. For information regarding indications for antiretroviral therapy and the combination and sequencing of specific agents, see chapter 6.

Nucleoside Reverse Transcriptase Inhibitors (NRTI)

Class side effects. All nucleoside reverse transcriptase inhibitor (NRTI) agents may be associated with the hepatic steatosis/lactic acidosis syndrome, which may be severe and fatal. *Additional notable side effects are listed under each agent.*

Abacavir (Ziagen)

> *Route of administration: Oral.*
> *How supplied*: 300-mg tablets; oral solution 20 mg/mL.
> *Notable side effects*: Life-threatening hypersensitivity reactions have been seen in as many as 5% of patients receiving abacavir. Patients should be screened for HLAB*5701 before starting any regimen containing abacavir as those screening positive are at highest risk for severe allergic

reactions. Patients developing a rash or any other signs of hypersensitivity while receiving this agent should not be rechallenged, and the drug should be permanently discontinued. . Bone marrow depression is occasionally seen.

Usual adult dosage: 300 mg bid or 600 mg daily.

Instructions to patient: Patients should be instructed to discontinue use and contact the provider promptly if rash appears. Patient should be informed of this to avoid inappropriate use by other providers. It may be taken with or without food.

Didanosine (Videx EC, ddl).

Route of administration: Oral, powder for suspension.

How supplied: 125-, 200-, 250-, 400-mg capsules; powder (Videx) for oral solutions (10 mg/mL).

Notable side effects: The most serious side effects associated with didanosine are pancreatitis and peripheral neuropathy, seen in 5–9% and 10–20% of patients respectively. Both of these toxicities have precluded the use didanosine in combination regimens with zalcitabine and, occasionally, with other NRTIs.

Usual adult dosage: If body weight > 60 kg, 400 mg once daily or 200 mg q12h (tablets), 250 mg q12h (powder); if body weight < 60 kg, 250 mg once daily or 125 mg q12h (tablets), 167 mg q12h (powder).

Instructions to patient: Didanosine should be taken on an empty stomach.

Lamivudine (Epivir, 3TC).

Route of administration: Oral.

How supplied: 150-, 300-mg tablets; oral solution 10 mg/mL.

Notable side effects: None. Lamivudine is generally the best tolerated of the NRTIs. Side effects (e.g., headache , diarrhea) are usually self-limited. Bone marrow depression and peripheral neuropathy, two adverse reactions seen with other nucleoside agents, are encountered infrequently with lamivudine.

Usual adult dosage: 150 mg twice daily or 300 mg daily.

Instructions to patient: Take with or without food.

Stavudine (Zerit, D4T).

Route of administration: Oral.

How supplied: 15, 20, 30, 40 mg; oral solution 1 mg/mL.

Notable side effects: Stavudine is chemically similar to zidovudine but differs in its side effect profile. While hematological toxicity is rarely seen, peripheral neuropathy, similar to that associated with didanosine and with zalcitabine is common, particularly among patients with CD4 cell counts below 100/mm^3, prior neuropathy and those on other agents associated with peripheral neuropathy. Once established, neuropathy may be difficult to treat and may persist for several weeks after the drug is discontinued. Tricyclic antidepressants, anticonvulsants such as dilantin or gabapentin, or, in extreme, narcotic analgesics may improve the pain of neuropathy.

Usual adult dosage: If body weight > 60 kg, 40 mg bid; if body weight < 60 kg, 30 mg bid.

Instructions to patient: May take with our without food.

Zalcitabine (Hivid, ddC).   Manufacture of this drug has been discontinued.

Zidovudine (Retrovir, AZT).

Route of administration: Oral, intravenous.

How supplied: 300-mg tablets; 100-mg capsules with blue band; syrup 50 mg/5 mL; IV infusion 10 mg/mL.

Notable side effects: The most important adverse effect of zidovudine therapy has been bone marrow depression manifesting as anemia and/or neutropenia. This is seen more frequently among patients at advanced stages of HIV infection, especially those with CD4 cell counts less than $100/mm^3$ and typically begins between 2 and 4 months after therapy is instituted. In general, bone marrow depression has become less common as the recommended dose of zidovudine for adults has been reduced from 1500–600 mg daily. Other common side effects seen with zidovudine include headache, insomnia, and myalgia. Less common, although occasionally severe, side effects include myopathy and neuropathy. All zidovudine-related toxicities typically resolve with withdrawal of the drug.

Usual adult dosage: 200 mg tid or 300 mg bid.

Nucleotide Reverse Transcriptase Inhibitors

Tenofovir (Viread, TDF)

Route of administration: Oral.

How supplied: 300-mg tablet.

Notable side effects: The most important side effects are renal insufficiency, Fanconi syndrome, and decreased bone mineral density. Headache, diarrhea, nausea, and vomiting may also occur. Because of its excellent activity against hepatitis B virus (HBV), flares of hepatitis B may be seen in infected individuals upon discontinuation of tenofovir.

Usual adult dosage: 300 mg once daily.

Instructions to patient: May be taken with or without food.

Nonnucleoside Reverse Transcriptase inhibitors

Delavirdine (Rescriptor).

> *Route of administration*: Oral.
> *How supplied*: 100-, 200-mg tablets.
> *Notable side effects*: The most frequent side effect associated with delavirdine is skin rash, which occurs in 18% of individuals. Prior sulfonamide-related rash and Hispanic ethnicity may be risk factors for delavirdine-associated rash.
> *Usual adult dose*: 400-mg tablets tid.
> *Instructions to patient*: Tablets should not be taken with antacids.

Efavirenz (Sustiva).

> *Route of administration*: Oral.
> *How supplied*: 50- and 200-mg capsules; 600-mg tablets.
> *Notable side effects*: Over 50% of patients taking efavirenz experience one or more neurological side effects such as insomnia, nightmares, hallucinations, dizziness, or confusion. Preexisting depression or psychosis may also be exacerbated. As is the case with nevirapine and delavirdine, skin rash is also commonly seen with efavirenz. Less frequent side effects include elevated lipid levels, liver function abnormalities, elevated serum amylase, nausea, and diarrhea. It has been associated with fetal neural tube defects in animal studies.
> *Usual adult dose*: 600 mg once daily.
> *Instructions to patient*: Efavirenz should be taken at bedtime and on empty stomach to minimize the impact of CNS side effects.

Etravirine (Intelence).

> *Route of administration*: Oral.
> *How supplied*: 100-mg tablets.
> *Notable side effects*: Rash, nausea, hepatic failure.
> *Usual adult dosage*: 200 mg bid.
> *Instructions to patient*: Should be taken following a meal.

Nevirapine (Viramune).

> *Route of administration*: Oral.
> *How supplied*: 200-mg tablets, 50 mg/5mL oral suspension.
> *Notable side effects*: Skin rashes, which can be severe in some cases, have been the most frequently reported side effect of nevirapine therapy (Merino, 1999).
>
> As is the case with delavirdine and efavirenz, skin rash appears to be more common among individuals of Hispanic heritage or with prior history of sulfa allergy. Liver function abnormalities as well as clinical

hepatitis, which may be severe, and cholestasis have also been described. Hepatitis more common in women with pretreatment CD4 cell counts above 250 cells/mm^3 and men with counts above 400 cells/mm^3.

Usual adult dose: Days 1–14: one 200-mg tablet qd; day 15 forward: one 200-mg tablet bid.

Protease Inhibitors

Class side effects/interactions. All protease inhibitors may cause gastrointestinal side effects such as nausea, vomiting and, especially, diarrhea. Hyperglycemia, insulin resistance, hyperlipidemia, and fat redistribution (the so-called lipodystrophy syndrome) have been associated with all of the drugs in this class and can limit their usefulness in some patients. Each drug is metabolized by the cytochrome P450 system, and a wide variety of drug interactions, some significant, have been reported. All agents, with the exception of nelfinavir, should be administered in combination with ritonavir. Kaletra contains a fixed combination of lopinavir and ritonavir and is not administered with additional ritonavir. *Additional notable side effects are listed under each agent.*

Atazanavir

Route of administration: Oral.

How supplied: 100-, 150-, 200-, 300-mg capsules.

Notable side effects: Conduction blocks (PR prolongation), elevated bilirubin, hyperglycemia, nephrolithiasis.

Usual adult dosage: 400 mg with 100 mg ritonavir daily (if atazanavir naïve); 300 mg with 100 mg ritonavir once daily (when given with tenofovir or in treatment-experienced patients); 400 mg with 100 mg ritonavir once daily (when given with efavirenz). May require dose adjustment in hepatic insufficiency.

Instructions to patient: None.

Darunavir

Route of administration: Oral.

How supplied: 75-, 150-, 400-, 600-mg tablets.

Notable side effects: Skin rash, especially in patients with hypersensitivity to sulfonamides, hepatotoxicity.

Usual adult dosage: 800 mg with 100 mg ritonavir once daily (therapy-naïve patients); 600 mg with 100 mg ritonavir twice daily (therapy-experienced patients).

Instructions to patient: Take with meals.

Fosamprenavir (Lexiva)

Route of administration: Oral.

How supplied: 700-mg tablet, 50 mg/mL oral suspension.

Notable side effects: Skin rash, nephrolithiasis.

Usual adult dosage: 1400 mg bid or 1400 mg combined with 100–200 mg ritonavir once daily or 700 mg combined with 100 mg ritonavir bid (therapy-naïve patients). Once-daily dosing not recommended for PI-experienced patients.

Instructions to patient: Take with or without meals.

Indinavir

Route of administration: Oral.

How supplied: 200-, 333-, 400-mg capsules.

Notable side effects: Kidney stones, elevation of indirect bilirubin, dry skin, brittle nails, nausea, vomiting, diarrhea.

Usual adult dosage: 800 mg tid or 800 mg with ritonavir 100–200 mg bid.

Instructions to patient: Indinavir should be taken with 12 ounces of fluid and without food. Good hydration should be maintained to help prevent the formation of kidney stones.

Lopinavir/norvir (Kaletra)

Route of administration: Oral.

How supplied: Lopinavir 200 mg/ritonavir 50 mg; lopinavir 100 mg/ritonavir 25 mg; oral solution.

Notable side effects: Diarrhea, headache, fatigue, nausea hyperlipidemia, hyperglycemia. Pancreatitis, including severe, has been reported.

Usual adult dosage: Lopinavir/ritonavir 400 mg/100 mg bid or 800 mg/200 mg once daily (for PI-naïve patients; once daily dosing not recommended in pregnancy or in patients receiving efavirenz, nevirapine).

For PI-experienced patients or when used with efavirenz: 500 mg/125 mg bid.

Instructions to patient: May take with or without food.

Nelfinavir (Viracept)

Route of administration: Oral.

How supplied: 250-mg, 625 mg tablets; powder for oral solution (50 mg per level scoopful).

Notable side effects: Diarrhea (typically resolves with continued use). Nelfinavir is generally the best tolerated of the protease inhibitors.

Usual adult dosage: 750 mg tid.

Instructions to patient: Nelfinavir should be taken with food.

Ritonavir (Norvir)

Route of administration: Oral.

How supplied: 100-mg capsules, liquid (600 mg/7.5 mL).

Notable side effects: Nausea, bitter aftertaste, circumoral paresthesias, diarrhea. Ritonavir is generally the most poorly-tolerated protease inhibitor when used in full therapeutic doses.

Usual adult dosage: 600 mg bid. Because it is often poorly tolerated in full dose, ritonavir is almost exclusively used in a subtherapeutic dose (100–400 mg bid) to increase the serum concentration of other protease inhibitors. If used alone, a dose escalation schedule (e.g. 300 mg bid with daily 100 mg bid increments to a maximum total dose of 600 mg bid).

Instructions to patient: Refrigerate, take with food when possible.

Saquinavir (Invirase)

Route of administration: Oral.

How supplied: 200-mg gel capsules, 500-mg tablets.

Notable side effects: Diarrhea, nausea, headache (all generally mild).

Usual adult dosage: 1000 mg with 100 mg ritonavir bid.

Instructions to patient: Should be taken with meals but not with vitamin E supplements (each capsule contains 109 units of vitamin E).

Tipranavir (Aptivus)

Route of administration: Oral.

How supplied: 250-mg capsules; 100 mg/mL oral solution.

Notable side effects: Hepatitis, skin rash, rare intracerebral hemorrhage.

Usual adult dosage: 500 mg with 200 mg ritonavir bid.

Instructions to patient: Refrigerate capsules, can be taken with or without food.

CCR5 Coreceptor Antagonist

Maraviroc (Selzentry)

Route of administration: Oral.

How supplied: 150-, 300-mg tablets.

Notable side effects: Abdominal pain, cough, myalgias, hepatotoxicity, orthostatic hypotension.

Usual adult dosage: 150 mg bid when combined with protease inhibitors (except tipranavir/ritonavir); 300 mg bid when combined with NRTIs, tipranavir/ritonavir; 600 mg bid when given with efavirenz without protease inhibitors.

Instructions to patient: Take with or without meals.

Integrase Inhibitor

Raltegravir (Isentress)

Route of administration: Oral.

How supplied: 400-mg tablets.

Notable side effects: Nausea, headache, diarrhea, elevation of CPK.
Usual adult dosage: 400 mg bid.
Instructions to patient: Take with or without meals.

Fusion Inhibitor

Efuvirtide (T20, Fuzeon)

Route of administration: Subcutaneous injection.
How supplied: Vial containing 108 mg of T20 to be reconstituted with 1.1 mL of sterile water for injection.
Usual adult dosage: 90 mg twice daily.
Notable side effects: Pain at injection site, hypersensitivity reactions.
Instructions to patient: Refrigerate after reconstitution.

Combination Antiretroviral Products

At the time of this writing, several products in addition to Kaletra (see above) combining antiretroviral agents in fixed amounts are available:

Combivir (zidovudine/lamivudine)
Trizivir (abacavir/zidovudine/lamivudine)
Truvada (tenofovir/emtracitabine)
Atripla (tenofovir/emtricitabine/efavirenz)
Epzicom (abacavir/lamivudine)

Appendix II

Drugs used to prevent and/or treat HIV-related infections: Including tuberculosis and viral hepatitis

DRUG COMPENDIUM

An ever-growing number of new and old agents have found roles in the therapy or prevention of HIV-related opportunistic infections. The medications discussed here are commonly used in the outpatient setting. This compendium is focused on the indications and use of these drugs in the setting of HIV infection, although many are used for a great variety of indications unrelated to HIV/AIDS. The doses provided are those for adults with normal renal function. *Please consult manufacturers' package inserts for dosage adjustments in patients with renal insufficiency and for full toxicity information.*

Antiviral Agents

(See below for agents used in therapy of hepatitis B and C.)

Acyclovir (Zovirax)

Routes of administration: Topical, oral, intravenous.
Indications: Therapy of mucocutaneous (oral, topical) or systemic (intravenous) herpes simplex infections, long-term suppression of mucocutaneous herpes simplex infections, therapy of localized or disseminated varicella zoster infection.
Notable side effects: Headache, rash, nausea, diarrhea, bone marrow depression; seizures, hepatic and renal toxic effects rarely.
Usual adult dosage:
Herpes simplex, localized genital or oral: topical—every 4 hr while awake; oral—200 mg every 4 hr while awake; intravenous—10 mg/kg daily in 3 divided doses.

Herpes simplex, generalized or visceral: intravenous as above.

Varicella zoster, localized: oral—800 mg every 4 hr while awake.

Varicella zoster, generalized or visceral: intravenous—10 to 12 mg/kg every 8 hr or 1 g tid orally.

Cidofovir (Vistide)

Routes of administration: Intravenous.

Indications: Cytomegaloviral infection, especially retinitis.

Notable side effects: Renal insufficiency, proteinuria, renal tubular acidosis, leucopenia.

Usual adult dosage: 5 mg/kg IV weekly for 2 wk followed by 5 mg/kg IV every 2 wk. Probenecid (2 g orally) and adequate hydration before each dose.

Famciclovir (Famvir)

Route of administration: Oral.

Indications: Genital herpes simplex and localized herpes zoster infections.

Notable side effects: Headache, nausea, vomiting diarrhea.

Usual adult dosage:

Herpes zoster 500 mg every 8 hr for 7 days.

Herpes simplex 125 mg bid for 5 days; 250 mg bid may be used in chronic suppression in patients with frequent episodes.

Fomivirsen (Vitravene)

Routes of administration: Intravitreal injection.

Indications: Cytomegaloviral retinitis in patients not responding to or intolerant of other forms of therapy.

Notable side effects: Ocular inflammation, increased intraocular pressure.

Usual adult dosage: 330 µg every 2 wk for 2 doses then once every 4 wk.

Foscarnet (Foscavir)

Route of administration: Intravenous.

Indications: Cytomegaloviral infection not responding to other therapies, herpes simplex infection resistant to acyclovir.

Notable side effects: Renal insufficiency, proteinuria, seizures, hypokalemia, hypocalcemia, hypomagnesemia, neuropathy, gastrointestinal tract upset, liver function abnormalities, headache.

Usual adult dosage: 60 mg/kg every 8 hr for 14 days followed by 90–120 mg/kg daily.

Ganciclovir (Cytovene)

Routes of administration: Oral, intravenous, intraocular implant.
Indications: Cytomegaloviral infection.
Notable side effects:
> *Systemic therapy*: Bone marrow depression, fever, abdominal pain, confusion (all more common and severe with intravenous than with oral therapy).
> *Intraocular implant*: Retinal detachment.

Usual adult dosage:
> *Induction therapy*: 5 mg/kg IV q12 h for 14 days.
> *Maintenance therapy*: 5mg/kg IV qd 5 times each week.
> *Oral*: 1 g tid with food.

Valacyclovir (Valtrex)

Route of administration: Oral.
Indications: Localized herpes zoster, genital herpes simplex.
Notable side effects: Similar to acyclovir. Hemolytic-uremic syndrome.
Usual adult dosage:
> Herpes zoster: 1 g 3 times daily for 7 days.
> Genital herpes simplex (initial): 1 g twice daily for 10 days.
> Genital herpes simplex (recurrent): 500 mg twice daily for 5 days.
> Genital herpes simplex (chronic suppressive therapy): 1 g once daily.

Antifungal Agents

Fluconazole (Diflucan)

Routes of administration: Oral, intravenous.
Indications: Oral, esophageal candidiasis; chronic suppressive therapy of cryptococcal infection.
Notable side effects: None (GI upset rare).
Usual adult dosage:
> Oral or esophageal candidiasis: 200 mg by mouth initial dose followed by 100 mg daily.
> Cryptococcosis or systemic candidiasis: 400 mg oral (or intravenous) induction followed by 200–400 mg daily.

Itraconazole (Sporanox)

Routes of administration: Oral, intravenous.
Indications: Histoplasmosis, blastomycosis, aspergillosis in patients intolerant of amphotericin B, oral candidiasis refractory to fluconazole.

Notable side effects: Nausea, abdominal discomfort.

Usual adult dosage: Oral 100–400 mg qd (oral); intravenous 200mg bid for 4 doses followed by 200 mg daily. Duration of therapy is dependent on indication.

Agents Used in the Prevention and Treatment of *Pneumocystis carinii* Infection and/or Toxoplasmosis

Atovaquone (Mepron)

Route of administration: Oral (liquid).

Instructions to patient: Take with meals.

Indications: Mild to moderate *P. carinii* pneumonia (PCP) (partial pressure of oxygen > 70 mmHG), prophylaxis of PCP in patients intolerant of trimethoprim-sulfamethoxazole. Primary or secondary prophylaxis of toxoplasmosis.

Notable side effects: GI upset, headache, rash, fever.

Usual adult dose:

> PCP: 750 mg bid for 21 days.
> Prophylaxis: 1500 mg once daily.
> Toxoplasmosis prophylaxis: 1500 mg qd (primary) 750 mg po q 6–12 h (secondary).

Clindamycin

Routes of administration: Oral, intravenous.

Indications: Treatment of PCP (in combination with primaquine) or toxoplasmosis (in combination with pyrimethamine) in patients intolerant of sulfa drugs.

Notable side effects: Diarrhea (including antibiotic-associated colitis), skin rash.

Usual adult dosage:

> PCP (mild): Clindamycin 350–400 mg po q6h + primaquine 15 mg base po qd for 21 days.
> PCP (moderate/severe): Clindamycin 600 mg IVq8h+ primaquine 30 mg base qd for 21 days.
> Toxoplasmosis: Clindamycin 600 mg po or IV q6h + pyrimethamine 200 mg po once followed by 75–100 mg daily.
> (Note that clindamycin/pyrimethamine is effect in the secondary prevention of toxoplamosis (clindamycin 300–450 mg po q 6-8h + pyrmethamine 25–75 po qd) but not PCP. Folinic acid (10–15 mg po qd) should always be given with pyrimethamine.)

Dapsone

Route of administration: Oral.

Indications: Therapy (with trimethoprim); primary or secondary prevention of *P. carinii* infection. Primary prevention of toxoplasmosis.

Notable side effects: Hypersensitivity reactions, blood dyscrasias.

Usual adult dosage:

PCP (mild): Dapsone 100 mg qd + trimethoprim 5mg/kg po tid for 21 days.

Prophylaxis: Dapsone 100 mg qd.

Prophylaxis (toxoplasmosis): dapsone 50 mg po qd + pyrimethamine 50 mg po weekly.

Pentamidine

Routes of administration: Aerosol, intramuscular, intravenous.

Indications: Therapy (parenteral) or primary or secondary prophylaxis (parenteral or aerosolized) of *P. carinii* infection.

Notable side effects:

Systemic therapy: Hypotension, hyperglycemia, renal insufficiency, bone marrow depression (rare).

Aerosol therapy: Bronchospasm.

Usual adult dosage:

PCP (therapy): 4 mg/kg intravenously daily for 14–21 days.

Pyrimethamine

Route of administration: Oral.

Indication: Toxoplasmosis, therapy or prevention (with sulfadiazine or clindamycin) or prevention (with dapsone).

Notable side effects: Folate deficiency, pancytopenia, hypersensitivity reactions.

Usual adult dosage: Varies with indication (see above).

Sulfadiazine

Route of administration: Oral.

Indications: Therapy (initial and chronic suppressive) for toxoplasmosis (with pyrimethamine).

Notable side effects: Hypersensitivity reactions, Stevens-Johnson syndrome, photosensitization, nephrolithiasis, bone marrow depression.

Usual adult dosage: 2–6 g in 4 divided doses.

Trimethoprim/sulfamethoxazole (TMP-SMX)

Routes of administration: Oral, intravenous.

Indications: Therapy, primary or secondary prophylaxis of PCP. Primary prophylaxis of toxoplasmosis.

Notable side effects: Hypersensitivity reactions, Stevens-Johnson syndrome, photosensitization, neutropenia, hepatitis.

Usual adult dosage:

Prophylaxis of PCP or toxoplasmosis: Double-strength tablet (160 mg trimethoprim, 800 mg sulfamethoxazole) every other day to twice daily.

Treatment of PCP: 15–20 mg/kg trimethoprim, 75–100 mg/kg sulfamethoxazole daily in 4 divided doses.

Agents Used Primarily in the Treatment and/or Prevention of Mycobacterial Infection

(See chap. 8 for treatment regimens for *Mycobacterium tuberculosis* infection.)

Azithromycin (Zithromax)

Routes of administration: Oral, intravenous.

Indications: Treatment and prevention of *Mycobacterium avium* complex (MAC) infection.

Notable side effects: Diarrhea, nausea, abdominal pain.

Usual adult dosage:

MAC infection: 500 mg po qd (as part of multidrug regimen) (see chap. 8).

MAC prevention: 1200 mg po weekly.

Ciprofloxacin/Ofloxacin

Route of administration: Oral, intravenous.

Indications: As components of combination regimens in the therapy of MAC infection (see chap. 8). Potential role as component of multidrug regimen in treatment of multidrug resistant TB.

Notable side effects: Nausea, vomiting, CNS effects, Achilles tendon rupture, QT prolongation.

Usual adult dose:

Ciprofloxacin 500–750 mg po bid.

Ofloxacin 200–400 mg po bid.

Clarithromycin

Route of administration: Oral.

Indication: Treatment (in combination regimens) and prevention of MAC infection. Treatment (with pyrimethamine) of toxoplasmosis in patients intolerant of standard therapy.

Notable side effects: Diarrhea, nausea, abdominal pain.
Usual adult dosage: 500 mg bid.

Ethambutol

Route of administration: Oral.
Indications: In combination therapy of *M. tuberculosis* or MAC infection (see chaps. 6 and 8).
Notable side effects: Optic neuritis.
Usual adult dosage: 25 mg/kg/day for 2 mo followed by 15 mg/kg/day.

Isoniazid

Route of administration: Oral, intramuscular, intravenous.
Indications: Single-drug therapy of latent tuberculosis; component of multidrug regimen in therapy of active tuberculosis.
Notable side effects: Hepatitis (may be severe), peripheral neuropathy, hypersensitivity reactions.
Usual adult dosage: 300 mg/day orally.

Moxifloxacin (Avelox)

Route of administration: Oral, intravenous.
Indications: Potential role as component of multidrug regimen in treatment of multidrug resistant TB.
Notable side effects: See ciprofloxacin.
Usual adult dosage: 400 mg daily (oral or intravenous).

Pyrazinamide

Route of administration: Oral.
Indication: Component of multidrug regimen in therapy of active tuberculosis or, with rifampin, short-course therapy of latent tuberculosis.
Notable side effects: Hepatitis, hyperuricemia.
Usual adult dosage: 15–30 mg/kg daily orally (maximum daily dose: 2 g).

Rifabutin

Route of administration: Oral.
Indications: Prevention or, in combination, regimens, treatment of MAC infection (see chap. 6)
Notable side effects: Myalgia, arthralgia, red urine, anterior uveitis when administered with clarithromycin.
Usual adult dosage: 300 mg, dose adjustments required when used with protease inhibitors (see chap. 8).

Rifampin

Route of administration: Oral, intravenous.
Indication: Component of multidrug regimen in therapy of active tuberculosis or with pyrazinamide in short-course therapy of latent tubcerculosis.
Notable side effects: Hepatitis, hypersensitivity reactions, orange discoloration of urine and tears; accelerates metabolism of methadone (may cause withdrawal symptoms), corticosteroids, oral hypoglycemic agents.
Usual adult dose: 600 mg daily; dose adjustments required when administered with protease inhibitors (see chap. 8).

Cycloserine (Seromycin)

Route of administration: Oral.
Indication: Component of multidrug regimen for resistant tuberculosis.
Notable side effects: Seizures, psychosis, peripheral neuropathy.
Usual adult dose: 15 mg/kg daily in 2–4 divided doses.

Ethionamide

Route of administration: Oral.
Indication: Component of multidrug regimen for resistant tuberculosis.
Notable side effects: GI upset, peripheral neuropathy.
Usual adult dose: 15–20 mg/kg daily in 1–3 doses.

Streptomycin

Route of administration: Intramuscular.
Indication: First-line treatment of tuberculosis.
Notable side effects: Ototoxicity, nephrotoxicity, peripheral neuropathy, neuromuscular blockade.
Usual adult dose: 15 mg/kg daily for initial 2–3 mo then 15 mg/kg 3 times weekly.

Amikacin

Route of administration: Intramuscular, intravenous.
Indication: Second-line treatment of tuberculosis.
Notable side effects: See streptomycin.
Usual adult dose: 7.5–10 mg/kg daily.

Capreomycin

Route of administration: Intramuscular, intravenous.
Indication: Second-line treatment of tuberculosis.
Notable side effects: See streptomycin.
Usual adult dose: 1 g daily.

Hepatitis B Agents

(See chap. 8 for treatment regimens and indications.)

Lamivudine

Route of administration: Oral.
Notable side effects: Headache, GI distress.
Usual adult dose: 100 mg daily (note that HIV dose is 150 mg twice daily or 300 mg daily).

Adefovir

Route of administration: Oral.
Notable side effects: Nephrotoxicity.
Usual adult dose: 10 mg daily.

Entecavir

Route of administration: Oral.
Notable side effects: Minimal.
Usual adult dose: 0.5 mg daily.

Telbivudine

Route of administration: Oral.
Notable side effects: Minimal.
Usual adult dose: 600 mg daily.

Tenofovir

Route of administration: Oral.
Notable side effects: Nephrotoxicity.
Usual adult dose: 300 mg daily.

Pegylated Interferon-α (Pegasys/α-2a, Peg-Intron/α-2b)

Route of administration: Subcutaneous.
Notable side effects: Depression (sometimes severe), worsening of other psychiatric disorders, flu-like syndrome, blood dyscrasias, thyroid dysfunction, GI upset, headache, myalgias, skin rash (sometimes severe).
Usual adult dose:
  Pegylated 40k interferon α-2a (Pegasys): 180 μg subcutaneously once weekly.
  Pegylated interferon α-2b ((PEG-Intron): 0.5–1.5 μg subcutaneously once weekly.

Hepatitis C Agents

(See chap. 8 for treatment regimens.)

Ribavirin

Route of administration: Oral.

Notable side effects: Hemolytic anemia; contraindicated in pregnancy or in women or men contemplating a pregnancy.

Usual adult dose:

Genotypes 1 or 4:
1000 mg daily if weight < 75 kg.
1200 mg daily if weight > 75 kg.

Genotypes 2 or 3:
800 mg daily.

Pegylated Interferons

See above.

Index

261

Primary infection
  women, 188
Process indicators, 210
Program structure, 200–205
  access to care, 203–205
    entry into care, 203–204
    record keeping, 204–205
    specialty referral, 204
  staffing, 200–203
    care management, 203
    clinical pharmacy staff, 202–203
    nurses, 201
    patient advisory groups, 203
    peer group intervention, 203
    physicians, 200–201
    social workers/service staff, 202
Progressive multifocal leukoencephalopathy
    (PML), 44, 49, 133
Prostate cancer, HIV and, 174
Prostate specific antigen (PSA) testing, 174
Protease inhibitors (PI), 105, 106
  efficacy, 109
  mode of action, 109
  mother to child transmission,
    prevention, 185–186
  patterns of use, 110
  resistance to, 110
Provider experience, 211
PSA. *See* Prostate specific antigen (PSA)
    testing
Pseudomonas aeruginosa, 57–58
Psoriasis, 29
Psoriatic arthritis, 67
Psychiatric disorders, 23–24, 72, 149
Psychosis, 149
Pulmonary disorders, 56–58
  mycobacterial infection. *See also*
    Mycobacterial infection
    atypical, 58–59
    tuberculosis, 58
  opportunistic infections
    bacterial pneumonia, 57–58
    coccidioidomycosis, 57
    cryptococcal infection, 56–57
    cytomegalovirus infection, 57
    histoplasmosis, 57
    Pneumocystis pneumonia, 56
    toxoplasmosis, 57

Pulmonary embolism, 92
Pulmonary hypertension, 60–61, 92
Pulmonary toxoplasmosis, 57
Pulmonary tuberculosis, 155–156, 158
Pyrazinamide, 137
Pyridoxine, 137, 157
Pyrimethamine, 130, 131

Quality indicators, 210–211
  hospitalization rates, 211
  opportunistic infections, prevention
    of, 211
  outcome indicators, 211
  process indicators, 210
  provider experience, 211
  volume indicators, 210
Quality management, HIV-infected
    individuals, 208–215
  consensus measures of quality, 212
    recommended measures, 212
  indicators, 209. *See also* Quality
    indicators
  resource-limited settings, 213–215
Quality of life, 170–172

Racial/ethnic patterns, 169
Radionuclide studies
  fever, 83–84
Raltegravir (Isentress), 110–111,
    248–249
Rapid antibody tests, 6
  advantage of, 17
RBV. *See* Ribavirin (RBV)
Rectal carcinoma, 31
Rectal examination, 31–32
Regimens, 110, 120
Reiter's syndrome, 66–67
Relapse, of former substance user, 149
Renal disorders, 64–65
  HIV-associated nephropathy, 65
Renal injury, 108
Reptiles, 39
Rescriptor. *See* Delavirdine
Resistance
  chemokine CCR5 receptor antagonists,
    111
  integrase strand inhibitors, 111